THE NEW EXECUTIVE BRAIN

Also by Elkhonon Goldberg

The Executive Brain: Frontal Lobes and the Civilized Mind

*The Wisdom Paradox: How Your Mind Can Grow
Stronger As Your Brain Grows Older*

THE NEW EXECUTIVE BRAIN

Frontal Lobes in a Complex World

Elkhonon Goldberg

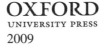

OXFORD
UNIVERSITY PRESS
2009

OXFORD
UNIVERSITY PRESS

Oxford University Press, Inc., publishes works that further
Oxford University's objective of excellence
in research, scholarship, and education.

Oxford   New York
Auckland   Cape Town   Dar es Salaam   Hong Kong   Karachi
Kuala Lumpur   Madrid   Melbourne   Mexico City   Nairobi
New Delhi   Shanghai   Taipei   Toronto

With offices in
Argentina   Austria   Brazil   Chile   Czech Republic   France   Greece
Guatemala   Hungary   Italy   Japan Poland   Portugal   Singapore
South Korea   Switzerland   Thailand   Turkey   Ukraine   Vietnam

Copyright © 2009 by Elkhonon Goldberg.

Published by Oxford University Press, Inc.
198 Madison Avenue, New York, New York 10016
www.oup.com

Oxford is a registered trademark of Oxford University Press

Library of Congress Cataloging-in-Publication Data

Goldberg, Elkhonon.
The new executive brain : frontal lobes in a complex world / Elkhonon Goldberg.
p. ; cm.
Includes bibliographical references and index.
ISBN: 978-0-19-532940-7
1. Frontal lobes. 2. Neuropsychology. I. Title.
[DNLM: 1. Frontal Lobe—physiology. 2. Brain Diseases—physiopathology.
3. Mental Processes—physiology. WL 307 G618n 2009]
QP382.F7G653 2009
612.8'25—dc22
2009006253

9 8 7 6 5 4 3 2 1
Printed in the United States of America
on acid-free paper

To my mentor and friend Alexandr Luria

Acknowledgments

My thanks go to Oxford University Press for ensuring the success of *The Executive Brain* and thus laying the ground for *The New Executive Brain*. My editor Craig Panner, assistant editor David D'Addona, and production editor Lynda Crawford, as well as the copy editor Jerri Hurlbutt, were all superb with their combination of a soft touch and a firm hand at every stage of my work on *The New Executive Brain*. Dmitri Bougakov has again been most helpful with numerous technical aspects of the book. Michael Carlisle was a source of wise advice on numerous issues, including the book's title. Nicholas (Colly) Myers kindly agreed to critically review the manuscript and his comments and insights are greatly appreciated. Richard Gallini provided the artwork for the book with patience and insight. Jeffrey Donaldson provided invaluable help with references. Larry Abbott, Sigurd Ackerman, Robert Bilder, John Caronna, Michael Cole, Colby Collier, Anna DiStefano, John Fawcett, Cecilia Gamburg, John Garland, Brian King, Lisa King, Sergey Knazev, Alex Martin, Allan Mirsky, Ralph Nixon, Peter Palmer, Kenneth Podell, Silvana Riggio, and Daniel Sodickson have provided valuable input. My dog Brit has been my constant and most agreeable companion throughout the process, never judgmental and never demanding, unless hungry.

I am particularly grateful to Vladimir and Kevin for giving me an opportunity to learn from their conditions; to those called Toby and Charlie as well as L. H. and S.F. for sharing their life stories and allowing me to describe them in this book; to Kevin's father for allowing me to write about his son; and to Robert Iacono for sharing his experience with cingulotomy.

I dedicate this book, as one before, to the memory of my mentor and friend Alexandr Romanovich Luria.

E. G.
New York, N.Y.

Contents

Foreword

We live in an increasingly complex and bewildering world of fast change and unprecedented problems. Leaving aside the familiar, long term issues relating to global warming, the more acute anxiety in the mind of many must surely be the scary and uncharted waters, at the time of writing, of the current economic crisis. Why should a financial meltdown be of any direct relevance to brain research? Interestingly enough, President Obama has suggested that there may be psychological factors at work—namely, greed and recklessness. Whilst the brain mechanisms underlying such quintessentially human traits would always have been of interest, surely there has never been a time quite like this, when the subject takes on a still sharper focus.

Perhaps it's no surprise, however, that Elkhonon Goldberg's book does not set out with the goal of solving the global recession, nor indeed of explaining how a particular mind-set might have contributed to it. Rather the journey on which he is about to take you, is towards a new perspective on one of the biggest remaining mysteries within the brain, a mystery that will fascinate not just the neuroscience cognoscenti in the field, but anyone curious to understand the human mind, especially at the moment.

You are about to uncover some of the secrets of the frontal lobes of the brain. These large areas, occupying as they do almost a third of the total outer layer of the human brain—almost twice as much as our nearest primate relative the Chimpanzee—present a real puzzle. We have known for a long time that, when damaged, the patient seems remarkably unaffected, at least with regard to basic functions of movement and the senses: the most famous example of frontal lobe damage occurred in the nineteenth century when a premature ignition of explosive drove a four-foot long iron rod through the temples of one Phineas Gage. As became apparent over the subsequent few months, the problem resulting from such damage was far from immediately obvious: a subtle change in character where, for example, the individual becomes far more distracted by the here and now, and far less concerned with consequences.

But since the 'hypo-frontal' syndrome is just that, a complex array of behaviors, the frontal lobes have become a kind of kitchen sink for many brain researchers, where virtually any sophisticated function that one wanted to house in a particular brain region could be obligingly accommodated by the frontal lobes: whatever a subject or patient might be asked to do, the frontal lobes would inevitably "light up," i.e. show activation in brain scans. This issue, the seduction of brain imaging techniques, and the misleading, misplaced simplicity of interpreting them is well articulated by Elkhonon. We see that, convenient though it might be to think of the brain in a modular fashion composed of centres for this or that sophisticated function, such thinking is as outdated as the old phrenology of the nineteenth century.

In this book, you'll discover a whole new take on how to tackle the problem of the frontal lobes. A helpful clue with which we start is to see that not only have the human brains in evolution undergone exaggerated expansion but, as so often in biology, such evolution is reflected in personal development with the frontal lobes not coming fully active until the third decade of life. Occupying, as it does, such as large part of our grey matter, yet at the same time, relatively irrelevant in early childhood, what could the frontal lobes be doing? Elkhonon shows how we cannot think of brain areas as independent mini-brains, but rather as massively interlinked with each other. As it happens, the frontal lobes are more connected to all other parts of the brain than any other region: hence we see how this sophisticated area is at the same time more sensitive and vulnerable in a whole host of diverse brain disorders ranging from neurological diseases to more ,subtle conditions such as schizophrenia and ADHD. There is even a recent, intriguing report showing a negative correlation with frontal lobe activity and Body Mass Index!

Given that we know that those with frontal damage are particularly reckless in gambling trials, and obese people too show a recklessness in a gambling task, it is hard to conceive of what the crucial common feature might be, linking childhood schizophrenia, gambling and indeed over-eating. My own thought has been that it is the domination of the sensory press of the external world over the checks and balances of past experiences and inter-related memories that is trumped in some way when the frontal area is not functioning flat out.

However, rather than pushing a particular, idiosyncratic theory such as I have just mentioned, Elkhonon offers the reader a rich and authoritative manual that enables you to develop your own thoughts. Not only is the journey therefore a richly rewarding one, where as the reader you will feel that you are actually making an intellectual voyage rather than merely assimilating disparate facts, but all the more readable as there is much personal narrative and anecdote. We researchers are so often thought of as dysfunctional nerds: so, it is really warming to see showcased personal triumphs, issues, problems and tributes, which makes not just the scientific struggle, but the scientists themselves, come truly alive.

But back to the seemingly unrelated world of politics and economics: Elkhonon ends by drawing an intriguing parallel between the development of nations and the development of the brain: he shows how the prefrontal lobes, by being effectively the crown of creation, are nonetheless an intrinsically weak force that has power only in the context of the many other brain areas to which it is connected and to which it thereby bestows cohesion. The reader may or may not agree with the thought-provoking analogies to the European Union: whilst such comparisons, valid though they may be, could well remain the province of dinner party conversations, my feeling is that Elkhonon's work contributes even more profoundly and immediately to an understanding of the world. He helps us understand crucial human issues such as sense of self and accountability. Such attributes must be of relevance surely, not just to the neuroscientist, but to anyone hoping to make the most of living in the twenty-first century.

Susan Greenfield
Oxford, April 2009

THE NEW EXECUTIVE BRAIN

1

Introduction

My earlier book *The Executive Brain* has lived 2 parallel lives in 12 languages: as a trade book for the general public interested in the brain, and as a text read by students, clinicians, and cognitive neuroscientists. *The New Executive Brain* is a successor book which reflects some of my own more recent thinking as well as the recent discoveries in the vibrant field of cognitive neuroscience. In writing this book I have tried to maintain a balance between it being sufficiently rigorous and informative to be of value to the scientific and professional audience, and sufficiently accessible and entertaining to the general readership.

I hope that *The New Executive Brain* will also enjoy two parallel lives. Currently, brain research is among the most vibrant and rapidly developing fields of scientific inquiry. In the last 8 years, myriad new developments have taken place, some of which I have tried to reflect here. In addition, numerous general-interest books about the brain have been published, with the brain, brain research, brain ailments such as ADHD and Alzheimer's disease, and brain remedies including various forms of cognitive enhancement and innovative pharmaceuticals becoming all the rage. Today members of the general educated public are vicarious participants in the incredible journey that neuroscience has become. For these readers my message is, enjoy! I hope that my book will help you take part in this journey.

To my colleague clinicians and scientists, my message is more nuanced, and it is best communicated after reading the book, rather than beforehand. So read it. I hope that you will find it thought provoking; don't rush to the Epilogue until you have finished the book.

Some of the chapters in *The New Executive Brain* are less technical and of general interest; they should appeal to both the general reader and professionals. Other chapters are somewhat more technical but still accessible to the general reader. They deal with broad issues of cognitive neuroscience that are of interest to scientists and clinicians as well as to lay readers interested in the workings of the brain and the mind. The book does not represent an attempt at an encyclopedic, textbook-like account of the frontal lobes. Rather, it is an idiosyncratic account of my own understanding of several central issues in cognitive neuroscience and of the personal context that led me to write about them.

In this book I explore the one part of the brain that makes individuals who they are and defines their identity; that encapsulates their drives, ambitions, personality, and essence: the frontal lobes of the brain. If other parts of the brain are damaged, neurological illness can result in the loss of language, memory, perception, or movement. Yet the essence of the individual, the personality core, usually remains intact. All this changes when illness strikes at the frontal lobes. What is lost then is no longer an attribute of your mind. It *is* your mind, your core, your self. The frontal lobes are the most uniquely human of all the brain structures, and they play a critical role in the success or failure of any human endeavor.

"Descartes' error," to borrow the elegant phrase of Antonio Damasio,[1] consisted in believing that the mind has a life of its own, independent of the body. Altough a literate society no longer believes in the Cartesian dualism between body and mind, we are still shedding the vestiges of the old misconception in stages. Today few educated people, no matter how unschooled in neurobiology, doubt that language, movement, perception, and memory all somehow reside in the brain. Yet ambition, drive, foresight, insight—those attributes that define one's personality and essence—are viewed by many as "extracranial," as if they were attributes of our clothes and not our biology. These elusive human qualities are also controlled by the brain, particularly by the frontal lobes. The prefrontal cortex is the current focus of much neuroscientific research, yet it is largely unknown to nonscientists.

The frontal lobes perform the most advanced and complex functions in all of the brain, the so-called executive functions. They are linked to intentionality, purposefulness, and complex decision making. They reach significant development only in humans; arguably, they make us human. The entire human evolution has been termed "the age of the frontal lobes." My teacher, Alexandr Luria, called the frontal lobes "the organ of civilization." This book is about the numerous roles frontal lobes play in cognition.

This book is about leadership. The frontal lobes are to the brain what a conductor is to an orchestra, a general is to an army, the chief executive officer is to a corporation. They coordinate and lead other neural structures in concerted action.

The frontal lobes are the brain's command post. We will examine how the leadership role has evolved in various facets of human society—and in the brain.

This book is about motivation, drive, and vision. These qualities and clarity about one's goals are central to success in any walk of life. You will discover how all these prerequisites of success are controlled by the frontal lobes, and how even subtle damage to the frontal lobes produces apathy, inertia, and indifference.

Self-awareness and awareness of others are also addressed in this book. Our ability to accomplish our goals depends on our ability to critically appraise our own actions and the actions of those around us. This ability rests with the frontal lobes. Damage to the frontal lobes produces debilitating blindness in judgement.

This book is also about talent and success. We readily recognize literary talent, musical talent, and athletic talent. But in a complex society such as ours, a different talent comes to the fore: leadership. Of all the forms of talent, the ability to lead, to compel other human beings to rally behind a person or cause, is the most mysterious and the most profound. In human history the leadership talent has had the greatest impact on the destinies of others and on personal success. This book highlights an intimate relationship between leadership and the frontal lobes. Of course, the converse of this is that poor frontal lobe function is especially devastating to an individual. Therefore, this book is also about failure.

Related to talent and success is creativity. Intelligence and creativity are inseparable, yet not the same; each of us has known people who are bright, intelligent, thoughtful—and barren. Creativity requires the ability to embrace novelty. We will examine the critical role of the frontal lobes in dealing with novelty.

This book is about men and women. Neuroscientists are only now beginning to study what people on the street have assumed all along, that men and women are different. Men and women approach things differently and have different cognitive styles. We will examine how these differences in cognitive styles reflect the gender differences in the frontal lobes.

This book is about society and history. All complex systems have certain features in common, and by learning about one system we learn about the others. We will examine analogies between the evolution of the brain and the development of complex societal structures, and derive certain lessons about our own society.

This book is also about social maturity and social responsibility. Frontal lobes define us as social beings. It is more than coincidence that the biological maturation of the frontal lobes takes place at the age that has been codified in virtually all developed cultures as the beginning of adulthood. Poor development of or damage to the frontal lobes may produce behavior devoid of social constraints and sense of responsibility. We will discuss how frontal lobe dysfunction may contribute to criminal behavior.

Relatedly, this book is about cognitive development and learning. Frontal lobes are critical for every successful learning process, for motivation and attention.

We have become increasingly aware of subtle disorders afflicting both children and adults—attention deficit disorder (ADD) and attention deficit hyperactivity disorder (ADHD).[2] This book describes how ADD and ADHD are caused by subtle dysfunction of the frontal lobes and the pathways connecting them to other parts of the brain.

This book is about aging. As we age, we become increasingly concerned about the degree of our mental astuteness. With increased public awareness of age-related cognitive decline, everyone is talking about memory loss, yet no one speaks of the loss of executive functions. Thus the frontal lobes' vulnerability to Alzheimer's disease and other dementias is addressed here.

The frontal lobes are also exceptionally fragile, making them vulnerable to neurological and psychiatric illness. Recent studies have shown that frontal lobe dysfunction is at the core of devastating disorders, such as schizophrenia and head trauma. Frontal lobes are also involved in Tourette's syndrome and obsessive-compulsive disorder.

Contemporary neuroscience is only now beginning to address the enhancing of cognitive functions and protection of the mind against decline. Some of the latest ideas and approaches are reviewed here.

Above all, this book is about the *brain*, the mysterious organ that is part of us, makes us who we are, and endows us with our powers and weighs us down with our weaknesses, the microcosm, the last frontier. In writing this book, I have made no attempt to be dispassionately encyclopedic; rather, my intent was to present a distinctly personal, original, and at times provocative viewpoint on a number of topics in neuropsychology and cognitive neuroscience. Although many of these points were published earlier in scientific journals, they do not necessarily represent the prevailing opinion in the field, and many of them remain distinctly partisan, controversial, my own.

Finally, this book is about *people*: about my patients, my friends, and my teachers, who in various ways and on both sides of the now-extinct Iron Curtain helped shape my interests and my career, thus making this book possible. The book is dedicated to Alexandr Romanovich Luria, the great neuropsychologist, whose legacy informed and shaped the field like nobody else's. For me he was, at various times, "my professor, my mentor, my friend, and my tyrant."[3] Our relationship was close and complex. In Chapter 2, I give a very personal account of one of the greatest psychologists of our time and of the extraordinarily difficult context in which he worked.

A friend of mine once remarked, succinctly and to the point: "Brain is great!" Among all the intellectual, quasi-intellectual, and pseudo-intellectual fads today, popular interest in the brain reigns supreme. It is shared by an enlightened general public driven by genuine curiosity about "science's last frontier"; by parents, eager for their children to succeed and dreading the prospect of failure; and by insatiable baby boomers, determined to remain in the driver's seat forever, but approaching the age when debilitating mental decline becomes a statistical possibility. To meet this unparalleled interest, scores of popular books have been written about memory, language, attention, emotion, cerebral hemispheres, and related subjects. Incredibly, though, one part of the brain has been completely ignored in this genre: the frontal lobes. This book has been written to fill that gap.

At the same time, the educated public is becoming disabused of the blissful Cartesian delusion that the body is frail but the mind is forever. As we live longer, are better educated, and get ahead by our brain rather than brawn, we are increasingly interested in our minds and concerned about losing them.

Our self-centered society's preoccupation with illness has created a complex tangle of reality, neurosis, and guilt, with doomsday overtones. Never too far from the center of our collective consciousness, this preoccupation has usually focused on one illness that encapsulated all our fears, thus becoming, in the words of Susan Sontag,[4] a metaphor. In recent history, first it was cancer, then acquired immune deficiency syndrome (AIDS). As the shock value and novelty of the metaphor du jour wore off and familiarity bred a (magical) sense of security, a new focus would arise: dementia became, appropriately, the new focus. Since, with age, dementia strikes a significant proportion of the population, the concern is basically rational but, like most fads, has taken on neurotic overtones.

As behooves a movement, the preoccupation with dementia has acquired its own metaphor, a metaphor within a metaphor, so to speak. This metaphor is *memory*. In the information society dominated by aging baby-boomers, there is a growing concern about forestalling cognitive decline and enhancing cognitive well-being. Memory clinics and memory-enhancing supplements proliferate. Major magazines are replete with features on memory. *Memory* has become the code name for the emerging mental fitness trend and the emerging preoccupation with losing one's mind, with dementia.

But cognition consists of many elements, memory being only one of them. Likewise, memory is one of many aspects of the mind central to our existence. Memory decline is only one of many ways in which the mind can be lost, just as Alzheimer's disease is but one of the several still incurable dementias and AIDS is one of several grave infectious diseases. Although undoubtedly fragile, memory is by no means the only, and possibly not even the most vulnerable, aspect of the mind, and memory loss is not the only way in which the mind can be lost. People often complain of deteriorating "memory," for lack of a better or more accurate term, when what really ails them is the decline of an entirely different aspect of cognition.

As this book will show, no other cognitive loss comes close to the loss of executive functions in the degree of devastation that it visits on one's mind and one's self. As we learn more about brain diseases, we are discovering that the frontal lobes are particularly affected in dementia, schizophrenia, traumatic head injury, attention deficit disorder, and a host of other disorders. The executive functions are affected in dementias both frequently and early.

Any future efforts to enhance cognitive longevity through mind-enhancing "cognotropic" pharmacology, cognitive exercise, or any other means will have to focus on the executive functions of the frontal lobes. This book reviews the emerging scientific methods designed to protect and enhance the mind in general and the executive functions of the frontal lobes in particular.

Finally, we will draw broad analogies between the development of the brain and development of other complex systems, such as digital computational devices and society. These analogies are based on the assumption that all complex systems have certain fundamental features in common and that understanding one complex system helps us understand the others.

I believe that ideas are best understood when considered in the context in which they arise. Therefore, interwoven with the discussion of various topics of cognitive neuroscience are personal vignettes about my teachers, my friends, myself, and the times in which we lived.

2

An End and a Beginning:

A Dedication

Petty gripes aside, we live in a forgiving world, where the margin of error is usually quite generous. I have always suspected that even in the highest reaches of power, decision making is a pretty sloppy process. Once in a while, however, situations arise in the life of a human being, and in a society, which allow no margin of error. These critical situations tax the decision maker's executive abilities to their utmost. At the age of 62, I can think of only one such situation in my life. For me, a student of executive functions, the experience had the dual significance of a personal drama and a practical study in the workings of the frontal lobes—my own.

On an early spring afternoon, my mentor, Alexandr Romanovich Luria, and I were immersed in a conversation that we had had a dozen times before. We were strolling away from Luria's Moscow apartment, up Frunze Street and on toward the Old Arbat.[1] We proceeded cautiously, because Luria had broken his leg and had developed a limp, slowing his usually brisk walking pace. Moscow was thawing after a frigid winter, and the plaza was getting crowded. But Luria was so imposingly professorial in his heavy, almost floor-length, navy cashmere coat with astrakhan collar and matching hat that the crowd gave way.

The year was 1972. The country had lived through Stalin's murderous years, through World War II, through more of Stalin's murderous years, and through Khrushchev's aborted thaw. People were no longer executed for dissent; they were merely jailed. The overriding public mood was no longer bone-chilling terror, but damp, resigned, stagnant hopelessness and indifference, a societal stupor of sorts. My mentor was 70 and I was 25. I was approaching the end of my *aspirantura*, a postgraduate course usually leading to a faculty position. We were talking about my future.

As on many occasions before, Alexandr Romanovich was saying that it was time for me to join the Party—the Communist Party of the Soviet Union. A party member himself, Luria offered to nominate me and to arrange the second nomination from Alexey Nikolayevich Leontyev, also an illustrious psychologist and our dean at the University of Moscow, with whom I was on generally cordial terms. Party membership was the first rung of the Soviet elite, an obligatory stepping-stone for any serious aspirations in life. It was understood that party membership was a sine qua non for any career advancement in the Soviet Union.

It was also understood that nominating me for party membership was a very generous gesture for both Luria and Leontyev. I was a Jew from Latvia, which was regarded as an untrustworthy province, and of "bourgeois" background. My father had spent 5 years in the Gulag as an "enemy of the people." I did not exactly adhere to the Soviet ideal. By vouching for me, Luria and Leontyev, the two paramount figures in Soviet psychology, ran the risk of irritating the university's party organization for pushing "another Jew" into the rarefied strata of the Soviet academic elite. But they were willing to do it, which meant that they wanted me to stay on at the University of Moscow as a junior faculty member. The two of them had protected me before by letting me get away with, or extricating me from, various situations, and they were prepared to support me again.

Again and again, however, I told Alexandr Romanovich that I was not going to join the party. On a dozen occasions over the past few years, whenever Luria brought it up, I would sidestep the subject, turning it into a joke, saying that I was too young, too immature, not yet ready. I did not want an open clash, and Luria did not force one. But this time he was speaking with finality. And this time I said that I was not going to join the party because *I did not want to*.

Alexandr Romanovich Luria was arguably the most important Soviet psychologist of his time. His multifaceted career included groundbreaking cross-cultural and developmental studies, mostly in collaboration with his mentor Lev Semyonovich Vygotsky, one of the greatest psychologists of the twentieth century. But it was his contribution to neuropsychology that earned him truly international acclaim. Universally regarded as a founding father of neuropsychology, he studied the neural basis of language, memory, and, of course, executive functions. Among his contemporaries, nobody contributed to the understanding of the complex relationship between the brain and cognition more than Luria, and for this he was revered on both sides of the Atlantic (Fig. 2.1).

Born in 1902 into the family of a prominent Jewish physician, he had lived through the cultural ferment of the beginning of the century, the volatile years

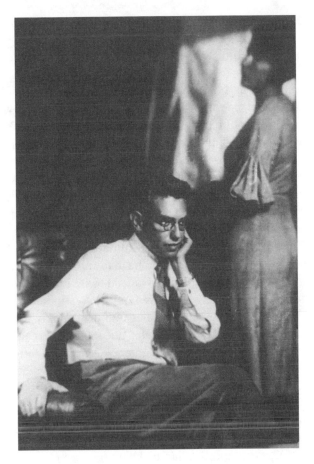

Figure 2.1 Alexandr Romanovich Luria and his wife Lana Pymenovna Luria, both in their early 30s. (Courtesy Dr. Lena Moskovich.)

of the Russian revolution, the civil war, Stalin's purges, World War II, a second round of Stalin's purges, and, finally, a relative thaw. He witnessed the names of his two closest friends and mentors, Lev Vygotsky and Nicholai Bernstein, besmirched and their life's work banned from existence by the state. At various points in his life he was on the verge of incarceration in Stalin's Gulag but, unlike many other Soviet intellectuals, was never actually imprisoned. His career was a peculiar blend of an intellectual odyssey driven by a genuine, natural unfolding of scientific inquiry and a survival course on the Soviet ideological minefield.

Coming from the westernmost edge of the Soviet empire, from the Baltic city of Riga, I grew up in a "European" environment. Unlike the families of my Moscow friends, my parents' generation did not grow up under the Soviets. I had some sense of European culture and European identity. Among my professors at the

University of Moscow, Luria was one of the very few who was recognizably European; this quality was one of the things that drew me to him. He was a multilingual, multitalented man of the world, completely at home with Western civilization.

But he was also a Soviet man used to making compromises in order to survive. I suspected that in the deepest recesses of his being there was a visceral fear of brutal, physical repression. I had known other people like him, and it seemed that the latent fear was forever with them, even when the circumstances had changed and the fear was no longer based in reality, until they died. This fear was the glue of the Soviet regime and, I imagine, the glue of any other repressive regime, until its collapse. This duality of inner intellectual freedom, even haughtiness, and everyday accommodation was rather common among the Soviet intelligentsia. I did not condemn Luria's party membership but I did not respect it either, and it was a source of nagging ambivalence in my attitude toward him. I sort of pitied him for that, an odd feeling for a student to have toward a revered mentor.

My relations with Alexandr Romanovich and his wife Lana Pymenovna, herself a noted scientist–oncologist, were virtually familial. Warm and generous people, they had the habit of drawing their associates into their family life, inviting them to their Moscow apartment and country dacha, and taking them along to art exhibits. The youngest among Luria's immediate associates, I was often the object of their semiparental supervision, ranging from finding me a good dentist to reminders to shine my shoes. As is normal in life, we were occasionally at loggerheads in little things, but we were very close.

Now, as I stated point blank that I was not joining the party, Luria halted in the middle of the street. With a tinge of resignation but also a matter-of-fact finality, he said: "Then, Kolya (my old Russian nickname), there is nothing I can do for you." And that was that. This could have been devastating under a different set of circumstances, but that day I felt relief. Unbeknownst to Alexandr Romanovich or almost anyone else, I had already made up my mind to leave the Soviet Union. By making party membership a precondition for his continued patronage, he freed me from any obligation I felt toward him, which may have interfered with my decision. After this conversation, the last hesitation had been removed, and the question was no longer if, but how.

The decision to leave the country had developed gradually and my motives were complex. I lived under an oppressive regime. Yet my personal career had not been impeded up to that point. The state practiced tacit anti-Semitism; it was known that unwritten quotas existed at universities, yet I studied at the best university in the land. It was known that generally the Jews were not welcome into the highest strata of the Soviet society, yet I did not experience anti-Semitism directed at me personally. Most of my closest friends were Russian, and in my immediate social circle the issue of ethnicity simply did not arise. I was surrounded with successful Jews of my parents' generation, which meant that a career was possible in the Soviet Union despite the tacit restrictions. Religious practices were curtailed and impeded; I grew up in a secular family and this was not an issue of personal concern.

Most of my friends understood that we lived in a society that was neither free nor affluent. Despite the Soviet grandstanding, there was a national sense of inferiority and a sense that the rest of the world was more vibrant, richer in opportunities. We were cut off from that world, the Iron Curtain being a palpable reality, and the larger world beckoned. Having grown up in Westernized Riga, I had no fear of that world.

Political indoctrination began in the Soviet Union practically from the nursery. My family, however, was a little enclave of passive dissent and I began to receive a healthy antidote against official propaganda very early in life. My father was sent to a labor camp when I was a year old. In a grim joke circulating around the country in those days, two inmates were chatting in a labor camp. "How much time did you get?" "Twenty years" "What did you do?" "I burned down a collective farm. And what did you do?" "Nothing" "How much time did you get?" "Fifteen years" "Rubbish. For nothing you get only ten."

My father was sentenced to 10 years in the Gulag in western Siberia. He was sentenced as part of what I called "sociocide," a systematic extermination of whole social groups: the intelligentsia, the foreign-educated, the former affluent class. A mere membership in one of these groups marked a person for persecution. My father was sent to a labor camp, and in the hallway of our apartment my mother kept two packed small suitcases, one for herself and one for me. Separate labor camps existed for the "wives of the enemies of the people," and special orphanages existed for the "children of the enemies of the people." Suitcases were packed and ready in many apartments across the land. The plainclothes agents of the state used to drive up in unmarked black cars (*voronki*, Russian for "little crows") without warning in the middle of the night, ring the doorbell, and give their victims 15 minutes to get ready, before taking them away for 5, 10, 20 years, or for good. One had to be prepared.

I grew up knowing that my father was far away, but not knowing where, exactly. The address on his letters was just a "post office box," and as a child I kept wondering why my father had chosen to live in a box, far away. When Stalin's death was announced in March 1953, somber music was played across the city through loudspeakers. People were weeping on the streets. My mother rushed to the apartment pulling me along, unable to contain her joy and afraid to reveal it in public. My mother had always been politically vocal, to the point of recklessness. It was dangerous to confide even in one's own children, since they were encouraged to report on their parents—and some did. One of them, a boy by the name of Pavlik Morozov, had become a national hero.

Within months, many prisoners of the Gulag were released ahead of time, my father among them. I recall my mother falling into the embrace of a skeleton-thin stranger on the train station platform in Riga. I was 6 years of age and had no memories of my father. Only then did I find out that the "box" was a labor camp, and what this meant. That was my first insight into the true nature of the state we lived in. Many years later my mother recalled that upon discovering the exact nature of my father's "box" I had thrown a fit of rage that frightened her by its intensity, screaming, "So this is what the Soviet Union is really all about!'

Life soon settled into normalcy. As I was growing up, I had no illusions about the state I lived in and had no attachment to it in a patriotic sense—far from it; by a certain age I developed a reasonably well-articulated sense that my whole Soviet existence was a regrettable accident of birth. Yet, on a day-to-day level I felt comfortable and often happy, and I "blended in." I was accepted by the University of Moscow and was on my way to joining the academic elite. But gradually the realization grew that there was no future for me in the Soviet Union, just as there was no future for the Soviet Union.

And now I was standing in the middle of Arbat, knowing that the last source of hesitation had been removed. An existential decision now awaited an executive solution. An attempt to leave the country required an intricate plan, and there was no guarantee of success. To get out, I had to outsmart the Soviet state. I knew that my frontal lobes were going to be heavily taxed during the months to come.

The "workers' paradise" was designed like a mousetrap: it was easier to get in than out. Soviet citizens could not leave the country at will, even temporarily. Permission to go abroad as a tourist or in an official capacity already implied an elite status. A whole family was almost never allowed to travel together; a hostage was always kept to prevent defection. Emigrating permanently was even more difficult. Until the early 1970s it was virtually unheard of. Then, as the consequence of détente and under the pressure from the United States Congress, limited emigration was allowed for Jews to go to Israel. By restricting emigration in this way, the authorities hoped that the precedent could be contained. In reality, however, once Jews were out of the country they were free to go where they chose. Many, myself included, chose the United States. This produced an ironic moment in the history of Russia, when being Jewish suddenly became an asset. I was a member of that all-of-a-sudden "privileged" minority. In that unique set of circumstances, my Jewishness provided a vehicle, more than an impetus, to attempt to get out. As is often the case in life, the relationship between a desire and an opportunity was a bit circular.

But there were many hurdles to jump. The Soviet state was brutally pragmatic. The greater the perceived value of the individual, the more difficult it was to get permission to leave the country. For the graduates of elite universities the chances approached zero. As a graduate of the Moscow State University, the Harvard of the East, I was a valued property of the state. People like me were not ordinarily allowed to emigrate. The slave-owning analogy extended further. Even if permission was granted in principle, the state exacted a ransom, which was determined on the basis of a person's educational level. My ransom would be particularly exorbitant.

My doctoral dissertation had been written and bound, and the oral defense was scheduled in a few months. It was clear that I could not apply for an exit visa while still at the University of Moscow. Anyone applying for an exit visa was made an instant persona non grata. Nobody would allow me to defend my dissertation under these circumstances. I would be immediately expelled from the university.

Delaying my application until after my defense seemed like a logical thing to do. But as I was beginning to plot my escape, it became clear that an advanced degree would jeopardize my chances. Reluctantly, I was reaching the conclusion that I would have to somehow sabotage my own defense. As the frontal lobe functions go, this was an extreme case of inhibiting an urge for immediate gratification. I had to sacrifice something that I had striven for for several years and that would have been mine, with an assured outcome, in a few months' time. The delayed gratification was the prospect of getting out of the country. In the hierarchy of goals (prioritizing one's objectives, another frontal lobe function), this was a higher goal.

The strategy was not without risk. By not receiving my doctorate, I was merely enhancing my chance of success in being allowed to emigrate but by no means assuring it. The equation was too murky to compute the gain in probabilities with any degree of precision. Whatever it was, the probability remained high that I would not be allowed to leave. In situations like this, people remained in lifelong limbo. Denied the request to leave the country, they were also denied the opportunity to reenter the mainstream of the Soviet society. They were fired from their positions and became pariahs, condemned to menial jobs on the fringes of society. But this is precisely why the doctorate no longer mattered. Refused the right to leave, I would be driving a taxi for a living with or without my doctorate.

There was another reason not to defend the dissertation: protecting my friends. My professors would be held responsible by the authorities for the "lack of political vigilance," for nurturing a future "traitor to the motherland." Bizarre as this vernacular sounded, it was actually used in the official political discourse in the Soviet Union. As my mentor, Alexandr Romanovich would be particularly affected. This had to be avoided.

Gradually, a plan took shape in my head. I would somehow avoid defending my dissertation. Then I would disappear from the Moscow State University as inconspicuously as possible and leave Moscow altogether. I would go to my native city of Riga and get the lowliest job possible. Then, after several months, or a year, I would apply for the exit visa. Then it would be out of my hands.

The exact timing of my application would have to depend on things not under my control. Détente was gathering steam. Henry Kissinger was in and out of the country. There were intimations in the press of an imminent visit by President Nixon.

In those situations the Soviets tended to put on their liberal face. I was determined to time my application to coincide with these events as precisely as possible. As I thought through the details of my plan, I had a strange sense of depersonalization, as if I were going through the plot of a novel about someone else's life. But this was to be my story, and it was self-inflicted.

I was trying to cover my tracks. Not that I believed that at the critical moment of decision the authorities would be ignorant of my past. No one could cover their tracks in the Soviet Union. Wherever you moved, you had to register with the local police. An internal file followed every Soviet citizen with every movement around the country. But I was counting on the indifferent and fundamentally brainless nature of the Soviet bureaucracy. By the 1970s, there were very few zealots left within the system. Things were done by the book. The book said that graduates of the University of Moscow and the like were valuable and should not be allowed to leave. The book also said that street-sweepers, cab drivers, and grocery clerks were dispensable and could be let go in the name of lip service to détente. But the book said nothing about Moscow State University graduates turned street-sweepers. My gamble was that the authorities, in their mechanical ways, would not ruminate over my file.

There was another element in my calculations. In a tacit way, I was communicating to the authorities that I was not afraid of them. By relinquishing voluntarily the prestige and promise of my university position and assuming a menial job, I was, in a way, preempting them. Of my own accord, I was visiting upon myself everything they would have done to me had I applied for the exit visa while still at the University of Moscow. By robbing them of the means of repercussion, I robbed them of their control over me. Jailing me was the only thing left to them. Not being an active dissident, I did not think that was likely. The less fear I showed, the more effort they knew it would take to intimidate me into retreat from my plan. With détente in the air and their eagerness to look "civil," they were likely to conclude that keeping me was not worth the effort. But there was no guarantee.

My first impulse was to sit down with Alexandr Romanovich and reveal my plan to him. But there were two compelling reasons not to do so. Although I was doing all I could to distance myself from him and thus minimize any possible repercussions of my actions for him, I could not be certain of his reaction. Whatever his true beliefs were, publicly he had always been a loyal, sometimes eagerly loyal, Soviet citizen. Was it only a patina, which he was careful not to drop? Did he truly believe what he said? I suspected that it was something in between, that a constant conscious dissonance between what you said and what you felt was too painful to endure. In many years of our close association, I was never able to have a candid political discussion with Alexandr Romanovich. Whenever I tried to draw him out, his response was a strident, almost frenzied "party line." The closest Luria had ever come to revealing his deeply buried discontent was through an occasional oblique muttering, "Vremena slozhnye, durakov mnogo" ("These are complex times, many fools around"). What was first adopted as protective mimicry in time became a form of "autohypnosis."

Ironically, the term *autohypnosis* was proposed in 1990, half-jokingly, by none other than Luria's own daughter Lena, over dinner at Nirvana, an Indian restaurant overlooking New York's Central Park. We were talking about her parents, both long deceased, and about other people of their generation. Like myself, Lena was fascinated by political autohypnosis as a psychological defense mechanism under tyranny. Luria's wife, Lana Pymenovna, was considerably less given to autohypnosis, and over the years we had had many candid conversations on forbidden subjects.

With this background, there was no guarantee that Luria would not report my intentions to the university authorities. According to the rules governing the system, this was actually expected of him, and ignoring the rule would be perceived as a serious transgression by a Soviet professor and party member in good standing. Informed about my plans, the university would find me a potential source of embarrassment and get rid of me immediately. I would find myself in limbo even before applying for the visa. That was particularly risky. Expelled from the university as "politically unsound," I would find it extremely difficult to get a job—any kind of job. Within the parameters of the Soviet mousetrap-state, this was a very dangerous position. A law on the books allowed the state to arrest and jail "parasites," or people without employment. This rarely enforced law was invoked when the authorities wanted to "get" someone—particularly the "politically unsound" trying to leave the country. For the sake of my plan and my teacher's soul, I could only hope that he would not turn me in, but there was no guarantee.

There was another, less self-centered reason not to confide in Alexandr Romanovich. Simply put, I was afraid that the shock of the news about my plans would trigger a heart attack right then and there. He did have a bad heart, and the visceral fear of the state could lead to an emotional reaction disproportionate to the reality of the situation. From every angle, Alexandr Romanovich was better off not knowing about my intentions. Only a few people knew about my plans. They were all trusted friends, despite their very different origins and persuasions.

And so I decided to resort to a white lie. Canceling an already scheduled oral defense was unheard of. I invented a story about a medical emergency in the family and the pressing need to get a job right away. My manifest plan was to move back to Riga, get a job, support my family until the "crisis" was over, and then come back to defend—in half a year or a year, with any luck. Luria was disturbed by the story, but through a tour de force I prevailed. I was able to disengage myself from the university without revealing, and thus jeopardizing, my plans.

I arrived in Riga and began to look for a job. This turned out to be very difficult, since I was obviously overqualified for the jobs I applied for. Finally, I was hired as a hospital orderly at a downtown city hospital—the lowest on the totem pole.

I was assigned to the emergency intensive care unit. The patients—car accidents, overdoses, stab wounds, rapes—gave me a new perspective on the city of my birth.

The patients were brought in by ambulance in the middle of the night. I reported for work at six in the morning, by which time some of them had already died. Identifying the dead on the filthy beds and counting them was my first order of the day. Six or seven was about average. My duty was to deliver the cadavers to the morgue. I carried them manually on a shaky stretcher with my "partner," Maria.

Maria was a toothless, perpetually drunk woman of 40 going on 65. Her command of Russian profanities was awesome. In those days, I was pretty foul-mouthed myself, yet I was humbled by her virtuosity. Every morning on arrival she checked out the medical autoclaves for ethanol used to sterilize medical instruments. This was her breakfast. By seven in the morning, when we were ready to load our cadavers, she was so drunk she could barely walk. She stumbled, tripped, and occasionally fell. Then I was stuck with two cadavers, a real one and a virtual one.

The rest of my activities were trivial by comparison: carrying bottles with medications, mopping floors, transferring patients—all the usual tasks orderlies do all over the world. It was a surreal experience. But after months of extreme cognitive exertion associated with critical decision making (this must have been the first time in my life when I discovered such a thing as cognitive exertion), there was calm, a hiatus, a semblance of stability, however fragile and bizarre. For the next few months, until I applied for my visa, there were no critical decisions to make. And when I applied, I would not be fired. Not from this job! I was resting my frontal lobes.

In due time, I applied for my exit visa, and a few months later I was summoned to receive the response. It was favorable. I was free to go. The uniformed woman who gave me the news had my file in front of her. She browsed through it and exclaimed with incredulity: "They are letting you go with a background like this!" I just shrugged my shoulders. There was no indignation in her voice, just bemusement. It was not her decision and she did not care. As I was walking down the street, I again had a sense of depersonalization, as if this was not happening to me but to someone I was watching from outside. My parents, who I suspect did not quite believe until the very end that my brazen plot would suceed, had the bitter-sweet experience of the impossible coming true, but supported me all the way and paid my state "emigration ransom," something I would not have been able to do on my own.

I flew to Moscow to say goodbyes. Like hundreds of times before, we were sitting together around the massive antique desk with brass lion heads in Luria's study. Two years had passed since our walk on the old Arbat. Alexandr Romanovich and I talked for many hours—six, seven, or more. Lana Pymenovna served tea and joined us intermittently. Luria was not offended by my white lie. He sounded relieved to have been left out of the whole affair. Finally he said, "I don't approve of *what* you are doing, but I thank you for *how* you have done it." It was understood that I could never contact him from abroad; I was now persona non grata. This was to be our last conversation. Alexandr Romanovich died 3 years later.

I came to the United States in the late summer of 1974 via a circuitous route of Vienna and Rome, and started from the beginning. The intellectual and stylistic continuity linking a pupil to his master was broken, and I found myself in my new homeland essentially on my own. This made things harder in the beginning, yet in retrospect, more gratifying. At the same time, the continuity was preserved through the numerous and enduring threads of my teacher's influences, which to this day permeate my career in ways both obvious and subtle. Exactly 35 years have passed since that uneasy farewell. My interest in the frontal lobes was seeded by Alexandr Romanovich and has remained among the most persistent themes of my career. And so this book is written in memory of Alexandr Romanovich Luria, the man who influenced my life in definitive ways, and of the complex times in which his career ended and mine began.

3

The Brain's Chief Executive:

The Frontal Lobes at a Glance

The Many Faces of Leadership

They arrive at work in limousines with smoked-glass windows; they ride to the top floors of the corporate headquarters in private elevators; their salaries are beyond the average person's imagination. An informal survey suggests that they are, on average, a few inches taller than the rest of us. Cloaked in mystique and regarded with awe, they are the chief executive officers—the CEO's of America.

Up the street from the soaring midtown Manhattan corporate head-quarters, at Carnegie Hall, a disheveled conductor rehearses his orchestra. A few blocks south, off Broadway, an exasperated stage director tries to get actors to grasp his interpretation of a famous play. They would seem to have little in common with the corporate baron, but they perform similar functions. To a naive observer, the CEO does not manufacture the company's product, just as the conductor does not make music, and the director does not act. Yet they direct the actions of those who manu-facture the product, play the music, or perform on stage. Without them there would be no product, no concert, no show.

The role of a leader sending others into action, instead of acting him- or herself, evolved in society relatively late. The history of early music makes no mention of the conductor, and there is no mention of a director in the

Greek theater. Early warfare was a clash of two hordes, each man fighting his own fight; the general came millennia later. And it was fairly recent in the history of warfare that the top military commander no longer inspired the troops with his personal frontline courage but guided the battle from the rear.[1]

The function of leadership acquires a distinct status and becomes separate only when the size and complexity of the organization (or the organism) crosses a certain threshold. Once the function of leadership has crystallized into a special-ized role, the wisdom of leadership is to maintain a delicate, dynamic balance between the autonomy of and control over the organism's parts. A wise leader knows when to step in and impose his or her will and when to step back and let the lieutenants display their own initiative.

The leader's role is elusive but critical. Let the leader lapse, however briefly, and disaster strikes. An orchestra will descend into cacophony, corporate deci-sion making will grind to a halt, and a great army will falter. In fact, some his-torians attribute the decisive defeat of Napoleon's Great Army at Waterloo to the emperor's flagging leadership due to a painful exacerbation of chronic illness.[2]

The leader's role is critical but elusive. I recall wondering, as a little boy, why the orchestra required that funny man on the podium waving his hands, since he did not contribute anything audible to the music being created before me. And I recall my friend's 3-year-old son describing his father's job as "sitting in the office and sharpening pencils" (his father was the chairman of a large department at a major university).

Likewise, early neurology texts contained elaborate descriptions of the roles played by other parts of the brain, but gave the frontal lobes barely a footnote. The implication was that the frontal lobes were there mostly for ornamental purposes. It took neuroscientists many years to even begin to appreciate the importance of the frontal lobes for cognition. When this finally did happen, a picture of particular complexity and elegance emerged. We will begin to examine it now.

The Executive Lobe

The human brain is the most complex natural system in the known universe; its complexity rivals and probably exceeds the complexity of the most intricate social and economic structures. It is science's new frontier. The 1990s were declared by the National Institutes of Health (NIH) the decade of the brain. Just as the first half of the twentieth century was the age of physics, and the second half of the twenti-eth century was the age of biology, so the beginning of the twenty-first century is the age of brain–mind science.

Like a large corporation, a large orchestra, or a large army, the brain consists of distinct components serving distinct functions. And like these large-scale human organizations, the brain has its CEO, its conductor, its general: the frontal lobes.

To be precise, this role is vested in but one part of the frontal lobes, the prefrontal cortex. It is a common shorthand, however, to use the term *frontal lobes*.

Like the exalted leadership roles in human society, the frontal lobes were late in coming. In evolution their development began to accelerate only with the great apes. As the seat of intentionality, foresight, and planning, the frontal lobes are the most uniquely "human" of all the components of the human brain. In 1928 the neurologist Tilney suggested that entire human evolution should be considered the "age of the frontal lobe."[3]

Like the functions of a CEO, the functions of the frontal lobes defy a soundbite definition. They are not invested with any single, ready-to-label function. A patient with frontal lobe disease will retain the ability to move around, use language, recognize objects, and even memorize information. Yet like a leaderless army, cognition disintegrates and ultimately collapses with the loss of the frontal lobes. In my native Russian language, there is an expression "bez tsarya v golovye"—"a head without the czar inside." This expression could have been invented to describe the effects of frontal lobe damage on behavior.

As if the royal connection was not enough, the frontal lobes have been invested also with divine aura. In his remarkable cultural–neuropsychological essay, Julian Jaynes advances the idea that internally generated executive commands were mistaken by primitive humans for externally originated voices of the gods.[4] Thus, by implication, the advent of executive functions at early stages of human civilization may have been responsible for the molding of religious beliefs.

Art historians have noted a curious detail in *The Creation of Adam*, Michelangelo's great fresco on the ceiling of the Sistine Chapel. God's mantle has the distinct shape of the outline of the brain, his feet rest on the brain stem, and his head is framed by the frontal lobe. God's finger, pointed toward Adam and making him human, projects from the prefrontal cortex. In the words of Julius Meier-Graefe, "There is more genius in the finger of God, calling Adam to life, than in the whole work of any of Michelangelo's forerunners."[5] No one knows whether the allegory was intended by Michelangelo, or whether the image is coincidental; it may well be the latter. But a more powerful symbol of the frontal lobes' profound humanizing effect can hardly be imagined. The frontal lobes are truly "the organ of civilization."

Because the frontal lobes are not linked to any single, easily defined function, early theories of brain organization denied them any role of consequence. In fact, the frontal lobes used to be known as "the silent lobes." Over the last decades, however, the frontal lobes have become the focus of intense scientific investigation. Still, our efforts to understand the functions of the frontal lobes, and particularly the prefrontal cortex, are very much a work in progress and, for lack of more precise concepts, we often lapse into poetic metaphor. The prefrontal cortex plays the central role in forming goals and objectives and then in devising plans of action required to attain these goals. It selects the cognitive skills required to implement the plans, coordinates these skills, and applies them in a correct order. Finally, the prefrontal cortex is responsible for evaluating our actions as success or failure relative to our intentions. The prefrontal cortex is also critical for forming abstract representations of the environment as well as of complex behaviors, as studies of extracellular recordings in monkeys have shown.[6,7]

Human cognition is forward looking, proactive rather than reactive. It is driven by goals, plans, aspirations, ambitions, and dreams, all of which pertain to the future and not to the past. These cognitive powers depend on the frontal lobes and evolve with them. In a broad sense, the frontal lobes are the organism's mechanism of liberating itself from the past and projecting into the future. The frontal lobes endow the organism with the ability to create neural models of things as a prerequisite for making things happen, models of something that does not yet exist but that one wants to bring into existence.

To conjure up an internal representation of the future, the brain must have an ability to take certain elements of prior experiences and reconfigure them in a way that in its totality does not correspond to any actual past experience. To accomplish this, the organism must go beyond the mere ability to *form* internal representations, the models of the world outside. It must acquire the ability to *manipulate* and *transform* these models. As a friend of mine, a gifted mathematician, has said, the organism must go beyond the ability to see the world *through* mental representations; it must acquire the ability to work *with* mental representations. A metaphor I sometimes use to explain the unique role of the prefrontal cortex in forging mental representations is one of the mermaid. You don't need your frontal lobes to conjure up the mental image of a human; nor do you need them to conjure up the mental image of a fish, since both are based on past experiences. But you do need your prefrontal cortex to conjure up the mental representation of a mermaid, since it is very unlikely that you have ever encountered one in real life.

One of the fundamental distinguishing features of human cognition, systematic tool-making, may be said to depend on this ability, since a tool does not exist in a ready-made form in the natural environment and has to be conjured in order to be made. To go even further, the development of the neural machinery capable of creating and holding images of the future, the frontal lobes, may be seen as a necessary prerequisite for tool making, and thus for the ascent of humankind and the launching of human civilization as it is frequently defined.

Moreover, the generative power of language to create new constructs may depend on this ability as well. The ability to manipulate and recombine internal representations critically depends on the prefrontal cortex, and the emergence of this ability parallels the evolution of the frontal lobes. The relationship between the emergence of language and the advent of the frontal lobes late in evolution is not commonly invoked, but it may be the generative capability conferred by the frontal lobes, more than the mysterious "language instinct,"[8] that made complex propositional structures possible. This point is also implicit in a review of the neurobiology of language, by Michael Ullman.[9] The critical role of the prefrontal cortex in making use of the "open-ended" generative capacity inherent in language was made dramatically clear in the functional magnetic resonance imaging (fMRI) study by a group of Dutch neuroscientists led by Peter Hagoort.[10] When normal subjects hear sentences with statements containing semantic violations ("trains are sour") or real-world violations (misstating the color of trains in the Netherlands), their left inferior prefrontal cortex becomes particularly active.

Therefore, the roughly contemporaneous development of executive functions and language was adaptively highly fortuitous. Language provided the means for building models, and the executive functions provided the means of manipulating them and conducting operations on the models. To parlay this into the language of biology, the advent of the frontal lobes was necessary to make use of the generative capability inherent in language. For the believers in drastic discontinuities as a major factor in evolution, the confluence between the development of language and executive functions may have been the definitive force behind the quantum leap that was the advent of humans.

Of all the mental processes, goal formation is the most actor-centered activity. Goal formation is about "I need" and not about "it is." So the emergence of the ability to formulate goals must have been inexorably linked to the emergence of the mental representation of "self." It should come as no surprise that the emergence of self-consciousness is also intricately linked to the evolution of the frontal lobes. All these functions can be thought of as metacognitive rather than cognitive, since they do not refer to any particular mental skill but provide an overarching organization for all of them. For this reason some authors refer to the functions of the frontal lobes as "executive functions," by analogy with the corporate CEO.

I find the analogy with the orchestra conductor even more revealing. But to fully appreciate the functions and the responsibilities of the conductor, we first need to learn more about the orchestra.

4

Architecture of the Brain:

A Primer

The Microscopic View

The brain consists of hundreds of billions of cells (*neurons* and *glial cells*), intricately interconnected by pathways (*dendrites* and *axons*). Several types of neurons and glial cells exist. Some of the pathways between neurons are local, branching within their immediate "neighborhoods." But others are long, interconnecting distant neural structures. These long pathways are covered with white fatty tissue, *myelin*, which facilitates the passage of the electric signals generated within the neurons (*action potentials*). The neurons and short local connections together comprise the *gray matter*, and the long myelinated pathways comprise the *white matter*. Every neuron is interconnected with a myriad of other neurons, resulting in intricate patterns of interactions. Thus a network of mind-boggling complexity is constructed of relatively simple elements.

The principle of achieving great complexity through multiple permutations of simple elements appears to be universal and is implemented in nature (and culture) in a variety of ways. Think, for instance, of language, in which thousands of words, sentences, and narratives are constructed out of a few dozen letters; or think of the genetic code—a virtually infinite number of variants can be achieved through the combination of a finite number of genes.

Although the signal generated within a neuron is electric, the communication between the neurons takes a chemical form. Intertwined and interwoven with the structural complexity described above are the brain's multiple biochemical systems. The biochemical substances, called *neurotransmitters* and *neuromodulators*, allow communication between neurons. An electric signal (*action potential*) is generated within the body of the neuron and travels along the axon until it reaches the terminal, the point of contact with a dendrite, a pathway leading to another neuron. At the point of contact there is a gap called the *synapse*. The arrival of the action potential releases small quantities of chemical substances (neurotransmitters), which travel across the synapse like rafts across a river and attach themselves to *receptors*, highly specialized molecules on the other side of the gap. This accomplished, the neurotransmitters are broken down in the synapse with the help of specialized enzymes. Meanwhile, the activation of postsynaptic receptors results in another electric event, a *postsynaptic potential*. A number of postsynaptic potentials occurring together result in another action potential, and the process is iterated thousands of thousands of times along both parallel and sequential pathways. This allows coding information of stupendous complexity.

We are constantly learning about new types of neurotransmitters and neuromodulators. To date, several dozens of them have been discovered: glutamate, gamma-aminobutyric acid (GABA), serotonin, acetylcholine, norepinephrine, and dopamine, to name a few. Some neurotransmitters, like glutamate or GABA, are found virtually everywhere in the brain. Other neurotransmitters, like dopamine, are restricted to certain parts of the brain. Each neurotransmitter can bind to several receptor types, some of which are ubiquitous and others, region-specific. Sometimes the term *neurotransmitter* is used inclusively to refer to all of the above. Often, however, more careful terminology is used, distinguishing between neurotransmitters and neuromodulators on the basis of their action time course and neuroanatomical distribution. Neurotransmitters, which include glutamate and GABA, are fast acting, and are in charge of local interactions throughout the brain. By contrast, neuromodulators, which include dopamine, norepinephrine, serotonin, and acetylcholine, are slower acting, are controlled by nuclei located in the brain stem, and exert their influence over distant brain regions via long axons. Dopamine in particular has been linked to the function of the frontal lobes and will figure prominently in much of the forthcoming discussion. Different types of dopamine receptors—D1, D2, and D4 among them—play different roles in the executive functions of the frontal lobes,[1] and pharmacoligical dysruption of their function interferes with important functions of the frontal lobes, such as working memory.[2] But it would be naïve to think that other neuromodulators do not play a role in mediating executive functions of the frontal lobes. Thus, it has been demonstrated that prefrontal serotonin depletion results in cognitive inflexibility, one of the most common consequences of frontal lobe dysfunction.[3] Our understanding of the biochemical bases of cognition in general and of the executive functions in particular is very much work in progress, still far from complete and awaiting new discoveries.

The brain can be thought of as the coupling of two highly complex organizations, structural and chemical. This coupling leads to an exponential increase in the system's overall complexity. This, in turn, is further increased by the ubiquitous feedback loops, with the activity of the signal source being modified by its target, both local and global, structural and biochemical. As a result, the brain can produce an infinite array of different activation patterns, corresponding to the infinite states of the outside world. The neuron represents a microscopic unit of the brain, and the pattern of connectivity between neurons represents the microscopic organization of the brain.

When the organism is exposed to a new pattern of signals from the outside world, the strengths of synaptic contacts (the ease of signal passage between neurons) and local biochemical and electrical properties gradually change in complex distributed constellations. This represents learning, as we understand it today.[4]

The Macroscopic View

Neurons are grouped into cohesive structures, *nuclei* and *regions*. Each structure consists of millions of neurons. The nuclei and regions represent the macroscopic units of the brain, and the pattern of connectivity between them represents the macroscopic organization of the brain. The brain is a highly interconnected system, and the architecture of the major connections between its nuclei and regions provides a useful aerial view of the whole system.

For heuristic purposes, I resort to the metaphor of a tree. A tree has a trunk and branches. Branches divide into limbs. At the end of the limbs sits fruit. In a way, the brain is organized in a similar manner. One can think of the brain as an arousal and activation tree. Its trunk is in charge of the general physiological arousal and activation necessary for the function of various brain structures, the fruit. This is the brain's anatomical pivot, the *brain stem*. Massive damage to the brain stem disrupts consciousness and may lead to coma.

Contained within the compact brain-stem core are numerous nuclei, which give rise to an intricate system of pathways. In many instances the nuclei and their projections are biochemically specific, linked to a particular neurotransmitter; in other instances they are biochemically complex, involving several neurotransmitters. These are the branches and limbs of the arousal tree. Each branch contains projections to a distinct part of the brain, ensuring its activation. A few decades ago it was common to refer to these branches collectively as the ascending reticular activating system (ARAS).[5] Today it is increasingly possible to identify its distinct neuroanatomical and biochemical components and to study these components separately. Damage to any given branch will not disrupt conscious-ness in a global sense, but will interfere with specific brain function. Each branch of the arousal tree projects into distinct components of the brain, each with its own set of functions.

A number of subcortical structures exist in the brain. In evolution, subcortical structures developed before the cortex, and for millions of years they guided the complex behaviors of various organisms. In contemporary living reptiles, and even birds, the neocortex is only minimally represented.[6] In a phylogenetically ancient, acortical brain two sets of structures could be identified: the *thalamus* and the *basal ganglia*. Early in evolution the central nervous system divided into two lateral halves. Therefore, each of the brain structures described here consists of a pair of twin halves: left and right.

Despite a certain functional overlap, the thalamus and the basal ganglia were invested with distinctly different functions. In the ancient, precortical brain the thalamus was mostly in charge of receiving and processing information from the external world, and the basal ganglia were in charge of motor behavior and action. Thus the distinction between perception and action seems to have been funda-mental in the brain's architecture from early on. The arousal tree divides into two major branches, one projecting separately into the subcortical machinery of perception (the *dorsal branch*), the other into one of action (the *ventral branch*).

Although often treated as a single structure, the thalamus is, in fact, a collection of many nuclei. Some of them are in charge of processing distinct types of sensory information: visual, auditory, tactile, and the like. Other thalamic nuclei are in charge of integrating various types of sensory information. A complex hierarchy of input integration is present in the thalamus. The dorsomedial thalamic nucleus is at the summit of this hierarchy, and it is closely interconnected with the prefron-tal cortex. Other thalamic nuclei, found around the midline, are nonspecific, in charge of various forms of activation.[7]

Closely linked to the thalamus is the *hypothalamus*. While the thalamus moni-tors the world outside, the hypothalamus monitors the organism's internal states and helps maintain them within the adaptive, homeostatic parameters. The hypo-thalamus is also a collection of distinct nuclei, each related to a distinct aspect of homeostasis: food intake, liquid intake, body temperature, and so on. Together, the thalamus and the hypothalamus are referred as the *diencephalon*.[8]

The basal ganglia include the caudate nuclei, the putamen, and globus pallidus. In the precortical brain these structures were central to the initiation of actions and control over movements. In the evolved mammalian brain, the basal ganglia are under particularly close control of the frontal lobes and work in collaboration with them. In fact, the collaboration is so close that I tend to think of the caudate nuclei as part of the greater frontal lobes.

A structure called the *amygdala* is also regarded as one of the basal ganglia, but it serves a somewhat different function. The amygdala regulates those interactions of the organism with the external world that are critical to the survival of the specimen and the species: decisions to attack or to escape, to copulate or not, to ingest or not. It provides rapid, precognitive, affective assessment of the situation in terms of its survival value.[9]

The *cerebellum* is a large structure attached to the back (or, as a neuroanatomist would say, to the dorsal aspect) of the brain stem. Its anatomy parallels in miniature the anatomy of the whole brain: a pivot called the *vermis* and two cerebellar cortical hemispheres, characterized by an astounding degree of structural homogeneity. The cerebellum is important in movements, particularly in coordinating fine movements with sensory information. But because of the sheer number of neurons in the cerebellum—about 50 billion, almost half of the total number of neurons in the brain—researchers have always been suspected that it is important for other functions as well. In particular, it has been shown that the cerebellum is closely linked to the frontal cortex and participates in complex planning.[10,11] This is consistent with the neuroanatomical findings that the subdivisions of the cerebellum interconnected with the dorsolateral prefrontal cortex seemed to co-evolve simultaneously with the dorsolateral prefrontal cortex. Magnetic resonance imaging (MRI) studies have shown that these parts of the cerebellum reach a disproportionately large size; and diffusion tensor imaging (DTI) studies have shown that they receive a disproportionately large number of fibers in humans compared to those in nonhuman primates.[12]

Relatively late in the evolution of the brain, the cortex began to emerge, first the archicortex, then the paleocortex.[13] They include the hippocampus and the cingulate cortex. The *hippocampus*, the "seahorse," is composed of two long structures hugging the inside of the temporal lobes (or in neuroanatomical terms, on their mesial aspects); so strictly speaking one should talk about *hippocampi*, since there are two of them – one in each hemisphere. The hippocampus plays a critical role in memory; the extent of this role is the real question. Some scientists believe that it is dedicated particularly to spatial learning.[14] I think that this is a narrow view prompted by animal experiments, where spatial learning is the only possible paradigm to study memory. Others believe that, in humans, the hippocampus is also implicated in verbal memory.[15] Although the exact role of the hippocampi in memory is still being debated, most neuroscientists no longer believe that the hippocampi are the actual "storehouses" of memories. Instead, the hippocampi likely facilitate the formation of neocortical circuits, which embody memories, by coactivating widely dispersed neocortical neurons in the absence of the actual external stimulation, thus allowing the Hebbian "fire-together-wire-together" principle to play itself out over time. As the neocortical memory representation becomes increasingly robust, the hippocampal participation recedes.[16,17,18,19]

The other part of the cortex, the *cingulate cortex*, hugs the inner surface of the hemispheres overlying the corpus callosum. Its function is not entirely clear, but it has been implicated in emotions. Together with the amygdala and hippocampi, the cingulate cortex comprises the so-called limbic system,[20] a somewhat outdated construct implying a functional unity among these structures, whose heuristic value has been increasingly challenged. The anterior cingulate cortex, presumed to deal with uncertainty, is closely linked to the prefrontal cortex.[21] In a sense, it is also part of the greater frontal lobes. A certain functional unity has been demonstrated between the left dorsolateral prefrontal cortex and the left anterior cingulate cortex, and the right dorsolateral prefrontal cortex and the right anterior cingulate cortex as they mediate distinctly lateralized braian functions.[22] The extent to which the dorsolateral perfrontal cortex and the anterior cingulate cortex are functionally interconnected will become clear throughout subsequent discussion.

Finally, the *neocortex* arrived on the evolutionary scene,[23] a thin mantle hugging the brain and wrinkled in walnutlike convolutions. The cortical mantle has its own intricate organization. It consists of six layers, each characterized by its own neuronal composition. Certain parts of the neocortex are organized into vertical "columns" cutting through the layers and representing distinct functional units. The arrival of the neocortex has radically changed the way information is processed and has endowed the brain with far greater computational powers and complexity. The division into two lateral twin systems continues within the cortex, giving rise to two cerebral hemispheres. The distinction between the perception and action systems is also retained at the neocortical level, the posterior (back) part of the cortex dedicated to perception and the anterior (front) part dedicated to action. But despite these divisions, the neocortex is much more heavily interconnected than its subcortical predecessors. As we will see later, this may have been its adaptive raison d'être (see Chapter 5, Autonomy and Control in the Brain).

The arrival of the neocortex radically changed the balance of power within the brain. The ancient subcortical structures, which used to discharge certain functions independently, now found themselves subordinated to the neocortex and assumed supporting functions in the shadow of the new level of neural organization. For a scientist trying to understand these functions this new relationship presents a source of confusion: what these subcortical structures had evolved to do before the advent of the cortex is probably not exactly what they do today, in the fully cortical brain. And so, paradoxically, our understanding of cortical functions is in many respects more precise than our understanding of the thalamic or basal ganglia functions, despite the fact that the cortex is, in some sense, more "advanced."

The neocortex consists of distinct regions, the *cytoarchitechtonic regions*, each characterized by its own type of neuronal composition and patterns of local connectivity. The neocortex performs diverse functions, yet no simple relationship exists between its different functions and cytoarchitectonic regions. The neocortex consists of four major lobes, each linked to its own type of information: the *occipital* lobe deals with visual information, the *temporal* lobe deals with sounds, the *parietal* lobe deals with tactile sensations, and the *frontal* lobe deals with movements.

At a very late stage of cortical evolution, two major developments took place: the emergence of language and a rapid ascent of the executive functions. As we will see, language acquired its place in the neocortex by attaching itself to various cortical areas in a highly distributed way. And the executive functions emerged as the brain's command post in the front portion of the frontal lobe, the *prefrontal cortex*. The frontal lobes underwent an explosive expansion at the late stage of evolution.

According to Korbinian Brodmann,[24] the prefrontal cortex or its analogues account for 29% of the total cortex in humans, 17% in the chimpanzee, 11.5% in the gibbon and the macaque, 8.5% in the lemur, 7% in the dog, and 3.5% in the cat (Fig. 4.1).

There are several ways of delineating the prefrontal cortex relative to other cortical areas. One such method is based on so-called cytoarchitectonic maps, maps of the cortex comprised of morphologically distinct, numbered brain regions (Fig. 4.2). These cortical regions are called "Brodmann areas," named after the author of the most commonly used cytoarchitectonic map.[25] According to this definition, the prefrontal cortex consists of Brodmann areas 8, 9, 10, 11, 12, 13, 44, 45, 46, and 47.[26] The prefrontal cortex is characterized by the predominance of the so-called granular neural cells, found mostly in layer IV.[27]

An alternative but roughly equivalent method of outlining the prefrontal cortex is through its subcortical projections. A particular subcortical structure is commonly used for this purpose: the *dorsomedial thalamic nucleus*, which is, in a sense, the point of convergence, or the "summit," of the integration occurring

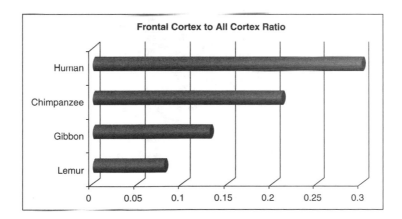

Figure 4.1 Ratio of frontal cortex to total cortex in different simian and primate species. Based on Brodmann (1909).

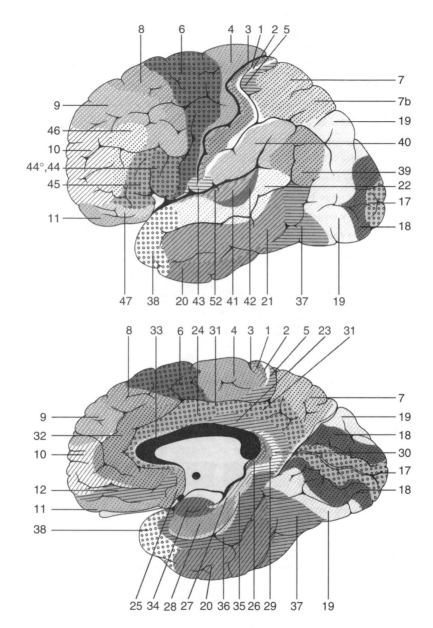

Figure 4.2 Cortical map with cytoarchitectonic regions after Brodmann. [Adapted from G. W. Roberts, P. N. Leigh, and D. R. Weinberger, *Neuropsychiatric Disorders* (London: Wolfe, 1993). Reprinted with permission.]

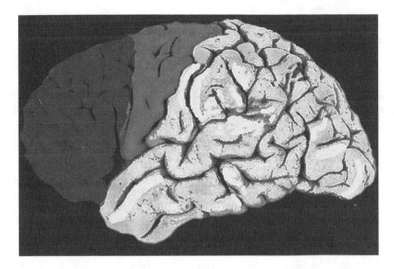

Figure 4.3 Prefrontal cortex (dark shading) in relationship to the frontal lobe (combined area of light and dark shading).

within the specific thalamic nuclei. The prefrontal cortex is then defined as the area receiving projections from the dorsomedial thalamic nucleus. The prefrontal cortex is sometimes delineated also through its biochemical pathways. According to that definition, the prefrontal cortex is defined as the area receiving projections from the mesocortical dopamine system. The various methods of delineating the prefrontal cortex outline roughly identical territories, shown in Figure 4.3.

In a curious parallel between the evolution of the brain and the evolution of brain science (we will revisit this subject more than once), interest in the prefrontal cortex was also late in coming. But then it gradually began to reveal its secrets to the great scientists and clinicians such as Hughlings Jackson[28] and Alexandr Luria,[29] and in the last few decades to researchers including Antonio Damasio,[30] Joaquin Fuster,[31] Patricia Goldman-Rakic,[32] and Donald Stuss and Frank Benson.[33]

The Command Post and Its Connections

A command post is only as good as its lines of communications with the combat units. True to its "executive" functions, the prefrontal cortex is probably the best-connected part of the brain. The prefrontal cortex is directly interconnected with virtually every distinct functional unit of the brain.[34,35] It is connected to the posterior association cortex, the highest station of perceptual integration, and also with the premotor cortex, basal ganglia, and the cerebellum, all involved in various aspects of motor control and movements. The prefrontal cortex is connected with the dorsomedial thalamic nucleus, the highest station of neural integration within the thalamus; with the hippocampus and related structures, known to be critical for memory; and with the cingulate cortex, presumed to be critical for emotion and dealing with uncertainty. In addition, this command post connects with the amygdala, which regulates most basic relations between the individual members of the species, and with the hypothalamus, in charge of control over the vital homeostatic functions. Last but far from least, it is connected with the brain stem nuclei in charge of activation and arousal.

Of all the structures in the brain, only the prefrontal cortex is embedded in such a richly networked pattern of neural pathways. This unique connectivity makes the frontal lobes singularly suited for coordinating and integrating the work of all the other brain structures—the conductor of the orchestra. The elaborate connectivity of the prefrontal cortex makes it ideally suited for combining diverse inputs into arbitrary associations; you don't necessarily need the prefrontal cortex to form the mental image of a human or of a fish, but you do need it to form the mental representation of a mermaid (an amalgamation of the two). Indeed, the prefrontal cortex is replete with neurons firing in a way that implies various "conjunctive" associations.[36] The far-reaching consequence of this propensity is the prefrontal cortex's generativity, its ability to form not only neural representations that are directly based in experience, but also those which are not. As we shall see, however, this extreme connectivity also puts the frontal lobes at particular risk for disease. As in political, economic, and military organizations, the leader is ultimately responsible for the subordinates' blunders. It is also worth noting that not every signal received by the brain through the sensory systems is communicated to the frontal lobes; a considerable degree of input filtering is evident.[37] Furthermore, increasing integration probably occurs in various parts of the prefrontal cortex in direct relationship to their proximity to the frontal poles, as we will find out in the next chapters.

We will see later that the prefrontal cortex, unique among the brain structures, seems to contain the map of the whole cortex, an assertion first made by Hughlings Jackson[38] at the end of the nineteenth century. It has been proposed that this property of the prefrontal cortex may be the critical prerequisite of consciousness, the "inner perception." Since many aspects of our mental world may, in principle, be the focus of our consciousness, it stands to reason that an area of convergence of all its neural substrates must exist. Developing the argument to its logical extreme, this leads to the provocative proposition that the evolution of consciousness, the highest expression of the developed brain, parallels the evolution of the prefrontal cortex. Indeed, certain experimental data have been used to argue that the concept of "self," which is deemed to be a critical attribute of the conscious mind, appears only in the great apes. And it is only in the great apes that the prefrontal cortex acquires a major place in the brain. The admittedly very limited rendition of self in these experiments entails putting a bright mark on a creature's forehead, placing the animal in front of the mirror, and examining its reactions. It is argued that most mammalian species in such experiments respond to their own mirror image as if it were a stranger, but a chimpanzee will attempt to remove the spot from its forehead, thus revealing its comprehension that the image in the mirror is one of its own self. I have to confess that when I attempted the experiment with my bull-mastiff Brit, he seemed to act less in the manner of a dog and more in the manner of a great ape, which he is definitely not, but then again, canines are olfactory creatures more than visual ones, which may have invalidated our bedroom mirror experiment.

Having touched upon the Pandora's box called "consciousness," I have no intention of actually opening it. I have always felt that there is less to the concept of consciousness than meets the eye. To me the possession of consciousness equals the possession of the neocortex, particularly of its association regions; and the phenomenon of conscious experience is nothing more and nothing less than the activation of a sufficiently extensive neocortical network for a sufficient length of time and at a sufficient level of intensity. In this I concur with Joaquin Fuster and Jeffrey Hawkins.[39,40] To put it in different terms, in order to be potentially available to consciousness, an experience has to be represented in the neocortex, and must most likely involve the heteromodal association cortices (prefrontal, inferoparietal, and inferotemporal) at least to some degree, even though probably not exclusively. And the conscious experience itself (or bringing an experience or a thought into the focus of consciousness) is the excitation of the corresponding network at a sufficient level of intensity, temporal duration, and spatial extent. This understanding of consciousness helps explain, in fact, predicts, among other things, that the representations stored in the left hemisphere are more readily available for consious experience (this assertion will be more clear from the following discussion, particularly in Chapter 14). Considered in such terms, consciousness is stripped of its status as the Holy Grail of neuroscience, with all the implications of having a mysterious, as yet hidden, specialized machinery. I realize that this assertion may upset a number of my colleagues and may even sound flippant, but this is what I honestly believe today, and nothing in the currently available neuroscientific literature has forced me to change my mind. Not being a politician running for a high office, however, I reserve the right to change my mind, and am in the process of thinking through a few experiments whose outcomes may compel me to do just that.

Why, then, have neuroscientists, and certainly the general public, been so committed to the concept of consciousness and to the axiomatic assumption of its centrality in the workings of the mind? My answer to this question is shockingly embarrassing in its implications: because old gods die hard. Instead of representing a leap forward, the quest for the mechanisms of consciousness represents a leap backward. The dualism of body and soul has been rejected in name but not in substance. We no longer talk about soul; we now call it consciousnes, just as in some circles people no longer talk about creation, they talk about "intelligent design." We may feel embarrassed by certain old, tired explanatory constructs, and feel intellectually obligated to discard them, but they are often too ingrained for us to truly purge them from our own mental makeup. We give them different names and sneak them right in through the back door. Like many recent converts, we continue to honor the old gods in secret—the god of soul in the guise of consciousness.

5

The Orchestra's Front Row:

The Cortex

Sounds and Players

To appreciate the role of the conductor, one must recognize the complexity of the orchestra. The brain orchestra consists of a large collection of players—the skills, competencies, and knowledge that comprise our mental world. And the neocortex indisputably includes the brain orchestra's most accomplished players.

Scientists have long been intrigued by the complexity and functional diversity of the brain, particularly its most advanced part, the cortex. Most of us have seen, in college textbooks or on junk-store shelves, old phrenological maps. Today they are mostly dismissed as bizarre quackery. Yet they reflect the state-of-the art understanding of brain organization around the early nineteenth century, when the father of phrenology, Franz Joseph Gall, published his influential work.[1] Phrenologists looked at the bumps on the surface of the skull and related them to individual mental abilities and personality traits. They then constructed elaborate maps of those relationships, placing specific mental attributes in specific parts of the brain.

From the standpoint of contemporary science, phrenological maps represented a false start. Like alchemy's relation to chemistry, phrenology belongs to the prehistory of neuroscience, rather than its early history.

Yet it was the first time that the cortex was considered as an ensemble of distinct parts, an orchestra rather than a single instrument, and an attempt was made to identify the players.

Phrenologists recognized that we are all in command of certain cognitive skills (reading, writing, computing), traits (courage, wisdom, recklessness), and attitudes (affection, contempt, hesitation). At first glance, the meaning of these words appears self-evident, and one might expect that each of these properties of the mind should have its distinct location in the brain, the dominant belief held a century and a half ago. But scientists have since learned that the way everyday human language labels mental traits and behaviors does not quite correspond to the way they are represented in the brain. Today, we still think of the cortex as consisting of many functionally distinct parts. Yet the scientific language we use to describe these distinct functions has changed substantially. Just compare the two maps in Figures 5.1 and 5.2. The first brain map was designed by Gall at the beginning of the nineteenth century. The second brain map was designed by the famous neurologist Kleist at the beginning of the twentieth century.[2] While obviously not current, the second map is much closer to the principles of neural organization as we understand them today.

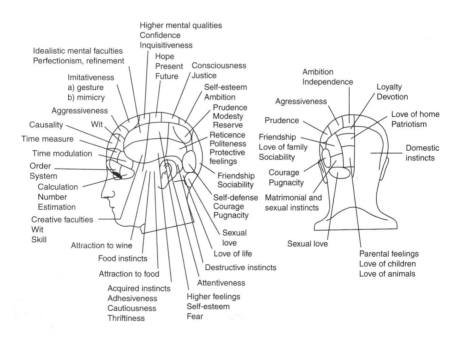

Figure 5.1 Phrenological map in the spirit of Gall [From *Higher Cortical Functions in Man, Second Edition*, by A. R. Luria. Copyright 1979 by Consultants Bureau Enterprises, Inc. and Basic Books, Inc. Reprinted with permission of Basic Books, a member of Perseus Books, L.L.C.]

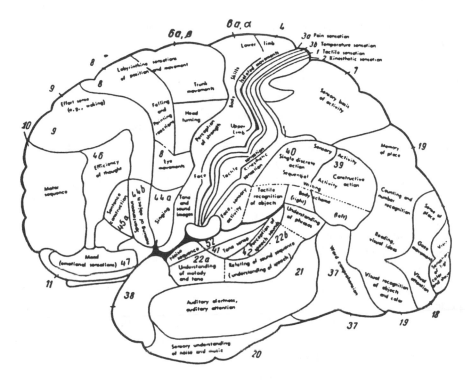

Figure 5.2 Cortical localization of functions after Kleist. [From *Higher Cortical Functions in Man, Second Edition,* by A. R. Luria. Copyright 1979 by Consultants Bureau Enterprises, Inc. and Basic Books, Inc. Reprinted with permission of Basic Books, a member of Perseus Books, L.L.C.]

The change in our understanding of the brain is reflected in these two maps. The difference between them represents more than the incremental growth of knowledge; it represents a paradigmatic shift, which took approximately a century to complete. In every field of knowledge, a profound difference exists between common-sense language and the scientific language used to describe its domain. Everyday language describes the world in terms of tables, chairs, stones, rivers, flowers, and trees. Early belief systems, the ancient precursors of science, attempted to explain the world by postulating a separate deity for every such everyday object.

By contrast, scientific language describes the world in terms of units not necessarily apparent through simple observation. The language of physics describes the world in terms of atoms and subatomic particles; the language of chemistry, in molecular terms. Brain science is currently where inorganic chemistry was in the days of Mendeleev, finding its organizing principles and working out the proper scientific language. The field is very much in flux—the transition from Gall's map to Kleist's map reflects this process. Phrenological traits such as acquisitiveness, veneration, or self-esteem may make immediate common sense, but they do not correspond to distinct structures of the brain.

Imagine yourself listening to complex music produced by an intricate array of unknown, and unseen, musical instruments, while trying to figure out what the instruments are, how many there are, and what each of them contributes to the totality of acoustic experience. You may hear loud tunes and quiet tunes, mellow tunes and piercing tunes, but how do these descriptions correspond to the actual composition of the orchestra? This is the challenge that generations of neuroscientists have had to meet, with limited and imprecise tools—a bit like the proverbial blind brahmins laboring to discern the nature of the elephant. The true "orchestra" of cognition is often difficult to understand in everyday terms. Really, what do things like "tactile recognition" in Kleist's map have to do with our everyday feelings, thoughts, and actions?

Assuming that a relationship exists between structure and function, our quest is aided somewhat by distinct features of brain morphology. The cortex consists of two hemispheres, and each hemisphere consists of four lobes: occipital, parietal, temporal, and frontal. Traditionally, the occipital lobe has been linked to visual information; the parietal lobe, to tactile information; the temporal lobe, to auditory information; and the frontal lobe, to motor functions. The left hemisphere has been linked to language and the right hemisphere to spatial processing. Over the last decades, however, many of these entrenched beliefs have been challenged by new findings and theories, which will be reviewed in the forthcoming sections of the book.

Noah's Predicament and the Landscapes of the Brain

Over the last few decades, hemispheric specialization has become a trendy topic in popular literature. It is common to talk about "right-brain" and "left-brain" therapies, "right-brain" and "left-brain" traits, "right-brain" and "left-brain" personalities. But it is important to realize that the two hemispheres have much more in common than what makes them different. The players sitting in similar positions on the two sides of the aisle play similar instruments. Hemispheric specialization is but two parallel variations on the same basic theme.

According to this theme, the occipital lobes are involved in vision; the temporal lobes, in auditory perception; and the parietal lobes, in tactile and somatosensory perception. But the human brain is more than a collection of narrowly dedicated sensory devices. We are able to recognize complex patterns, comprehend language, and analyze mathematical relationships. What is the neural basis of these and other complex mental functions? As we will see, the orchestra consists of many players whose contributions to the ensemble defy simple definitions and whose seating arrangement is both complex and fluid—truly a game of musical chairs.

Neuroscientists have traditionally relied on the effects of brain lesions to understand how the normal brain works. In its most simplistic form, the logic of such inquiry goes as follows. Suppose damage to brain area A impairs cognitive function *A* but not cognitive functions *B*, *C*, or *D*. By contrast, damage to area B impairs cognitive function *B* but not cognitive functions *A*, *C*, or *D*; and so on. We may then conclude that brain area A is responsible for cognitive function *A*, brain area B for cognitive function *B*, and so on (see Fig. 5.3).

The method used to reach this conclusion is called the *principle of double dissociation*. This time-honored method is at the heart of classical neuropsychology. It has contributed to our understanding of complex relations between the brain and cognition more than any other method to date. However, it is flawed in more than one way. In a highly interactive brain, damage to one area may affect the workings of other areas. An injured brain undergoes various forms of natural reorganization (*plasticity*), which makes it a rather spurious model of normal function. Despite these flaws, the lesion method has provided a wealth of useful information about the brain, and all our current theories of brain function are to some degree based on this information.

The effects of brain damage on cognition help answer not only the "where" questions but also the "what" questions. By observing the multiple ways in which cognition may disintegrate, we begin to understand how nature "splits" mental functions into specific cognitive operations, and how these operations are mapped on the brain.

Over the last few years, the advent of powerful functional neuroimaging methods has changed the way cognitive neuroscience is done. As noted previously, these

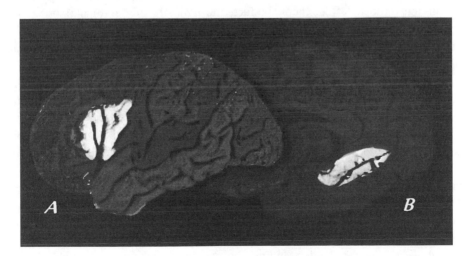

Figure 5.3 Double dissociation. (*A*) Broca's area: certain aspects of language impaired, facial recognition spared. (*B*) Fusiform cortex: certain aspects of facial recognition impaired, language spared.

methods include positron emission tomography (PET), single photon emission computerized tomography (SPECT), and particularly functional magnetic resonance imaging (fMRI). Based on various physical principles, from radioactive substance emission to local magnetic field changes, these methods have one thing in common: they allow us to observe directly the patterns of physiological activity in different parts of the brain as subjects are engaged in various cognitive tasks. A prominent American psychologist, Michael Posner, likened the impact of functional neuroimaging on cognitive neuroscience to the impact of the telescope on astronomy. Just as the invention of the telescope at the beginning of the seventeenth century made direct observation of the macrocosm possible, the introduction of functional neuroimaging at the end of the twentieth century enabled us to directly observe the workings of the mind for the first time in history.

Functional neuroimaging has its limitations. Most of its methods do not measure neural activity directly. Instead, they involve proxy measures, or "markers": blood flow, glucose metabolism, and so on. Strong evidence exists, however, that these markers accurately reflect the levels of neural activity. Another limitation has to do with our ability to identify the sources of activation, relating different aspects of this activation to specific mental operations. Neuroscientists are developing increasingly powerful statistical methods for solving this problem.

Yet another problem involves the relationship between task difficulty and task effortfulness, and the strength of the signal registered in the imaging device (fMRI, PET, or SPECT). With task familiarization and task mastery, signal strength usually drops.[3] In principle, this may mean that a highly automatic, effortless, "easy" task will fail to generate a detectable signal. But easy and effortless cognitive tasks are not extracranial. They too occur within our heads, and brain lesions continue to affect them. In fact, the *majority* of our mental processes are effortless and automatic, conducted, as it were, on autopilot. By contrast, the effortful and consciously controlled cognitive tasks represent only a minor portion of our mental life.

A real possibility exists that the currently available resolution of functional neuroimaging devices limits our imaging capability to the relatively "effortful" tasks, whereas "effortless" automatic tasks fail to generate a detectable signal. Most relatively complex cognitive activation tasks used in experiments probably consist of both effortful and effortless cognitive components. Therefore, their activation "landscapes" may be deceptive in that they reflect isolated peaks with invisible valleys in between. What you see may be far less than what you get. Trying to surmise the brain activation pattern of a cognitive task based on functional neuroimaging data may be like Noah trying to surmise the landscape of Mesopotamia after the Great Flood by staring at the peak of Mount Ararat protruding above the water. Understanding the relationship between signal strength and difficulty level in rigorously quantitative tasks will help interpret the fMRI and PET cognitive activation data. The available neuroimaging technologies are invaluable tools of cognitive neuroscience, as long as we are aware of their limitations and do not take the findings too uncritically and literally.

The introduction of new scientific methods is always exciting. At the same time, it threatens the stability of established assumptions. Most scientific discoveries expand and elaborate previously accumulated knowledge, rather than refuting it. The points of discontinuity in the flow of scientific progress are relatively rare. When they occur, and the old assumptions are refuted in favor of radically different ones, we say that a "paradigm shift" has taken place. The historians of science have hotly debated the relationship between the advances in scientific methods and conceptual breakthroughs. What drives what? Not every new scientific method, revolutionary though it may be, leads to an instant conceptual paradigm shift. The good news is that the recent functional neuroimaging findings from fMRI, PET, and magnetoencephalography (MEG) studies have by and large confirmed the earlier insights based on lesion studies and on traditional electroencephalography (EEG). The bad news is that major conceptual breakthroughs have yet to follow.

Neuropaganism: Module Madness

In the early 1980s Gall and his phrenology enjoyed an odd revival under the name of "modularity."[4] Brain lesions sometimes produce very particular and narrow cognitive deficits. They may affect the names of objects belonging to a specific category (e.g., flowers or animals) but spare all the other object names. Or they may impair the recognition of a specific class of objects but not other objects. For years, neuropsychologists have been enthralled by such phenomena, known as "strong dissociations." Some of the reported strong dissociations were uncanny. In one study a patient who was unable to name a peach or an orange had no difficulty naming an abacus and a sphinx!

Strong dissociations are rare, and most clinicians encounter not a single such case in the course of their careers. Nonetheless, many scientists felt that strong dissociations were particularly interesting and informative for understanding the brain mechanisms of cognition. Neuropsychological discovery and theory building became extremely dependent on the search for such "interesting cases" and their theoretical value has become an article of faith. The large numbers of mundane cases required for sorting through and extracting the precious few strong dissociations were dismissed as uninformative.

This circular pursuit has led to the conclusion that the cortex consists of distinct modules, each in charge of a highly specific cognitive function. The assumption was that the modules are encapsulated, separated by distinct borders and with very limited interactions. The cases with highly specific cognitive deficits were interpreted as the breakdown of narrowly dedicated modules, and the existence of such cases was taken as proof of the existence of these modules.

In this scheme of things, the cortex is understood as a mosaic of numerous parts separated by distinct borders with restricted communications between them. Each module is invested with a highly specific function. Searching for strong dissociations was accepted as the foremost method of identifying the mysterious modules. For each newly reported strong dissociation a new module was postulated, and the list was growing. This approach was remarkably similar to that at the heyday of phrenology, except that the strong dissociations caused by brain lesions had replaced the bumps on the skull as the leading source of insight.

The fallacy of this approach becomes apparent if one realizes that for every case of strong dissociations there are hundreds of cases of weak dissociations, where many functions are impaired together, albeit to different degrees. By making an a priori decision that these far more numerous cases are unimportant and only the strong dissociations are important, one inevitably drifts toward a bias in favor of the modular model of the brain.

In reality, the modular theory explains very little, since by lacking the ability to reduce multitudes of specific facts to simplifying general principles it fails the basic requirement of any scientific theory. Like the belief systems of antiquity, it merely relabels its domain by inventing a new deity for each thing—a neuropaganism of sorts. Nonetheless, like every simplistic notion, it has the seductiveness and illusory appeal of instant explainability, by introducing a new module for every new observation! In a book review written a number of years ago, I referred to this lack of intellectual subtlety and parsimony inherent in the modular theory of the neocortex as the "intellectual equivalent of Visigoth invasion."[5] When more parsimony is practiced, it often becomes clear that certain cognitive operations arise as emergent properties within complex networks, rather than representing specialized, dedicated modules. For example, Jonathan Cohen and his colleagues have demonstrated that a phenomenon akin to attentional disengagement arises in a neural net model naturally, without requiring a specialized, built-in "disengage" operator.[6] So the rush to postulating a specialized neural device for every observed phenomenon is often unnecessary and superfluous.

Given the extreme rarity of strong dissociations, they are likely to reflect the idiosyncrasies of individual cognitive styles and backgrounds and have little to do with the invariant principles of brain organization. If this is so, then the rare strong dissociations are nothing but uninterpretable statistical aberrations.

Consider the following: I am a native Russian speaker who learned English in my teens. My proficiency in both languages varies depending on the circumstances and is replete with strong dissociations. The effects of fatigue, inebriation, or illness have distinct, and opposite, effects on my ability to communicate in the two languages. In English my command of concrete lexicon (e.g., household objects, which I learned as a child) becomes very tentative, but my command of abstract lexicon (e.g., scientific terminology, which I learned as an adult) remains intact. In Russian the opposite happens: I begin to stumble in my attempts to convey high-level concepts but my everyday language remains invulnerable. Certain parts of the lexicon (e.g., names of flowers and fishes) are equally impaired in both languages, since I had never learned them in either language. A good friend of mine, an eminent psychologist from southern California, is a native English speaker with an excellent command of Russian. He reports equally strong state-dependent dissociations, similar in character but not in specifics, in both languages.

Should either of us have the bad luck of suffering a stroke, cognitive neuropsychological theory may be affected differently, depending on which of us would be examined and in which language. Strong dissociations would be promptly documented and reported, all due to utterly idiosyncratic circumstances of our respective personal histories, absurdly irrelevant to anything of neuroscientific importance.

Arguably, bilingualism is relatively uncommon. However, other unusual cognitive factors may play a role in different individuals. In combination these exceptions may account for most strong dissociations. Every individual cognitive profile is a landscape consisting of peaks (strong points) and valleys (weak points), and the disparities in altitudes may be quite dramatic. My near-complete ignorance of fish and flower names in my native Russian language is a case in point.

The effect of an extensive neurological disorder on a vastly uneven cognitive landscape can be compared with a flood that submerges the valleys but spares the peaks. Graded differences between the individual strengths and weaknesses will assume the appearance of strong dissociations and the trusting neuropsychologist will be swept by the sea of artifacts.

Are particular cortical areas assigned very narrow and specific functions? Or is human association cortex a relatively general-purpose device capable of assuming a broad range of functions? The modular view of the neocortex implies a high degree of regional specificity, but how strong is the evidence that such specificity exists? At least for higher-order functions, most claims of such specificity have been challenged by evidence that it is merely a special case of a broader underlying function. Take phonological processing, for instance. It is linked to a region of the left temporal lobe known as planum temporale, but so is the ability to recognize nonverbal environmental sounds in terms of their sources. Our ability to recognize unique acoustic stimuli as speech sounds and our ability to recognize barking as coming from a dog and meowing as coming from a cat are supported by the same brain structure.[7] Planum temporale in the left hemisphere is critical for phonological processing, but it is not narrowly dedicated to it. Instead, it appears that this part of the brain is critical for categorical analysis of any auditory signal. Our ability to recognize a unique auditory signal as a member of a familiar class of signals—verbal and nonverbal alike—is supported by the the left planum temporale. Functional neuroimaging studies have shown that the left planum temporale is activated in normal subjects both when phonological discriminations are made and when environmental sounds are matched with their sources. Likewise, when the left planum temporale is affected by a lesion, both the deficit of phonological processing (*sensory aphasia*) and the deficit of identifying sources of environmental sounds (*auditory associative agnosia*) are evident.[8] Clearly, in the context of our lives, the ability to understand language is generally more important than the ability to differentiate dog barking from cat meowing, so it is only natural that the former is emphasized and the latter is often ignored in characterizing the functions of the left temporal lobe. But as scientists trying to understand the function of this part of the brain we must be interested in identifying the underlying common thread: the fundamental functional property of which the phonological processing and the ability to recognize environmental sounds are but two special cases.

Facial recognition is another case in point. It has been linked to a different part of the temporal lobe, the so-called fusiform cortex in the right hemisphere. But the same part of the brain has also been implicated in recognizing unique exemplars of other classes of stimuli: unique horses, unique cows, or unique cars. Studies of the effects of brain damage lead to similar conclusions. Damage to the fusiform cortex results in *prosopagnosia* (deficit of facial recognition),[9] but in people normally adept at recognizing unique members of other visual categories (e.g., ranchers adept at telling apart individual cows) this ability erodes following damage to the same part of the brain.[10] Of course, under most circumstances and for most people, the ability to recognize human faces is a much more important ability than telling apart horses or cows, unless, of course, you are a cowboy or a rancher. But as in the previous example, it is important for a neuroscientist to go beyond the phenomena and to uncover the underlying general principle, with facial recognition and the recognition of unique exemplars of other classes of visual images being but special cases.

For instance, it would be important to address the following questions through cogent experimental designs:

1. Is this area responsible for facial recognition only, or is it involved in processing other information? If the latter is true, it is not likely to be modular.
2. Is it equally involved in processing any face, or does the nature of its involvement vary depending on such factors as the degree of familiarity with a given face? If the latter is true, it is not likely to be modular.
3. Is this area equally involved in any tasks of facial discrimination, or does the nature of its involvement depend on the specific task (e.g., unique face identification as belonging to Joe Blow, or generic facial identification as being Caucasian vs. Oriental)? If the latter is true, it is not likely to be modular.
4. Does the exact anatomy of this region change with age? Specifically, does its relative representation in the right hemisphere vs. the left hemisphere

change with age? Does it become more (or less) circumscribed with age? If the answers to these questions are "yes," it is not likely to be modular.

Whether you believe that facial recognition is modular or not will depend on how you answer these questions. Similar questions must be asked, and experiments designed, for any other cognitive function presumed to have a modular representation.

In weighing the arguments for and against the modular conception of the neocortex, it is important to distinguish between what I call *a priori, preordained* modularity and *a posteriori, resultant* modularity. By a priori modularity I mean the notion of hard-wired, narrowly preordained functional designation of different parts of association neocortex. I find it very difficult to accept its existence and my polemic ire is directly mostly against this extreme notion. I proposed the gradiental theory of the functional neocortical organization,[11] which will be discussed in the following section, as an alternative to this extreme notion. At the same time, it is entirely possible that certain tightly integrated neuronal groupings emerge over time, as a result of a certain cognitive history of an individual. This is what I call *resultant, a posteriori* modularity. Predictably, such resultant modularity will be different from a priori modularity (had it existed) in several important ways. It will exhibit less uniformity and a greater degree of individual differences and, most importantly, it will change over time as a result of the individual cognitive history. Because of the privileged association between well-established cognitive routines and the left hemisphere, such resultant a posteriori modularity is more likely to arise in the left hemisphere than in the right hemisphere. By contrast, the right hemisphere is the more amodular between the two.

The distinction between a priori and a posteriori modularity is a critical one, and the reader should keep this in mind in order to avoid the impression of contradictions in the book. My critique of modularity in this book and elsewhere in my writings is directed specifically at the notion of a priori modularity. To the extent that I will be attributing certain modular properties to various parts of the neocortex in the discussion to follow, I will be talking about a posteriori modularity. I realize that the introduction of two parallel defenitions of modulary, a priori and a posteriori, may sound like an unnecessary complication, but it captures an important, perhaps even fundamental, aspect of spatiotemporal dynamics of learning in the brain. I think that whenever modular concepts are invoked in characterizing brain function, it is necessary to specify the postulated nature of modularity in question: a priori or a posteriori. While this distinction has not been commonly emphasized in the past, I hope that it will become an important part of any discourse about the functional brain organization.

Because I don't believe in strong a priori modularity in the association cortex, I am less concerned than many other neuropsychologists and cognitive neuroscientists about precise neocortical localization and distinct boundaries between functionally dedicated regions. First, I don't believe that such boundaries exist in a strict sense. They arose as heuristic expedients (like a histogram to capture the properties of an integral), and then people began to take the modules literally, at which point they were turned into an obfuscating epistemological nightmare. Second, the cortical functional distributions (and the resultant modules, if they exist) change over time and differ from person to person, thus both fluidity and variability are to be expected. This is why I follow the reports claiming very specific functional designations of different prefrontal regions within a hemisphere[12] with great interest, but also with a degree of caution.

Cognitive Gradients and Cognitive Hierarchies

A didactic ploy is often used to explain the organization of the neocortex. The ploy is simplistic but heuristically powerful. It is based on the notion of a three-level hierarchy in the neocortex.

In the posterior aspect of the hemisphere, the first level of the hierarchy consists of primary sensory projection areas. They are organized in a "stimulotopic" fashion, which roughly means a point-to-point projection of the stimulus field into the cortical field. The projections are continuous (or as a mathematician would say, "homeomorphic"). This means that the adjacent points of the stimulus field project into the adjacent points of the cortical space. The primary sensory projection areas include the retinotopic visual cortex of the occipital lobe, the somatotopic somatosensory cortex of the parietal lobe, and the "frequency-topic" auditory cortex of the temporal lobe. In the frontal lobe, the first level of the hierarchy is represented by the motor cortex, which is also somatotopic. The mapping between the stimulus spaces and the primary projection areas is topologically correct but metrically distorted. Different cortical territories are allocated to different parts of the stimulus space not on the basis of their relative sizes, but on the basis of their relative importance.

The second level of the hierarchy consists of cortical areas involved in more complex information processing. These areas are no longer organized in a stimulotopic fashion. However, each of these areas is still linked to a particular modality. These cortical areas, called *modality-specific association cortices*, are adjacent to the primary projection cortical areas.

Finally, the third level of the hierarchy consists of the cortical regions that appear at the latest stages of the evolution of the brain and are presumed to be central to the most complex aspects of information processing. They are not linked to any single modality. Instead, the function of these cortical areas is to integrate the inputs coming from many modalities. They are called *heteromodal association cortices* and include the inferotemporal cortex, inferoparietal cortex, and, of course, the prefrontal cortex.

When the effects of brain lesions are examined realistically and without strident preconceptions, a very different view from the modular picture of the brain emerges.

Damage to adjacent parts of the cortex produces similar, albeit not identical, cognitive deficits. This pattern implies that adjacent regions of the neocortex perform similar cognitive functions, and that a gradual transition from one cognitive function to another corresponds to a gradual, continuous trajectory along the cortical surface. The way cognition is distributed throughout the cortex is graduated and continuous, not modular and encapsulated. This pattern of organization, which I have labeled "gradiental," applies particularly to the heteromodal association cortex, probably less so to the modality-specific association cortex, and least of all to the primary projection cortex, which retains strongly modular properties.

The concept of the cognitive gradient first occurred to me in the late 1960s, when I began to take courses in neuropsychology. Together with other students, I was being exposed to a potpourri of neuropsychological syndromes, an endless and disparate laundry list. I began to feel that I needed an autodidactic device enabling me to organize these neuropsychological syndromes into a coherent, simplifying scheme. The gradiental model served this purpose admirably, since it allowed me to interpolate syndromes rather than memorize them by rote. Then I came to realize that the gradiental notion of cortical functional organization is also a powerful conceptual and explanatory tool in thinking about the brain and brain disorders—far more powerful than the prevailing view of the cortex as consisting of discrete functional regions. Among other things, my gradients enabled me to accurately predict the effects of particular brain lesions before empirically observing these effects, and I enjoyed the game. It also helped explain how different parts of the neocortex acquired their functions. I began to think of my gradients as the neuropsychological analogue of the Mendeleev periodic table of elements.

The first person I shared my gradiental theory with was Ekhtibar Dzafarov from Baku (now the capital of independent Azerbaijan on the Caspian Sea). Ekhtibar, a fellow student a few years my junior at the Psychology Department of the Moscow State University, was a protégé of mine. A brilliant polymath and mathematical prodigy, Ekhtibar was a study in cultural contradictions. He had a creative and rigorous mind thoroughly at home with Western philosophy and literature, yet he retained his Eastern mores.

Through happenstance, I was probably responsible for Ekhtibar's admission to the university. Graduate students were often asked to interview freshmen applicants as part of the admissions procedure. The dean's office alerted us to the particular attraction the Psychology Department presumably held for "mentally unstable" applicants. In light of this concern and in the spirit of the culture in which we lived, we were instructed to watch out for "psychotic" applicants and to surreptitiously mark their files with a Magic Marker—a kiss of death for the applicant's dreams of attending Moscow State University.

And so I was sitting one sweltering July afternoon in a non–air-conditioned office of the Moscow State University old campus on Manezhnaya Square, forcing myself to listen to an inarticulate young applicant across the desk, my attention wandering. Meanwhile, my friend Natasha Kalita at the adjacent desk was interviewing an impeccably dressed, lanky southerner with jet-black hair. The young man, appearing still in his teens, spoke excellent Russian but with an unmistakable accent of the Caucasus. As I began to eavesdrop on their conversation to relieve the boredom, the young southerner was talking about the Goedel theorem, while Natasha's increasingly glassy eyes betrayed total incomprehension. As the southerner moved on to the Turing machine, I saw Natasha's hand reach for the Magic Marker. But I already sensed a kindred spirit and very quickly told Natasha to swap. She took over my incoherent lout and I completed the interview with the young southerner.

I wrote a glowing review and Ekhtibar became a psychology freshman, probably the brightest in the department. Following that encounter he attached himself to me and saw me as his protector. We quickly developed intellectual respect for each other and became each other's sounding boards for our more far-fetched ideas and theories.

When a few years later I was ready to leave the country, Ekhtibar flew from Moscow to Riga to say goodbye. We spent an evening in quiet conversation in the living room of my parents' third-floor apartment. As a persona non grata and a "traitor to my country," I suspected that the apartment was bugged, and so we made sure that the telephone (presumed by most Soviet citizens to be the most common device used for apartment bugging) was removed from the room and disabled. Many years later Ekhtibar told me that on his return from Riga his parents were summoned by the KGB (Komitet Gosudarstvennoi Bezopasnosti, Committee of State Security), warned about their son's unsavory associations with politically objectionable characters like myself, and had the content of our farewell conversation recited to them in great detail as a proof of the KGB's omniscience. I have no idea how they taped us. I can only guess that a van was parked on the street next to the building, filled with eavesdropping equipment. Although I had few illusions left about my old country's rulers, I found the story mind-boggling, sad more than outrageous. I was not a prominent dissident; by any rational standard, I was a political nobody. Yet this is how resources were being spent in the country not known for its wealth, barely a decade and a half before its final collapse under its own weight.

And so it was Ekhtibar to whom I first divulged my homespun gradiental theory, which deviated sharply from everything we were taught about the brain. This was done in style, over Georgian red wine at lunch, while beholding a sweeping panorama of Moscow from the rooftop restaurant of the Ministry of Defense Hotel next to the university campus, colloquially known among students as "the Pentagon." The choice of venue was ironic, since I was in the middle of evading, with Luria's connivance, the Soviet military draft, a rather dangerous endeavor in that time and place.

Ekhtibar was impressed and endorsed the idea. So I decided to take it higher up and the next day discussed it with Alexandr Romanovich. I had always thought of my gradiental model as a direct and immediate derivation from Luria's own approach to brain–behavior relations. But to my surprise he did not see it that way and basically dismissed it in favor of the more traditional "localizationist" premise. One of many good things about Luria was that it was possible to disagree with him in a scientific debate without risking the erosion of the personal relationship. Even when he did not share your ideas, he did not feel threatened by them. His attitude was never one of irritation; it ranged from enthusiasm to benign indifference, and this is precisely what it was this time.

I wrote my gradiental theory only 15 years later, in 1986, when I was privileged to spend a year as a visiting scholar at the Institute for Advanced Studies of the Hebrew University of Jerusalem. Ironically, the think tank in which I was invited to participate was devoted to modularity of cognition. The other members of the groups—distinguished neuropsychologists and cognitive neuroscientists from all over the world—were all propoponents of the modular point of view, and I was the *enfant terrible* of the group, arguing vociferously a contrarian point of view. Our intellectual disagreements did not stand in the way of an exceptionally warm and stimulating environment. We all became, and remain, close personal friends, and I look back to the year in Jerusalem as one of the happiest in my life.

When the journal article in which I introduced the concept of a cognitive "cortical gradient" was finally published in 1989[13] and then published again as a book chapter,[14] it was largely ignored by the scientific community. The process of getting the 1989 paper accepted was itself deflating. It was rejected with scathing reviews as nonsensical by a leading journal, where I felt it belonged. It was finally published in a journal in which it was less likely to make an impact and, indeed, it didn't. The notion of modularity was too entrenched and simplistically appealing at the time. In fact, my decision to leave full-time academia, after so many years, for private practice was to a large extent triggered by this and a few other failures to make a dent in what I rightly or wrongly perceived as a mediocre Zeitgeist of the field. Since I had failed to break it, and to be "successful" by the standard academic yardsticks I would have had to be part of the "majority club," I felt that I should not make my career beholden to the trends that I could not in all honesty respect, let alone abide. Sometime later the members of the Jerusalem think tank were asked to contribute to a special journal issue on modularity. As befits a bad boy, I titled my paper "Rise and Fall of Modular Orthodoxy," prophesizing, by way of a parting shot, its imminent demise.[15]

Indeed, by the late 1990s modularity was in retreat. The last spasm of prescientific neuropsychology was coming to an end and the gradiental view of the cerebral cortex was on the ascendancy. At least in the United States, this happened to a large extent due to the computational work by Jay McClelland,[16] Martha Farah,[17] and others guided by the intuition inspired by the neural-net paradigm, the same intuition that had informed my own thinking since my Moscow University student days. This, I believe, represents a true paradigm shift in cognitive neuroscience, and like every paradigm shift it entailed an uphill battle. In a remarkable essay, "Scotoma: Forgetting and Neglect in Science," Oliver Sacks likens the recent changes in our views about the brain to the paradigm shift in physics at the turn of the twentieth century.[18] That was the time when the Newtonian physics of discrete bodies was supplanted by the new physics of fields—electric, magnetic, and gravitational.

As I argue later in this book, the notion of modularity is not entirely misplaced. Modularity probably accurately captures an archaic principle of neural organization, which was supplanted later in evolution with the gradiental principle. If this is so, then an uncanny parallel exists between the evolution of the brain and the intellectual evolution of how we think about the brain. Both the evolution of the brain itself and the evolution of our theories about the brain were characterized by a paradigm shift from modular to interactive.

The current tools of genomics may offer a powerful new tool for helping resolve the modularity–gradient controversy, at least to a degree. A growing body of research exists mapping regional gene expression in the brain.[19] It would be very interesting to overlap the maps of functional organization with the maps of regional gene expression for the neocortex as well as for other parts of the brain, and to examine the degree of agreement between these two kinds of maps. The a priori modularity premise would predict that functionally different brain regions should correspond to regions with different gene-expression patterns. By contrast, the emergent gradient premise would predict a relative absence of such strong correspondences.

A Thing Is a Thing

The gradiental principle is best understood by examining two fundamental aspects of our mental world: perception and language. Consider two alternative ways in which the mental representations of things may be coded. In the first version, various categories of things (fruit, flowers, clothes, tools, etc.) are coded as separate "modules," each occupying a distinct, circumscribed location in the cortex. In the second version, the representation of every category of things is distributed according to its various sensory components: visual, tactile, auditory, and so on.

The first possibility is consistent with the modular principle of cerebral organization. In fact, the proponents of this principle usually quote cases of perceptual or naming difficulties affecting specific, isolated categories of things. As noted earlier, such cases are extremely rare, but they do exist. The second possibility is consistent with the gradiental, continuous principle of cortical organization.

To help decide which of the two alternatives is closer to truth, we turn to a peculiar class of neurological disorders, *associative agnosias*.

Imagine walking into a department store. You find yourself surrounded by hundreds of objects, most of them unique in at least some respect. How likely is it that you have already seen that particular pattern on a tie, that particular cut of a dress, or that particular shape of a vase? You have probably not encountered the exact replicas of any of these objects before. Nonetheless, you immediately recognize them as members of certain familiar categories: a tie, a dress, and a vase. Paradoxically, these objects are instantly familiar, despite the fact that, strictly speaking, they are novel.

Categorical perception, the ability to identify unique exemplars as members of generic categories, is a fundamental cognitive ability without which we would be unable to navigate the world around us. We take this ability for granted, and in most cases we exercise it automatically, effortlessly, and instantaneously. But in brain disease this fundamental ability may become severely impaired, even when the basic senses (vision, audition, touch) are unaffected, as in associative agnosias.[20]

Our knowledge of the outside world is multimedia in nature. We can evoke the visual image of the tree's green crown as well as the sound of the leaves ruffled by the wind, the scent of its flowers in bloom, and the rough feel of the bark under our fingers. How does the ability to recognize common objects suffer in associative agnosias? Do the various attributes of the mental representation of an object share a similar fate? Does the perceptual breakdown in associative agnosias occur according to whole objects or according to its sensory dimensions?

Research into the effects of brain damage on cognition has shown that in agnosias the ability to perceive objects is never destroyed completely. It is usually limited to certain sensory systems without affecting the others. Consequently, different partial agnosias have been identified and named. A patient with *visual object agnosia* is unable to recognize a common object visually but will immediately recognize it on touch. A patient with *pure object astereognosia* is unable to recognize the same common object on touch but will recognize it visually. A patient with *associative auditory agnosia* is unable to recognize a common object by its characteristic sound (e.g., a dog by its barking) but will have no trouble recognizing it either visually or by touch.[21]

So none of these forms of agnosia eliminates our ability to perceive an object completely, but only partially. In each form of agnosia, the deficit is usually limited to a distinct sensory modality (visual, auditory, or tactile); and in that and only that modality is the patient's perception severely impaired. By the same token, this partial deficit is usually not limited to a particular class of objects (such as items of clothing or household tools) but affects all types of objects to some degree. Yet the patient is not blind, deaf, or numb. While the agnosias are definitely linked to particular sensory systems, sensations are not themselves affected. The deficit involves the interpretation of sensory information, rather than its reception.

What is the neuroanatomy of associative agnosias? The cortical territories whose damage leads to these agnosias are adjacent to the areas in charge of sensory inputs as they arrive in the cortex. The territory of visual object agnosia abuts the visual cortex of the occipital lobe, the territory of associative auditory agnosia abuts the auditory cortex of the temporal lobe, and the territory of pure object astereognosia abuts the somatosensory cortex of the parietal lobe.

From this it follows that the mental representation of a thing is not modular. It is distributed, since its different sensory components are represented in different parts of the cortex. And it is gradiental, since the regions of these partial representations are continuous upon the areas of corresponding sensory modalities.

A Word to a Thing

Consider two alternative ways in which the knowledge of word meaning may be coded in the brain:

1. Representation of word meanings is modular in nature. All word meanings are bundled together and separated from the cerebral representation of the real physical world that they denote.
2. Representation of word meanings is distributed. It is distributed in close neuroanatomical proximity to the cerebral representations of the corresponding aspects of the physical world. This would mean that the meanings of different types of words are coded in different parts of the cortex.

Although most representations of things and events involve multiple sensory modalities, some are more dependent on certain sensory modalities than on others. In humans, mental representations of physical objects depend mostly on the visual modality and only secondarily on other sensory modalities. This is reflected in the idiom "to bring an image before the mind's eye"—not the "mind's ear" or the "mind's nose." You can test this yourself by asking a friend to describe a common object. The odds are that the description will focus on what the object looks like and only later, when pressed, on what it sounds, smells, and feels like. By contrast, a talking dog (a relatively more olfactory creature) would almost certainly invent the idiom "to bring before the mind's nose." At the same time, mental representations of physical actions—walking, running, hitting—are less visual and more motor and tactile or proprioceptive in nature.

Objects are represented in language by nouns, and not just any nouns but concrete nouns. *Chair* is an object word, but *independence* is not. Actions are represented in language by verbs, specifically by concrete verbs. *Run* is an action word, but *equivocate* is not. What are the cortical representations of object words and action words like? Are they represented together in a distinct part of the cortex, or are their representations distributed, according to their meaning, throughout different parts of the cortex?

Lesion studies of patients suggest that the cortical mapping of language is decidedly distributed. The breakdown of naming is usually not global but partial. The loss of object words (*anomia for nouns*) is caused by damage to the part of the temporal lobe adjacent to the visual occipital lobe. In these cases action words are relatively spared. By contrast, the loss of action words (*anomia for verbs*) is caused by damage to the frontal lobe, just in front of the motor cortex. This suggests that the cortical representation of object words is closely linked to the cortical representation of objects themselves, and the cortical representation of action words is closely linked to the cortical representation of actions themselves.[22]

Studies with healthy subjects using functional neuroimaging methods support this conclusion. Alex Martin and his colleagues at the National Institute of Mental Health reviewed a large number of such studies and concluded that both the cortical representation of objects and the cortical representation of word meanings denoting objects are highly distributed.[23] Various features of these representations are stored close to the sensory and motor areas that participated in acquiring information about these objects. For instance, the naming of animals activated the left occipital areas, whereas the naming of tools activated the left premotor regions in charge of right hand movements.[24] This is depicted in Figure 5.4.

Again, a decidedly nonmodular, distributed, and continuous picture of cortical functional organization arises, consistent with the gradiental model. The knowledge of word meaning is not stored in the brain as a separate, compact module. Different aspects of word meaning are distributed in close relationship to those aspects of physical reality which they denote.

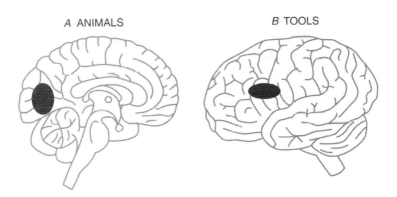

Figure 5.4 Distributed cortical representation of language. The cortical representation of word meaning denoting the objects are highly distributed. Various features of these representations are stored close to those sensory and motor areas that participated in acquiring information about the objects. (*A*) Area of increased blood flow when subjects name drawings of animals compared to when naming tools. (*B*) Area of increased blood flow when subjects name drawings of tools compared to when naming animals. [Adapted from Martin, Wiggs, Ungerleider, and Haxby (1996).[24] Reprinted by permission from *Nature*, copyright 1996 by Macmillan Magazines Ltd.]

Paradoxically, some of the findings commonly quoted by the proponents of modularity fit more naturally into the gradiental model of the cortex. The ability to name living things is more likely to be lost following brain damage than is the ability to name inanimate objects.[25] Of all the findings often mentioned in support of the modular view of the brain, this one is among the most robust and replicable. Yet simple common sense suggests a different, non-modular explanation.

Most inanimate objects we come into contact with are man-made. Man-made objects are created for a purpose; we do things with them. In most cases, this implies that the mental representations of inanimate objects have an additional aspect: the representation of actions implicit in the objects. This aspect is for the most part absent in the mental representations of living things. As a result, the mental representations of inanimate things are more widely distributed, involve more parts of the brain, and are therefore less vulnerable to the effects of brain damage.

Like the mental representations of the physical world itself, the mental representation of language *denoting* the physical world is distributed. A close relationship, in fact a close parallelism, exists between these two neural records. They seem to be coupled, one attached to the other. This makes both evolutionary and aesthetic sense; the neural blueprint is both parsimonious and elegant. And it adheres perfectly to the gradiental principle of functional cortical organization.

Cortical Gradients in the Frontal Lobes

For the posterior parts of the hemispheres, the gradients are represented by relatively continuous functional distributions along the occipitotemporal, temporoparietal, and occipitoparietal axes. Each axis is bounded at its extremes by a pair of primary sensory projection areas. As one moves away from these extreme points, one encounters areas in charge of higher-order processing within the corresponding modalities (*modality-specific association cortex*), and as one approaches the middle of the axis, one encounters areas in charge of functional fusion between the respective modalities (*heteromodal association cortex*). Superimposed on this general setup are hemispheric differences along the lines of previous discussion.[26]

But can one think about the frontal lobes in gradiental terms? At a very coarse level of analysis, the progression from motor cortex, to premotor cortex, to prefrontal cortex lends itself rather naturally to such understanding. But once you reach the prefrontal cortex, the situation becomes murkier. Intuitively, one is tempted to think that as one moves within the prefrontal convexity toward the frontal poles, one moves up the hierarchy of cognitive control, from more specific to more abstract and generalized levels—something akin to the hierarchy of receptive fields of increasing generality, but for action instead of perception.

The attempt to identify the levels of such a hierarchy of executive control was exactly what I undertook for my master's thesis at the Moscow State University in the late 1960s. This was years before neuroimaging, such as computerized axial tomography (CAT) let alone magnetic resonance imaging (MRI), became available, so my sophomoric exercise was sorely lacking in neuroanatomical precision. Nonetheless, the results were intriguing. Already in the United States, I presented them at one of the very early meetings of The International Neuropsychological Society in 1975 and published them a few years later.[27]

The study involved patients with prefrontal lesions of various etiologies and was conducted at the Burdenko Institute of Neurosurgery in Moscow, where Alexandr Luria had his laboratory. I was interested in motor perseverations, which I elicited by asking patients to draw simple geometric forms following verbal commands delivered in rapid succession ("draw a cross . . . circle . . . cross . . . square . . .") according to a set of protocols that I designed. The idea was to use perseveration as markers of executive breakdown at various levels of the cognitive hierarchy.

It was clear that several distinct forms of perseveration could be elicited, not all of them "motor." They could be distinguished on the basis of the unit of behavior that exhibited perseveration. These ranged from a simple movement to a motor sequence, to certain abstract topological features of geometric forms, to whole categories of action (the most abstract level). I termed these different types of phenomena "hyperkinetic perseveration," "perseveration of elements," "perseveration of features," and "perseveration of activities" (see Figure 8.3 later in the text, when I revisit the phenomena in a somewhat different context and describe them in more detail). These different perseveration clearly corresponded to breakdowns at different stages of the process and at different levels of the putative cognitive hierarchy that guided them. Perseveration of activity suggested the breakdown of selection of the general modus operandi ("Am I supposed to write or to draw?") and of the ability to switch from one activity to another. Perseveration of features suggested the breakdown of accessing the appropriate semantic category ("Is it a closed form or an open form?") and of the ability to switch from one semantic category to another within a given activity. Perseveration of elements suggested the breakdown of generating the appropriate motor sequence necessary to actually implement the selection made at an earlier stage and of the ability to make transitions from one such sequence to another. Finally, hyperkinetic perseveration suggested the breakdown of executing individual motor acts within the sequence and of the ability to switch from one individual motor act to another within a given sequence.[28]

Having interpreted the various perseveration types hierarchically, I was hoping to use them as markers of the cognitive structure of the underlying normal hierarchy of frontal lobe control characterized by an increasing degree of integration as one gets closer to the frontal poles. It all made conceptual sense cognitively and also neuroanatomically. I was quite convinced that different perseveration types reflected dysfunction at different points along the premotor–frontopolar axis. Hypothetically, hyperkinetic perseveration was supposed to reflect premotor dysfunction, and perseveration of activities was supposed to relfect dysfunction of the areas around the frontal poles, with the perseveration of elements and features somewhere in the middle of this continuum. This was precisely what I was hoping to find: a one-to-one relationship between the perseveration type and lesion location along the premotor–frontopolar continuum. In principle, that was entirely possible, since some of my patients had bilateral frontopolar resection following severe traumatic injury. But unfortunately for me, my lofty hypotheses had to remain so, since my clinical material was too mushy to allow precise neuroanatomical interpretation; the lesions were too massive and the neuroimaging methods nonexistent. In most of my patients several types of perseveration co-occurred, which further complicated the interpretation. It was noteworthy, however, that in the cases of massive frontal lobe damage and multiple perseveration types a clear pattern of recovery was evident over time: lower-level perseveration recovered first and higher-order perseveration much later.[29] This seemed to be consistent with their hierarchic interpretation and conceptually mapped well on the premotor–frontopolar axis, but still fell far short of the direct neuroanatomical interpretation I had hoped for.

Such a direct neuroanatomical interpretation was made possible many years later with the advent of functional neuroimaging. Jordan Grafman and his colleagues at The National Institutes of Health have shown in an fMRI study that, when a cognitive task is characterized by a hierarchy of goals, the regions around the frontal poles are activated only when the subjects have to keep in mind the main goal while performing subordinate goals.[30] Joshua Hoffman and his colleagues at University of California, Berkeley have showed in an fMRI study of healthy subjects that the selection of action is associated with the activation in different regions within the prefrontal convexity in increasing proximity to the frontal poles as the selection requirements become increasingly abstract. Hoffman and colleagues then gave tasks similar to those used in the fMRI study to a group of patients with focal frontal lesions. Consistently, the breakdown of higher-order abstraction based selection was associated with lesions closer to the frontal poles.[31] A somewhat similar set of findings was presented in an fMRI study by Etienne Koechlin and colleagues,[32] who introduced the notion of a hierarchic "cascade of executive processes." The postulated hierrarchy of control operates at the level of stimuli, perceptual context, and the temporal episode, and it is mediated by Brodmann areas 6 (premotor), 44/45 (inferior frontal), and 46 (middle prefrontal), respectively. This hierarchy seems very similar to the one implicit in the relationship between the "perseveration of elements," "perseveration of features," and "perseveration of activities" that I described many years earlier. In a related study, Koechlin and Hyafil have demonstrated that the anterior prefrontal cortex is critical for juggling between more than one concurrent behavioral tasks or mental plans.[33] A similar conclusion was reached by Narender Ramnani and Adrian Owen, who proposed that Brodmann area 10 is critical for integrating the outcomes of several cognitive operations in the context of a superordinate goal.[34] Ramnani and Owen also refer to the peculiar feature of frontopolar anatomy. Anterior prefrontal cortex is bidirectionally interconnected with heteromodal association regions of the posterior cortex but not with modality-specific regions. Furthermore, the anterior prefrontal cortex is characterized by a higher number of dendritic spines per cell and by high spine density, and at the same time by a lower density of cell bodies than is typical for other prefrontal regions. In combination, these features of gross pathway architecture and microcircuitry make the anterior preforntal cortex particularly well-equipped for a very broad integration of inputs.[35]

So it appears that a clear demonstration of the hierarchical nature of the functional organization of the prefrontal cortex, which eluded my low-tech attempts almost half-a-century ago, has been finally made possible by the state-of-the-art functional neuroimaging methods. It also appears that the functional organization of the frontal lobes is aligned along a cognitive gradient of an increasing abstraction and complexity of cognitive control, extending from the motor cortex to the frontal poles.

Autonomy and Control in the Brain

The frontal lobes are the instrument, and the agent, of control within the central nervous system. It would appear that their advent, late in evolution, should mark a more constrained brain organization. In reality, however, the situation is complex. Several countercurrents unfolded in the evolution of the brain, balancing each other. The evolutionary pressures behind the development of the frontal lobes were probably driven by the increasing degrees of freedom in brain organization and by the impending potential for chaos within it.

Since the early 1980s, the functional organization of the brain has been the focus of intense scientific debate. Two radically different blueprints have been considered. The first blueprint is based on the concept of modularity.[36] As discussed earlier, a modular system consists of autonomous units, each invested with a relatively complex function and relatively insulated from the others. Separate modules provide inputs to and receive inputs from one another, but they exert little or no influence over each other's inner workings. The interaction between modules is limited and gated through a relatively small number of information channels.

The alternative blueprint is a massively parallel, interconnected brain.[37] Here, the units are smaller, invested with far simpler functions, but far more numerous. They are closely interconnected and interact continuously through multiple channels.

The notion of modularity is a high-tech revival of eighteenth-century phrenology. Not only does it presuppose distinct borders between discrete units, but it also suggests their functional prededication. According to this view, a very specific function is rigidly preordained for each such unit.

By contrast, the notion of a massively interconnected brain owes its ascendancy, in a somewhat circular way, to the formal neural networks, or neural nets, which were themselves inspired by the biological nervous system. *Neural nets* are dynamic models of the brain. They were first introduced in the 1940s,[38] but the advent of computers gave them a recent boost. A neural net is an assembly of a large number of simple interconnected elements, expressed as a computer program. The properties of the elements and connections emulate, in a simplified way, the properties of the real, biological neurons and of the axons and dendrites that interconnect them. By running the program on the computer, the "behavior" of the model challenged with various tasks can be examined, and this allows the examiner to infer the dynamic properties of the real brain. With "experience," the formal neural nets acquire a rich array of properties, which were not explicitly programmed into them from the outset—the "emergent" properties. The patterns of their connection strengths change, so that various parts of the net form the "representations" of various incoming types of information.

Brain modeling with neural nets is one of the most powerful tools of cognitive neuroscience today. The studies of the emergent properties, together with the clinical data about the effects of brain lesions and the methods of functional neuroimaging looking at regional interactions, offer a glimpse into an alternative, amodular principle of brain organization. Earlier in the book, I referred to this principle as "gradiental." According to the gradiental principle, massive continuous interactions take place in the brain, while relatively little is preordained about the function of its parts. Instead, it is assumed that the functional roles of various cortical regions *emerge* according to certain basic gradients.[39]

Both the modular and the gradiental concepts have advocates and detractors. Both of them capture important properties of the brain. Modularity is best applicable to an old structure from an evolutionary standpoint, the thalamus, an assemblage of neuronal collections (nuclei). The interactive principle is best applied to a relatively recent evolutionary innovation in the brain, the neocortex. In particular, the interactive principle of organization captures the properties of the most recently evolved part of the neocortex, the so-called heteromodal association cortex, which is critical for the most advanced mental processes. Reptiles and birds are thalamic creatures with little cortical development.[40] This was probably also true for the dinosaurs. Mammals, by contrast, have a developed cortex, which is superimposed on and overrides the thalamus.

The thalamus and the neocortex are closely interconnected. The thalamus is often viewed as the precursor of the cortex, containing in a rudimentary way most of its functions. While functionally close, the thalamus and the neocortex differ radically in neuroanatomical structure. The thalamus consists of distinct nuclei, interconnected with a limited number of pathways as the only routes of communication. By contrast, the neocortex is a sheet without distinct internal borders, with rich pathways interconnecting most areas with most others.

If the thalamus is a close prototype of the cortex, then what were the evolutionary pressures for the emergence of the neocortex? What in evolution promoted the introduction of a fundamentally new principle of neural organization, rather than the refinement of an already existing one? Why was the emergence of a neural sheet, the neocortex, adaptively preferable to sticking with the thalamic principle by having more and larger nuclei? The question is admittedly a teleological one, looking for a purpose where there may be none. But we ask teleological questions all the time, putting them in quotation marks so to speak, as intellectual shorthand in our quest for understanding the evolution of complex systems, biological, economic, and social alike.

The probable answer to our teleological question is that different principles of neural organization are optimal for different levels of complexity. Up to a point, modular organization is optimal. But once a certain level of complexity is required, the transition toward a heavily interconnected net consisting of a large number of simpler (but diverse in kind) interactive elements becomes necessary to ensure adaptive success. Throughout evolution, the emphasis has shifted from the brain invested with rigid, fixed functions (the thalamus) to the brain capable of flexible adaptation (the cortex). This was reflected in the explosive neocortical evolution in the mammals.

For sheer combinatorial reasons, the neocortex permits orders-of-magnitude greater numbers of specific connectivity patterns than does a system organized according to the modular principle. Therefore, it is capable of processing a far greater degree of complexity. Furthermore, because the transition from one connectivity pattern to another may occur rapidly in the neocortex, it is characterized by a truly *dynamic topology*.

The advent of the neocortex has resulted in dethroning the thalamus from its place at the summit of the neurocognitive hierarchy and in placing it in a role that is in some sense subordinate to the neocortex. Therefore, the function of the thalamus in the developed mammalian brain is different from that for which it had originally evolved. This may be one of the reasons why the role of the thalamus in cognition has proved to be somewhat elusive and resistant to scientific investigation. One intriguing possibility is that the thalamus provides shortcuts in the communications among widely dispersed neocortical regions. In terms of the sheer number of intervening synaptic contacts, the distance between neocortical regions X and Y may be shorter via the thalamus than via a pathway contained within the neocortex.[41]

The transition from the thalamic to the cortical principle of brain organization marks a drastic increase of all possible interaction patterns among different brain structures, neuronal groupings, and individual neurons. With this development, the ability to select the most effective pattern in a specific situation becomes particularly important. But the growing degree of freedom available to the brain *in principle* had to be balanced with an effective mechanism of constraining it *at any given time*; otherwise there would be the neural equivalent of chaos.

At the latest stage of cortical evolution the frontal lobes developed to meet this "need." The type of control provided by the frontal lobes is probably weak, superimposed on a high degree of autonomy of other brain structures. At the same time, the frontal lobe control is "global," coordinating and constraining the activities of a vast array of neural structures at any given time and over time. The frontal lobes do not have the specific knowledge or expertise for all the necessary challenges facing the organism. What they have, however, is the ability to "find" the areas of the brain in possession of this knowledge and expertise for any specific challenge, and to string them together in complex configurations according to the need.

As a neurofuturistic exercise, suppose the evolution of the brain were to continue (in itself a far-from-obvious proposition, although one finding some recent support). Will it continue along the path of increasingly complex and elaborate neural nets, or will a qualitatively new principle of biocomputation emerge? An extrapolation based on the foregoing discussion predicts an emergence of a qualitatively more complex and dynamically interconnected network consisting of an order-of-magnitude larger number of smaller components. It is possible, for instance, to envision such a network built of various molecules, rather than neurons, as the basic components.

The principle of man-made molecular biocomputation is already being explored as the basis for the paradigmatic shift in computer design. Life may end up imitating art, the evolution of biological computational systems emulating the evolution of artificial computational devices. But then again, it may be precisely the evolution of man-made computational devices that, together with already existing cultural devices of knowledge accumulation and transmission, will make biological evolution of the brain superfluous.

6

Novelty, Routines, and Cerebral Hemispheres

A False Start

That one hemisphere (in most cases, left) is more intimately linked to language than the other has been known for many years. Paul Pierre Broca[1] and Carl Wernicke[2] demonstrated in the second half of the nineteenth century that isolated lesions of the left hemisphere drastically interfere with language. Aphasias (language disturbances) are commonly seen following left-hemispheric strokes but not right-hemispheric strokes.

The basic facts linking language to the left hemisphere are not in dispute. The question arises, however, whether the close association with language is the central attribute of the left hemisphere or a special case, a consequence of a more fundamental principle of brain organization. Any attempt to characterize the function of one hemisphere through language and the other through spatial processing leads to an unsettling conclusion. Since language, at least in its narrow definition, is a uniquely human attribute, any dichotomy based on language is applicable only to humans. Does this mean that no hemispheric specialization exists in animals? The scarcity of work on hemispheric specialization in non-human species suggests that this is still the prevailing assumption among neuroscientists.

But the assumption of human uniqueness of hemispheric specialization is counterintuitive, since we usually expect at least some degree of evolutionary continuity in traits. While many instances of evolutionary discontinuity undoubtedly exist, the working hypothesis in any scientific inquiry should be one of continuity. This was pointed out to me many years ago by none other than my own father, by profession an engineer, basically unschooled in psychology (and thus unencumbered with its preconceptions) but possessing general broad culture, a rigorous logical mind, and common sense.

The assumption of human uniqueness of hemispheric specialization also flies in the face of our general belief in the relationship between structure and function. The two cerebral hemispheres are not mirror images of each other. The right frontal lobe is wider than and protrudes over the left frontal lobe. The left occipital lobe is wider than and protrudes over the right occipital lobe. This double asymmetry is called the *Yakovlevian torque*, after the prominent Harvard neuroanatomist P. Yakovlev, who discovered it.[3] While the existence of this morphological asymmtetry has been know for some time, it has been further characterized more recently with quantitative magnetic resonance imaging (MRI) morphometry[4] The frontal cortex is thicker in the right hemisphere than in the left hemisphere.[5] But the Yakovlevian torque is present already in fossil humans, and many hemispheric asymmetries are present in the great apes.[6] Gender differences and hemispheric asymmetries in cortical thickness are present in the rat.[7] Planum temporale, a structure within the temporal lobe, is larger in the left hemisphere than in the right hemisphere in humans.[8,9] Traditionally, this asymmetry has been linked to language. Subsequent research has shown, however, that the sylvian fissure and, in particular, planum temporale, structures in the temporal lobe that are traditionally associated with language, are also asymmetric in orangutans, gorillas,[10] and chimpanzees,[11] just as they are in humans.

Differences between the two hemispheres are also apparent at the cellular level. So-called spindle cells, found mostly in the frontal and anterior cingulate cortex and characterized by particularly long axons, are far more numerous in the right hemisphere than in the left hemisphere. This asymmetry is not unique to humans either and is present across a wide range of mammalian species, particularly in the simians. Consistent with this is the finding by Torkel Klingberg and colleagues that the white matter is organized in a more regular manner in the right than in the left frontal lobes in both children and adults.[12]

Brain biochemistry is also asymmetric. The neuromodulator dopamine is somewhat more prevalent in the left hemisphere of various species, including the rat[13] and the mouse.[14] By contrast, the neuromodulator norepinephrine is more prevalent in the right hemisphere.[15] Neurohormonal estrogen receptors are more prevalent in the right hemisphere than left hemisphere.[16] These biochemical differences are already present in several nonhuman species.[17] In fetal monkeys, androgen receptor concentration in the frontal lobes is asymmetric in males but symmetric in females.[18] At the molecular level hemispheric differences were found in NMDA receptors between the left and right hippocampi.[19]

Thus it appears that the two hemispheres are different both structurally and bio-chemically in several animal species. It is therefore logical to suspect that the functions of the two hemispheres are also different in animals. Indeed, functional differences between the two hemispheres have been demonstrated in the monkey[20] and even in the sheep.[21] But in animals these differences cannot be based on language, since animals do not possess language, at least not in its narrow definition. It is clear that a more fundamental distinction is needed to capture the difference between the functions of the two hemispheres. Ideally, it would not refute the association between language and the left hemisphere, but embrace it as a special case.

Despite the fact that the language–visuospatial dichotomy of hemispheric specialization remains the mainstay of clinical neuropsychology, at least as an explanatory shorthand, there has been a growing realization that conceptually it fails to capture the whole story. A plethora of alternative formulations have been proposed, notably linking the left hemisphere to "analytic" processes and the right hemisphere to "holistic" processes; or the left hemisphere to "sequential" processing and the right hemisphere to "simultaneous" processes. But as I argue in *The Wisdom Paradox*, these dichotomies are too difficult to operationalize and thus to falsify, for them to be useful instruments of science.[22]

The New Paradigm

The idea that guided my approach to cerebral hemispheres was born 40 years ago in Moscow. As a student at the University of Moscow, I spent a lot of time at the Bourdenko Institute of Neurosurgery, where Luria had a laboratory. I became friendly with a few pediatric neurosurgeons, and over the bland fare of the hospital cafeteria they often spun their surgical tales. One tale sounded particularly puzzling. In very young children, damage to the right hemisphere was extremely devastating and damage to the left hemisphere was relatively inconsequential. Although these claims were not substantiated by formal research, they provided a hypothetical situation in need of explanation, an exercise in mental gymnastics I could not resist. Many years later the American developmental neuropsychologist Elizabeth Bates conducted formal studies in children that basically supported the hunch of my Russian neurosurgeon friends.[23]

The claim was directly opposite what is supposed to happen in an adult brain. In adults, the left hemisphere is frequently called the "dominant" hemisphere and is presumed to be particularly important. Neurosurgeons are often reluctant to operate on the left hemisphere for fear of affecting language. The right hemisphere, by contrast, is often presumed to be more expendable. In the old literature it was referred to as the "minor hemisphere." Neurosurgeons are generally more comfortable operating on the right hemisphere, and electroconvulsive shock therapy (ECT) is often administered to the right but not the left hemisphere.

Is it possible that the left hemisphere is dedicated to language and is therefore "silent" until language is fully developed? That could explain the lack of adverse effect of left-hemispheric damage in children, but could not explain the particularly severe adverse effect of right-hemispheric damage. Also, my neurosurgeon friends kept telling me that even when left-hemispheric damage affected the areas not commonly implicated in language, the consequences in children were quite benign.

It appeared that some sort of broad transfer of functions was taking place between the two hemispheres, from right to left, throughout development, and that this transfer was not limited to the acquisition of language. This observation gave rise to the idea that the difference between the two cerebral hemispheres revolves around the difference between cognitive novelty and cognitive routines. Is it possible that the right hemisphere is particularly adept at processing novel information and the left hemisphere is particularly adept at processing routinized, familiar information? I imported this idea with me when I moved to the United States in 1974. In 1981 my friend Louis Costa and I published a theoretical paper, for the first time linking the right hemisphere to cognitive novelty and the left hemisphere to cognitive routines.[24]

The Nobel Prize–winning psychologist Herbert Simon believes that learning involves the accumulation of easy-to-recognize patterns of all kinds.[25] Is it possible that the left hemisphere is the repository of such patterns?

Novelty and familiarity are the defining characteristics in the mental life of any creature capable of learning. In simple instinctive behaviors the triggering stimulus is instantly "familiar" and the degree of familiarity does not change with exposure. The organism's response is well formed from the outset and remains the same through the life span. The assumption is that the neural machinery controlling the stimulus response remains unaltered by experience. An example of such behavior is found in simple reflexes. When your nose itches, you scratch it automatically and unthinkingly. This response is not a result of learning and will not change throughout your life span.

The brains of higher animals, including humans, are endowed with a powerful capacity for learning. Unlike instinctive behavior, learning, by definition, is change. The organism encounters a situation for which it has no ready-made effective response. With repeated exposures to similar situations over time, appropriate response strategies emerge. The length of time or the number of exposures required for the emergence of effective solutions is vastly variable. The process is sometimes condensed in a single exposure (the so-called Aha! reaction). But invariably, the transition is from an absence of effective behavior to the emergence of effective behavior. This process is called "learning" and the emergent (or taught) behavior is called "learned behavior." At an early stage of every learning process the organism is faced with *novelty*, and the end stage of the learning process can be thought of as *routinization* or familiarity. The transition from novelty to routinization is the universal cycle of our inner world. It is the rhythm of our mental processes unfolding on various time scales.

The role of learning and learned behaviors increases throughout evolution, at the relative expense of instinctive behaviors. Is it possible that the emergence of structural and chemical differences between the two hemispheres was driven by the evolutionary pressures to enhance learning? In other words, is it possible that the existence of two different, separate but interconnected systems, one for novelty and the other one for routines, facilitates learning?

An experimental answer to this question would require comparing the learning abilities of two types of organisms: one with and one without two hemispheres, but otherwise of equal complexity. Since hemispheric duality is a universal attribute of all the advanced species, the experiment will never be staged. The best the investigator might be able to do is to plot the evolutionary growth curves of learning abilities and of hemispheric differentiation, hoping to see a parallel. But plotting such curves is an imprecise enterprise, based on arbitrary assumptions.

The arsenal of science, however, is not limited to experimental and empirical methods. While still the mainstay of science, experimental methods are intrinsically limited, thus most developed disciplines acquire a theoretical arm. A theory is a simplified model of some aspect of reality, which is usually constructed in a formal, often mathematical, language. Instead of direct experimentation, a model can be examined formally, or computationally, by deducing some of its properties from other properties. With the advent of powerful computers, it has become possible to combine deductive and experimental methods in a single computational approach. A model of the object in question is created in the form of a computer program, which is then run on the computer, simulating behavior. In this way, experiments can be designed with the model, and the dynamic properties of the model can be examined through studying its actual behavior. Of all the new developments in cognitive neuroscience, the advent of computational methods is particularly promising.

Especially exciting among them are formal neural nets. Composed of large ensembles of relatively simple units, neural nets are extremely brainlike. They can accumulate and store information about their environment (*inputs*), provided that they get feedback about their behavior. They truly learn.

Neural nets are being used increasingly to model and better understand the processes in the real brain. Stephen Grossberg, one of the pioneers of neural-net modeling, discovered that computational efficiency is indeed enhanced by splitting the system into two parts, one dealing with novel inputs and the other with routine inputs.[26] Other computational theories have also recognized the distinction between exploratory behavior in novel situations and cognitive routines in stationary situations. Although none of these theories have explicitly linked these two processes to the two cerebral hemispheres, they provide an additional argument that the emergence of such a split in evolution would confer a computational advantage on the brain.

Linking novelty to the right hemisphere and cognitive routines to the left hemisphere forces an entirely new way of looking at the brain. The traditional understanding of hemispheric roles in cognition is static and generic. Certain functions, like language, were thought to be invariably linked to the left hemisphere. Other functions, like spatial processing, were presumed to be linked to the right hemisphere in an equally inviolable fashion. A standard textbook on neuropsychology or behavioral neurology lists a fixed mapping of function into structure without much regard for any dynamic changes in the nature of this mapping. What happened to the Heraclitian wisdom that "it is impossible to step into the same river twice"? The dynamic nature of brain processes has been accepted as the cornerstone of neurobiology, and dynamic changes in the brain that are associated with learning have been demonstrated even in rodents.[27] While honored in most branches of neurobiology, this seemingly self-evident truth was ignored in human neuropsychology for many years. Furthermore, traditional neuropsychology and behavioral neurology tacitly assume that functional mapping of the brain is the same in all individuals, regardless of their education, vocation, or life experience. But this, too, defies common sense. Can a portrait photographer and a musician be using exactly the same parts of the brain to look at faces and listen to music?

Novelty and routinization are relative, however. What is novel for me today will become routine tomorrow, in a month, or in a year. Therefore, the relationship between the two hemispheres must be dynamic, characterized by a gradual shift in the locus of cognitive control over a task from the right hemisphere to the left hemisphere. This temporospatial dynamics is depicted in Figure 6.1. Furthermore, what is novel to me may be familiar to you, and vice versa. Therefore, the functional relationship between the two hemispheres is somewhat different in different people.

By the right-to-left information transfer I do not mean a literal transposition of information. More likely, mental representations develop interactively in both hemispheres, but the rates of their formation differ. They form more efficiently in the right hemisphere at early stages of learning a cognitive skill, but the relative rate reverses in favor of the left hemisphere during the late stages. We do not yet fully understand the neural machinery behind these differences, but we are in a position to formulate certain plausible hypotheses. Suppose that the left hemisphere forms and stores representations that are generic in the sense that they capture shared features of a whole class of specific things or situations, yet at the same time specific in that each representation captures the shared properties of a relatively narrow class of situations. By definition, a huge number of such representations will be required to capture the sum total of one's experiences and knowledge. By contrast, the right hemisphere forms and stores much coarser

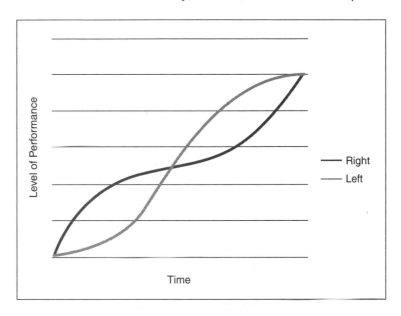

Figure 6.1 Transition from novelty to routinization in the course of learning a task. Right hemisphere is dominant at early learning stages, while the task is novel. Left hemisphere is dominant once task-appropriate cognitive strategies are firmly in place. This is a heuristic conceptual diagram not corresponding to any particular experiment, but rather intended to convey the general idea first formulated in Goldberg and Costa, 1981.[24]

representations, each of which captures the shared properties of a much broader class of situations. It stands to reason that the right hemisphere will contain much fewer such representations than the left hemisphere. One may even contemplate an extreme case, whereby the association cortex of the right hemisphere does not contain specific representations at all, but rather consists of a single relatively undifferentiated network capturing, in some sense, the averaged properties of all prior experiences.

When an individual is faced with a relatively familiar cognitive task, it is likely to resonate with a specific representation in the left hemisphere. But when an individual is faced with a relatively novel cognitive task, it is more likely to resonate with one of the coarser representations in the right hemisphere, precisely because these representations are less bounded and less specific. As the individual gains experience and expertise with the new type of cognitive task, very different things will happen in the two hemisphere. In the left hemisphere a new, relatively narrow-scope representation will be formed to capture the specific properties of the new type of cognitive challenge. By contrast, the right hemisphere will react in a far less drastic way and a mere updating of the larger-scale coarse network will take place.

In my book *The Wisdom Paradox*, the ways in which the two hemispheres represent the same data set are compared to the two alternative representations used in descriptive statistics to summarize a data set: as a mean and standard deviation summarizing all of the data (the right hemisphere) or as a scatter plot diagram with each point summarizing a specific subset of data (the left hemisphere).[28] Clearly, the arrival of a new data set will result in the two representations being updated in very different ways. In a scatter plot diagram a new data point will be added without erasing any of the previously entered data points (a new specific representation formed in the left hemisphere alongside the previously formed ones, which remain unperturbed). By contrast, the mean and standard deviation will be recalculated and replaced by slightly different values (an existing global coarse representation modified in the right hemisphere in its entirety). To use a grooves-in-the sand analogy, the right hemisphere consists of a large network of such grooves of varying degrees of depth, but all gravitating toward medium depth. By contrast, the left hemisphere consists of a collection of grooves clustered into separate mini-nets, each being quite deep within itself but with very shallow grooves connecting the mini-nets. This difference between the network organization in the left and right hemispheres is depicted in Figure 6.2.

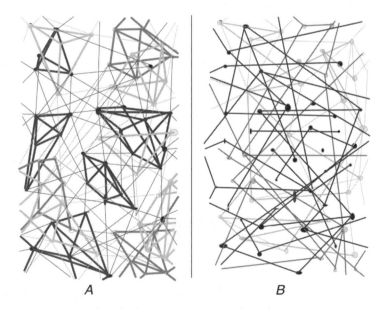

A   B

Figure 6.2 The difference between network organization in the left and right hemispheres. Neural network is more modularized in the left hemisphere (*A*) and less modularized in the right hemisphere (*B*). See text for further explanation. This heuristic representation is intended to convey a general idea rather than any realistic neuroanatomical properties.

This account of the different ways in which similar inputs are encoded in the two hemispheres leads to an interesting prediction. The information stored in the left hemisphere is more readily available to conscious experience, since it is stored in better-articulated networks (see discussion of the nature of consciousness in Chapter 4). It also relates to our earlier discussion of the differences between a priori and a posteriori modularity. To the extent that the left hemisphere is organized in a more modular fashion, this modularity is a posteriori rather than a priori. Another interesting prediction emanating from this account is that the right hemisphere is better able to deal with genuinely novel situations. Since the right-hemispheric network is relatively unbounded, any initial activation is likely to spread more widely than in the left hemisphere, and thus more likely to "hit upon" an effective way of dealing with a situation not previously encountered.[29]

Of course, all these considerations are highly intuitive. Nonetheless, I hope that these intuitions are sufficiently well articulated to serve as heuristics leading to more rigorous experimentation and modeling than those prompted by the more traditional characterization of the right-hemispheric processing mode as "global," and the left-hemispheric processing mode as "local." Some further elaboration of possible modeling approaches will be presented in Chapter 14.

We now reach an interesting conclusion: the right hemisphere, the novelty hemisphere, is modified by experience at a much slower rate than the left hemisphere, the hemisphere of established cognitive routines. The conclusion may seem counterintuitive at first glance, since the right hemisphere is the novelty hemisphere and the left hemisphere is the hemisphere of established cognitive routines. But at a deeper level of analysis, the slow-changing right hemisphere is better suited for dealing with novelty precisely because it contains an averaged default representation capturing certain shared, and thus poorly differentiated, features of many prior experiences. When the specific knowledge about the situation at hand is lacking, you fare best by doing whatever worked in the largest number of prior experiences. But once you have figured out the properties of the specific situation at hand, you tailor your response accordingly and store the newly gained experience.

My own conclusion about the two hemispheres updating mental representations at different rates was strongly influenced by our own experimental results from studies on actor-centered decision making in patients with lateralized frontal lesions (see Chapter 7).[30] An additional source of convergent evidence comes from computational work. Using neural net models, Stefano Fusi and colleagues have demonstrated that the computational efficiency of a network will be enhanced by a variable, as opposed to constant, rate of synaptic proliferation.[31] In other words, different learning situations call for different rates of synaptic modification. Is it possible that nature took care of this requirement by coupling two systems (hemispheres) that are generally similar, albeit not identical, in organization but characterized by different learning rates? Such an arrangement would benefit the combined system within a particularly broad range of learning situations by allowing it to switch between the leading roles of one or the other hemipshere.

The ways in which these functional differences between the two hemispheres may emerge as a consequence of the neuroanatomical differences between the two hemispheres is discussed in very broad terms in Chapter 14 of this book and elsewhere.[32] Meanwhile, let's continue our discussion at a strictly functional, macroscopic level. How do the two hemispheres interact in the course of response selection? Suppose the two hemispheres arrive at different response selection choices. Then a competitive relationship exists between the two hemispheres, most likely mediated by the inhibitory pathways of the corpus callosum and the anterior comissures. Suppose also that some sort of "working memory" window keeps track of the recent history of successes and failures (let's say over i previous trials). Suppose also that some criterion of success is set by the system, which we will call m $(0 < m < i)$. Then the system operates in the following fashion: when the number of successful trial n exceeds m $(0 < m < n < i)$, then the left hemisphere wins, since this implies that the specific representations that inhabit it have been adequate in guiding the decision-making process at hand. By contrast, when the number of successful trials within the working-memory window falls short of the criterion $(0 < n < m < i)$, then the right hemisphere wins, since this implies that none of the situation-specific representations housed in the left hemisphere was up to the job and the global default representation housed in the right hemisphere had to be invoked. We will discuss further the neural machinery and its microcircuitry responsible for the these macroscopic functional differences between the two hemispheres in Chapter 14 of this book.

Depending on education, vocation, and life history, what is novel for one individual is routine for another. Therefore, the roles of the two hemispheres in cognition are dynamic, relative, and individualized. And even more important, the distinction between novelty and routinization can be applied to any creature capable of learning, and hemispheric differences based on this distinction may already exist in nonhuman species. At least this possibility can be experimentally explored and the evolutionary continuity across species ascertained. This is by far a more compelling framework of scientific inquiry. Such demonstration of evolutionary continuities has indeed been provided by Giorgio Vallortigara and his colleagues, who report a differential association of the two hemispheres with novelty and with familiarity in several species.[33]

The history of science is replete with false starts. Scientific progress, however, is not based on a wholesale refutation of old claims with the arrival of new ones. This indeed would have meant hopelessly circular movement. It is more constructive when a new theory or discovery embraces old knowledge as a special case under a more general concept. The novelty–routinization theory of hemispheric specialization does not imply that the traditional notions linking language to the left hemisphere are wrong. Instead, it embraces them as a special case of a uniquely human way of representing information through a well-articulated routinized code, language.

I expected our 1981 article[34] presenting the novelty–routinization hypothesis of hemispheric specialization for the first time to make a big impact on the field, but this did not happen. It is not as if the paper went completely unnoticed. Several important neuroscientists and neuropsychologists considered it an important break-through. Notable among them were the late Joseph Bogen, the neurosurgeon who together with Roger Sperry pioneered the studies of callossomized patients;[35] the Canadian developmental neuropsychologist Byron Rourke, whose subsequent work on nonverbal learning disabilities was substantially based on the novelty–routinization hypothesis of hemispheric specialization;[36] and Gerald Turkewitz, also a developmental neuropsychologist whose numerous interesting insights remained relatively unnoticed in the field. It appeared that to the extent that our novelty–routinization hypothesis made an impact, it was among the developmental neuroscientists, whose work and observations lent themselves to an appreciation of the dynamic changes in cognition over time. But the rest of neuropsychology did not budge and it continued to embrace the static and misguided notions of brain–behavioral relations. Only very recently has the interest in the contrast between cognitive novelty and cognitive routine resurfaced, under the ruberic of "explora-tion vs. exploitation." This development is discussed further in Chapter 12.

The Evidence

In science even the most plausible and aesthetically appealing hypothesis must be put to an empirical test. Much of the evidence to support the dynamic relationship between the two hemispheres was obtained with rather simple tools. These tools exploited the basic properties of neural wiring. The majority of sensory path-ways in the brain are crossed: information from the left half of the outside world is delivered primarily to the right hemisphere, and information from the right half of the outside world is delivered primarily to the left hemisphere. This is true for tactile, visual, and, to a lesser extent, acoustic information. Of course, under normal circumstances the two hemispheres interact and share information owing to the massive fiber bundles connecting them, called the *corpus callosum* and the *commissures*. However, by delivering information very briefly to one side of the sensory field, it is possible to engage a single hemisphere, the one opposite the side of the input.

This can be accomplished with rather simple devices. One of them, the tachis-toscope, is a simple visual projection device exploiting this principle. For better or worse, the tachistoscope is probably responsible for more information about the workings of the two hemispheres than any other method. For acoustic information this is accomplished with a dichotic listening device, essentially a tape deck with two earphones.[37]

Much of the research with these methods has revolved around the restatement and elaboration of the static concept about the roles of the two hemispheres. Precious few breakthroughs have been made. Most research was aimed merely at extending the laundry lists of left-hemispheric functions and right-hemispheric functions. However, some of the findings led to provocatively unexpected conclusions, which violated the established "truth."

Music processing and perception of faces figure prominently on the right-hemispheric list. Traditionally, prosopagnosia (impairment of facial recognition) and amusia (impairment of melody recognition) have been regarded as symptoms of right-hemispheric damage following stroke or other conditions. Yet the classic experiment by Bever and Chiarello demonstrated a striking relationship between the side of musical processing and musical expertise.[38] Musically naive people process music mostly with the right hemisphere. Trained musicians, however, process music mostly with the left hemisphere. Since most people are musically naive, the old notion linking music to the right hemisphere is supported, but only in a weak, limited sense; the notion of an intrinsic, obligatory link between music and hemispheric specialization is no longer tenable. Instead, the side of processing musical information appears to be relative, determined by the degree of musical training and prior exposure to music. Similar findings have been reported for faces. Obscure faces are processed mostly by the right hemisphere, in keeping with the traditional views. But familiar faces are processed mostly by the left hemisphere.[39] Again we see relativity based on the novelty–routinization distinction.

The transition from cognitive novelty to cognitive routinization and the associated transition from the right hemispheric to left hemispheric superiority documented in these studies reflects the natural histories of learning and occurs on a time scale of years. A similar right-to-left transition of "cognitive gravity" can be demonstrated on a more brief time scale, one compatible with the constrains of a laboratory experiment.

Further confirmation of the novelty–routinization principle of hemispheric specialization comes from dynamic laboratory simulations of the learning process in the laboratory. In these simulations, a totally novel task is created, of the sort never experienced by the subject before and not even related to his or her prior experiences. The subject then gets extensive exposure to the task in a lengthy experiment extending over several hours or even days. Using the tachistoscopic and dichotic methods, it was possible to demonstrate that in the beginning the right hemisphere outperformed the left hemisphere. With repeated exposure to the task, however, the pattern was reversed, the left hemisphere emerging as the more accomplished one. This could be demonstrated for both auditory and visual stimuli, for nonverbal geometric forms and for verbal stimuli, as long as the task entailed an uncommon use of language. Thus, the right-to-left shift of hemispheric control appears to be a universal phenomenon, which can be demonstrated for a broad range of learning tasks, nonverbal and verbal alike, at various time scales ranging from years and possible decades to hours and possibly minutes. The novelty–routinization dimension appears to override all the other variables in determining the hemispheric affiliation of a task.

Compelling as the tachistoscopic and dichotic studies were, they required that the stimuli be presented under conditions bearing little resemblance to the way information is delivered in real life. The evidence was indirect, since it was inferred rather than directly observed in the brain. The evidence was also imprecise, since the tachistoscopic and dichotic methods are inherently incapable of revealing the exact neuroanatomy of information processing within the hemisphere. How relevant were these findings to real-life processes? It was important to demonstrate the dynamics of hemispheric interaction in more natural situations.

A dynamic theory of brain–behavior relations requires dynamic experimental tools. Truly appropriate research methodology to address the dynamic aspects of brain–behavior relations have become available only with the advent of functional neuroimaging. The dynamics of learning curves can be studied by imaging "snapshots" at various stages of the learning curve with much of the training taking place off-line between the snapshots.

A growing number of functional neuroimaging studies are using this methodology with modern technologies, such as functional magnetic resonance imaging (fMRI), positron emission tomography (PET), magnetoencephalography (MEG), and single photon emission computerized tomography (SPECT). The evidence obtained with these methods also demonstrates an intimate link between the right hemisphere and novelty and between the left hemisphere and routinization.

Alex Martin and his colleagues at the National Institute of Mental Health provided a particularly compelling demonstration of this kind.[40] Using PET, they studied changes in blood flow patterns while subjects learned various types of information: meaningful words, nonsense words, real objects, and nonsense objects. Each type of information was presented twice, but each time with unique items. During the first presentation, when the task was novel, the right mesiotemporal structures were particularly activated, but this activation decreased during the second exposure. By contrast, the level of activation was constant in the left mesiotemporal structures, shown in Figure 6.3. The findings are important, because blood flow level reflects the level of neural activation.

In Martin's study the right-to-left shift of activation was pervasive across all the four types of information, verbal and nonverbal alike. This means that the association of the right hemisphere with novelty and left hemisphere with routinization does not depend of the nature of information, but is universal. Furthermore, the right-to-left activation shift was present despite the fact that specific items were not repeated across the two successive trials. Thus the changes in the activation patterns reflect general aspects of learning, rather than specific item learning.

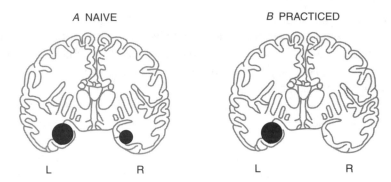

Figure 6.3 Changes in regional brain activation as a function of task familiarization. The right hemisphere is particularly active when the task is novel (*A*), but its activation level decreases with practice (*B*). [Adapted from Martin, Wiggs, and Weisberg (1997).[40] Reprinted by permission of Wiley-Liss, Inc., a subsidiary of John Wiley & Sons, Inc.]

Similar findings have been reported by a group of British neuroscientists.[41] Both for faces and for symbols, exposure to unfamiliar stimuli was associated with an enhancement of right occipital (fusiform) activation. By contrast, increasing familiarity was associated with a decrease in right occipital activation and increase in left occipital activation. As in Martin's study, the novelty–familiarity effect is present regardless of the nature of the stimulus. It holds for both symbols (which in the orthodox scheme of things should be linked to the left hemisphere) and faces (which in the same scheme should be linked to the right hemisphere).

Using PET, Gold and his colleagues examined the changes in regional cerebral blood flow (rCBF) patterns in the course of learning a complex "frontal lobe" task (a combination of delayed response and delayed alternation) in healthy subjects.[42] Early (naive) and late (practiced) stages of the learning curve were compared. Frontal lobe activation was evident at both stages, but it was considerably greater at the early stage than at the late stage. Particularly noteworthy was the change of relative activation. At the early stage, rCBF activation was greater in the right than in the left prefrontal regions. At the late stage the pattern was reversed, showing a greater rCBF activation of the left than right prefrontal structures. This was accompanied by an overall decrease in prefrontal activation.

Shadmehr and Holcomb studied the PET rCBF correlates of learning a complex motor skill requiring subject to predict and master the behavior of a robotic device.[43] An increase in activity during early learning stages, relative to the baseline condition, was noted in the right prefrontal cortex (middle frontal gyrus). By contrast, increase in activity during the late, relative to early, training stages was noted in the left posterior parietal cortex, left dorsal premotor cortex, and right anterior cerebellar cortex.

Haier and his colleagues studied PET glucose metabolic rate (GMR) correlates of learning a popular spatial puzzle game (Tetris).[44] After 4 to 8 weeks of daily practice on Tetris, GMR in cortical surface regions decreased despite a more than sevenfold improvement in performance. Subjects who improved their Tetris performance the most showed the largest GMR decreases after practice in several areas.

Berns, Cohen, and Mintun studied the PET rCBF correlates of learning, and relearning, rule-governed systems of relations ("grammars").[45] Grammar A was introduced first followed by Grammar B. The difference between the two grammars was too subtle for the subjects to be aware of the transition. Serial neuroimaging snapshots were taken in the course of learning Grammar A and then Grammar B. The learning of Grammar A was characterized by an initial surge of activation in the right ventral striatum, left premotor, and left anterior cingulate structures with subsequent decrease in activation. By contrast, a gradual increase of activation was noted in the right dorsolateral prefrontal and right posterior parietal regions. The introduction of Grammar B led to a second surge of activation in the left premotor, left anterior cingulate, and right ventral striatum regions, with subsequent decline.

Raichle and his colleagues studied PET rCBF correlates of a linguistic task (finding appropriate verbs for visually presented nouns).[46] A list of nouns was first introduced (naive condition), then, after considerable practice, replaced with a new list (novel condition). Naive performance was characterized by a particular activation of the anterior cingulate, left prefrontal, left temporal, and right cerebellar cortices. The activation virtually disappeared following practice and was partly restored during the novel condition, with the introduction of a new noun list. Additional analysis revealed prominent right cerebellar activation during the naive and novel conditions, but not after practice. By contrast, significant left medial occipital activation was present after practice, but not during the naive or novel conditions. So even linguistic tasks are processed with some degree of reliance on the right hemisphere, as long as the task is novel. A somewhat similar relationship can be demonstrated between the linguistic task's difficulty (and, thus, presumably an incomplete routinization) and the right hemisphere: a task requiring longer processing time engages the right hemisphere to a greater degree.[47]

Tulving and his colleagues studied PET rCBF correlates of novelty and familiarity in facial recognition.[48] Familiarity was associated with the activation in a broad network of frontal and parieto-occipital regions bilaterally. Novelty was associated with the activation in a broad network of temporal, parietal, and occipital regions bilaterally. Additionally, novelty was associated with a distinctly asymmetric, right but not left, activation of the hippocampal and parahippocampal structures.

Broadly similar findings have been obtained using fMRI. Greater right inferior frontal and right inferior parietal activation has been reported in subjects engaging in a complementary (different) rather than imitative (same) action.[49] In a study comparing the mechanisms of "exploration" (novelty seeking) with those of "exploitation" (the use of previously acquired knowledge in an ambiguous gambling situation), Nathaniel Daw and his colleagues found particular activation in the *right* anterior frontopolar regions associated with exploratory behaviors.[50] By contrast, perceptual decision making involving "easy" targets (presumably unequivocally and readily recognizable as members of known categories) is guided by the *left* dorsolateral prefrontal regions, according to a study conducted in Leslie Ungerleider's laboratory at the National Institute of Mental Health.[51]

A particularly elegant demonstration of the right-to-left shift of the "center of cognitive gravity" is found in the study by a group of Japanese neuroscientists using gamma EEG frequency as an index of cognitive activation in a modified version of our actor-centered preference task[52] (the Cognitive Bias Task is described later in Chapter 7 of this book and elsewhere[53]). The findings are particularly remarkable because they are essentially two-dimensional, demonstrating both right-to-left and frontal-to-posterior shift of the center of cognitive gravity with task familiarization (see Fig. 6.4). The meaning of this finding will be made more clear in the next chapter, where we review the relationship between novelty and the frontal lobes.

A similar two-dimensional right-frontal to left-parietal shift has been reported by Robert Knight and his associates in an event-related potential study of practicing a novel visuomotor task.[54]

Over the last few years, several dichotomies have become prominent in the computational and neuroimaging communities that broadly approximate the distinction between cognitive novelty and cognitive routinization. The distinction

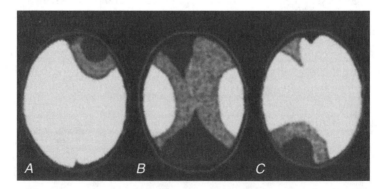

Figure 6.4 Shift of cortical gamma EEG activation with task familiarization. Darker shading corresponds to greater activation level. (*A*) Initial exposure to the task. The right frontal regions are particularly active. (*B*) Halfway through experiment—frontal activation has shifted to the left; posterior regions are active in both hemispheres. (*C*) Toward the end of the experiment—posterior regions of the left hemisphere are particularly active. [Adapted with permission from Kamiya et al. (2002).][52]

between exploration and exploitation is one of them. Another one, which specifically applies to the frontal lobes and related structures, is the distinction between
the "critic" and the "actor." The critic is in charge of learning to predict future
rewards, and the actor is in charge of using this knowledge in guiding behavior.
J. O'Doherty and colleagues conducted an fMRI study aiming to dissociate the
two, and concluded that the critic was mediated by the ventral striatum (putament
bilaterally and the right nucleus accumbens), whereas the actor was mediated by
the dorsal striatum (the left anterior caudate nucleus).[55] The ventral–dorsal distinction is certainly an interesting one. It resonates with the general, much older notion
that the orbitofrontal structures are critical for the personal value-appraisal functions and the prefrontal convexity is critical for navigating the external world. But
I was equally intrigued by the lateralized nature of O'Doherty's findings, though
not emphasized by the authors, linking the explorer critic mostly to the right forebrain, and the implementer actor mostly to the left forebrain.

This body of evidence presents a cohesive picture, with impressive consistency
existing between the old "low-tech" tachistoscopic and dichotic methods and the
state-of-the-art methods of functional neuroimaging. It appears that the cerebral
orchestra is divided into two groups of players. Those sitting on the right side of the
aisle are quicker at basic mastery of the new repertoire, but in the long run, with due
practice, those on the left side come closer to perfection. In the corporate analogy,
the large organization that is the brain appears to consist of two major divisions: one
dealing with relatively new projects, the other running established, ongoing production lines. In reality each cerebral hemisphere is involved in all the cognitive
processes, but their *relative degree of involvement* varies according to the novelty–
routinization principle.

A convergence of evidence in support of this broad conclusion comes from
several areas of neuroscience. In addition to the neuropsychological and neuroimaging evidence described above, behavioral–biochemical evidence points in the
same direction. Dopaminergic pathways are more prominent in the left hemisphere
and stimulation of the dopamine system in animal models produces stereotypic,
repetitive behaviors reinforced in prior experience. By contrast, noradrenergic
pathways are more prominent in the right hemisphere *and* stimulation of the
noradrenergic system produces exploratory, novelty-seeking behaviors,[56] whereas
pharmacological suppression of the noradrenergic system facilitates response
inhibition.[57] In a broadly similar vein, a computational argument was made by
Steven Grossberg[58] and others that the computational power of a neural net is
enhanced by separating within it the mechanisms of new knowledge acquisition
and old knowledge conservation.[59]

Findings of pathology point in the same direction. In conditions characterized
by a pathological augmentation of orienting response, as in post-traumatic stress
disorder, the associated electrophysiological activity is mostly lateralized to the
right hemisphere.[60]

The shift of the locus of cognitive control from the right to the left hemisphere occurs on many time scales: from minutes or hours, as in the experiments using within-experimental learning, to years and decades, as in learning complex skills and codes, including language. This shift may even be discerned on the scale transcending the life of an individual. It can be argued that the whole history of human civilization has been characterized by a relative shift of the cognitive emphasis from the right hemisphere to the left hemisphere, owing to the accumulation of ready-made cognitive "templates" of various kinds. These cognitive templates are stored externally through various cultural means, including language, and are internalized by individuals in the course of learning as cognitive "prefabricates" of sorts. Any attempt to translate Vygotskian cultural–historical psychology[61] into neuroanatomical terms will inevitably lead to this conclusion. In a more poetic, metaphorical vein, a somewhat similar conclusion was reached by Julian Jaynes in his rendition of the "bicameral mind" with the "voices of gods" emanating from the right hemisphere to guide our ancestors as they nagivated novel situations three millennia ago.[62]

Lessons for Clinicians

On a more mundane but in many ways more immediately relevant level of the nuts and bolts of clinical practice, the previous discussion raises some important questions about the principles of neuropsychological diagnostic test design, as well as about the design of cognitive activation tasks used increasingly for clinical diagnosis with fMRI and other functional neuroimaging techniques. It is common for such procedures to consist of multiple items processed by the subject over time. Think of the six categories on the Wisconsin Card Sorting Task; the five trials on the California Verbal Learning Test; or the 30 trials on the Benton Line Orientation Test.[63] The tacit assumption behind the interpretation of such tests is that the underlying functional neuroanatomy remains static and unchangeable throughout test administration. But the review presented earlier strongly challenges this assumption, leading to the inconvenient conclusion that averaging across all test items and arriving at a single score may not be such a great idea. Instead, a new generation of tests, or at least a new set of norms for old tests, should be created, segmenting the item sequence into several subsets and scoring each of them separately. The neuroanatomical implications of different segment scores will then be different.

This certainly complicates the business of clinical neuropsychological diagnosis. The argument against segmenting the experimental sequences into temporal components is sometimes made that this practice decreases the data point sample size and thus renders the data less stable. But this argument only works if you assume that all the data points in the sample are drawn from the same population. To the extent that by a "population" we mean all the data points representing the contribution of static functional neuroanatomy, the argument does not hold water, because the underlying functional neuroanatomy changes over time, during the testing procedure. Then merging all the data points obtained at vastly different points in the testing (or experimental) sequence becomes like throwing in a bunch of blood pressure values to increase the sample of IQ scores.

The novelty–routinization principle of hemispheric specialization represents a rather radical departure from much that has been regarded axiomatic in neuropsychology for many years. Understandably, a skeptical reader may ask: How do we reconcile the ideas expressed in this chapter with the decades of experimental findings claiming to demonstrate the link between verbal tasks and the left hemisphere, and the visuospatial tasks and the right hemisphere? These findings are not limited to the low-tech tachistoschopes of the 1960s; they include also cutting-edge, state-of-the-art functional neuroimaging tools.[64] Were they all wrong? It would be both presumptuous and folly for me to even remotely imply that they were, and it certainly is not my intent. But one must be reminded that there are precious few factorially pure tasks in clinical neuropsychology or, for that matter, in cognitive neuroscience. As a result, the verbal–nonverbal dimension is more than likely to be confounded with the novelty–familiarity dimension. The tasks that we call "verbal" are also likely to be more familiar; and the tasks we call "nonverbal" or "visuospatial" are also likely to be relatively novel. So even though there is no reason to believe that the huge corpus of findings obtained during the heyday of "hemispheric specialization" in the second half of the twentieth century is factually wrong, the interpretation of these findings may very well have been misleading.

Agnosias and Hemispheres

Studies of agnosias help us further understand the nature of hemispheric specialization. Earlier we introduced the novelty–routinization principle and argued that it captures the fundamental functional differences between the hemispheres. But a hemisphere is a big place. How is the novelty–routinization principle expressed in different parts of the cerebral hemispheres? Clearly, the extent of hemispheric specialization increases as one moves from the primary sensory and motor projection areas, where cortical mapping is basically contralaterally symmetric, to association cortices, where the functional differences between the hemispheres become increasingly profound. In the posterior cortex (occipital, temporal, and parietal lobes), these differences can be understood by considering how different types of agnosias are caused by damage to one or the other cerebral hemisphere.

Before going into the neuroanatomical discussion, let's engage our common sense and examine the difference between two important types of perceptual tasks. Consider these two examples. In the first instance, you walk into an unfamiliar conference room feeling tired, slump into an equally unfamilar chair (designed in a particularly arcane, unusual style), pick up an unfamiliar pen (designed in an equally over-the-top, artsy style) from the table, and begin to take notes on a presentation made by an unfamilar person in an unfamiliar voice with a slight, unfamiliar accent. How do you know that a chair is a chair and that a pen is a pen? You have never seen this particular chair or pen before, you may not even have encountered their particular designs before altogether, and it is certainly not written on the chair that it is a chair. You have just accomplished—effortlessly, instantly, and unselfconsciously—an amazing perceptual feat that may have confounded a computer. You recognized several unfamiliar unique objects as member of certain familiar object categories. You engaged in an act of pattern recognition. The same is true for your ability to understand the presentation despite the fact that both the presenter's voice and his accent are unique and unfamiliar to you. This notwithstanding, you were able to interpret unique and unfamiliar acoustic signals as members of familiar classes—speech sounds, words, and sentences.

In the second instance you bump into a person in the hallway later that day and instantly recognize him as the morning speaker; in fact, you recognized him even before he turned the corner by hearing his voice. He seems to have recognized you too, even though the earlier encounter was a fleeting one and there were many people, all strangers, in the conference room, and you exchanged casual nods of recognition. This, too, has been accomplished instantaneously and effotlessly, but this perceptual task is very different from the one described earlier.

In the first instance you recognized unique exemplars as members of generic categories. Clearly, for this process to take place, a mental representation of the category had to be stored somewhere in your head before you encountered the unique exemplar in question. An illiterate native of the Amazon jungle who had never encountered a pen before would not recognize a new one either. So the perceptual process in question is top-down in the sense that it presupposes the existence of a previously formed, somewhat generalized mental representation that guides your recognition of a unique exemplar as a category member. But because the task is not to recognize the object in all its unique attributes, but merely in term of its category membership, it does not require that you form a mental account of all its attributes, only of those germane to the category membership. If someone were to ask you about the color of the pen or of the chair in question, you very likely would not remember it because you didn't pay attention to these superfluous attributes.

In the second instance, the cognitive task was entirely different. You didn't recognize the stranger's face merely as a human face, or the stranger's voice merely as a human voice. You recognized him as his own self, as the unique examplar of humanity whom you had encountered briefly sometime earlier that day. This is not a task of identifying a unique exemplar as a member of a generic category, but a task of perceptual constancy. And even though the knowledge of category membership (that it was a human being and not a camel or an elephant) helped, it was not a sine qua non. You could have recognized even a totally meaningless blob of matter as its own self under varying conditions of observation, or a totally meaningless sound as probably belonging to the same source without even knowing what exactly that source was. Unlike in the first example, there is no obligatory, generic, previously formed mental representation stored in long-term memory to guide your recognition process.

The two examples represent two very different aspects of perception, which may be closely intertwined in real life but are neuroanatomically distinct. The first example represents our ability to recognize unique exemplars as members of generic categories. It depends on the availability of previously formed generalized, high-order, long-term mental representation and is mediated mostly by the left hemisphere. The second example represents our ability to recognize unique exemplars (objects, sounds, faces) as their own selves under ever-changing conditions of sensory input. It does not depend, or at least not nearly to the same degree, on the availability of previously formed generalized, high-order mental representations and is mediated mostly by the right hemisphere.

How do we know all this? Because of the different effects of damage to the left or the right hemisphere on perception. Damage to the left hemisphere results in various forms of an inability to recognize unique exemplars as members of generic categoris. We already know that this damage may take various forms, that it is usually modality-specific, and that different modalities (visual, auditory, or somatosensory) may be affected following damage to different parts of the hemisphere. But the damage invariably involves the left hemisophere. By contrast, damage to the right hemisphere results in various forms of inability to recognize unique exemplars as their own selves under changing sensory conditions. This damage may also take a variety of forms and is usually modality-specific, and different modalities may be affected following damage to different parts of the hemisphere. But here the damage invariably involves the right hemisphere.

Disorders of the ability to recognize unique exemplars as members of generic categories are called *associative agnosias*. Disorders of the ability to recognize unique exemplars as their own selves or as different unique exemplars of the same category are called *aperceptive agnosias*. Either form of agnosia can be caused by bilateral damage to the posterior association cortex; but when the damage is lateralized to the left hemisphere only associative agnosia is observed, and when the damage is lateralized to the right hemisphere only apperceptive agnosia is observed (see Table 6.1).[65] A more detailed discussion of various forms of perceptual disorders in relationship to hemispheric specialization can be found in an old paper of mine on associative agnosias.[66]

As an example, a middle-aged woman woke up one morning, walked into the bathroom, looked around, saw various objects (a toothbrush, a soap bar, a mirror), and did not know what they were. But she was able to recognze them when she touched the objects. The woman became scared, got an inkling that something was

Table 6.1 Neuroanatomy of Associative and Apperceptive Agnosias: Literature Review

Type of Agnosia	References, by Lesion Site		
	Left	Bilateral	Right
Associative Agnosias			
Visual object	Bauer and Rubens (1985)[67]	Hécaen and Albert (1978)[68]	
	Hécaen and de Ajuruguerra (1956)[69]	Hoff and Pötzl (1935)[70]	
	Hécaen et al. (1974)[71]	von Stauffenberg (1918)[72]	
	Nielsen (1937, 1946)[73,74]		
Pure	Foix (1922)[75]		
Astereognosia	Goldstein (1916)[76]		
	Lehrmitte and de Ajuruguerra (1938)[77]		
Semantic	Faglioni et al. (1969)[78]		
Associative	Kleist (1928)[79]		
Auditory	Spinnler and Vignolo (1966)[80]		
	Vignolo (1982)[81]		
Apperceptive Agnosias			
Visual		Damasio (1985)[82]	Benton and Van Allen (1968)[83]
		Damasio et al. (1982)[84]	Meadows (1974)[85]
		De Renzi et al. (1969)[86]	Warrington (1982)[87]
			Warrington and James (1967, 1988)[88,89]
			Warrington and Taylor (1973)[90]
Auditory			Faglioni et al. (1969)[91]

Source: E. Goldberg and W. Barr. Three possible mechanisms of unawareness of deficit. In: G. Prigatano and D. Schacter (eds.) *Awareness of Deficit: Theoretical and Clinical Issues*. (New York: Oxford University Press, 1991), 152–175.

medically wrong, and had herself driven to a local emergency room. A computerized tomography (CT) scan was performed and a left occipitotemporal stroke was discovered, which must have taken place during the night. This was a typical case of associative agnosia in the visual modality—visual object agnosia. Sometime later she was referred to me for a neuropsychological evaluation and became my patient.

So the functional differences between the posterior aspects of the two hemispheres can be characterized by two contrasting perceptual leitmotifs. For the left hemisphere it is the top-down process driven by previously formed generic representations allowing a class membership assignation of unique exemplars. For the right hemisphere it is a bottom-up process driven more by ad-hoc computations aimed at establishing similarities. In some sense the former process is more akin to perceptual deduction and the latter one to perceptual induction. A die-hard neuropsychological orthodox might say that the associative agnosias of the left hemisphere are secondary to language impairment, but this argument does not hold much water. First, associative agnosias may be present without language impairment and language impairment may be present without associative agnosia—the proverbial double dissociation. Second, as we already know, associative agnosias are modality-specific, something that the language-based explanation would have a hard time accounting for. Finally, but perhaps most important, categorical perception whose breakdown results in associative agnosias exists in other species in the absence of language. My bullmastiff Brit is able to distinguish between a doorman, even an unfamiliar doorman, and the rest of humanity in an uncannily unfailing way. How he does this, I do not know. So in principle the distinction between associative and aperceptive agnosias is applicable to other species as well. Whether their respective neuroanatomies are lateralized the way they are in humans is a fascinating question.

In light of these considerations, it may be particularly interesting to design animal models of the two classes of perceptual processes described above (identifying unique exemplars as members of generic categories, and identifying unique exempars as their own selves under changing sensory conditions) to find out, using functional neuroimaging, extracellular recording, or lesion methodology, whether they are mediated by different hemispheres. If that is the case, then the next step would be to examine the relationship between hemispheric specialization and handedness (call it "pawedness" if you wish). The question is a perfectly reasonable one, since most individual mammals have distinct pawedness that is stable in a given animal throughout its life span. The righ/left pawedness ratio in most (perhaps all) nonhuman species is not nearly as skewed as in humans and is much closer to 50/50.

Executive Deficit and Hemispheres

Damage to the frontal lobes often produces two classes of symptoms: perseveration and field-dependent behaviors, which in most severe cases may take the form of echo behaviors.[92] I will discuss both types of symptoms in considerable detail later in Chapter 10 of this book. For now suffice it to say that the term *perseveration* refers to a pathological inability to make a complete transition from one activity to a different one, so that some elements of a previous activity intrude maladaptively into the ongoing one. One can think of perseveration as a deficit of cognitive flexibility. By contrast, the term *field-dependent behavior* refers to an inability to stick to an ongoing task in a focused way and to withstand the effect of incidental distractions from the environment. One can think of field-dependent behavior as a deficit of the stability of mental operations. In extreme cases this deficit may take the form of *echopraxia* (physical imitation of other people's behavior) or *echolalia* (verbal imitation of other people's utterances).

In the clinical neuropsychological literature, perseveration and field-dependent behavior are traditionally viewed as two distinct classes of symptoms, each resulting from the breakdown of a distinct aspect of the executive control mediated by the frontal lobes. Furthermore, the existence of these two distinct classes of symptoms is often invoked as proof of the existence of two distinct aspects of executive control: the ability to guide behavior by internal representations, and the ability to shift cognitive sets in response to changing contingencies. These two aspects of executive control are sometimes referred to as "stability" vs. "plasticity," which are presumed to be in some sort of dynamic balance in normal cognition. Following frontal lobe damage this balance may be impaired, leading to perseveration (excessive stability of mental operations) or to field-dependent behavior (excessive plasticity of mental operations).[93]

The mechanisms of cognitive stability vs. cognitive plasticity mediated by the frontal lobes remain a matter of intense research and debate in cognitive and computational neurosciences, giving rise to the concept of "dynamic bystability"—an organism's ability to maintain a certain set of mental activities in a robust, "stable" way and then make a relatively abrupt transition to another set of mental activities, which in turn will be maintained in an equally robust, stable way.[94] Various mechanisms have been proposed to account for dynamic bistability. One such mechanism involves the dual nature of dopamine modulation.[95] As we already know, several dopamine recptors exist, and they appear to operate in different ways. It has been proposed that D1 receptors respond to low concentrations of dopamine and their activation produces "robust" maintanence of the organism's current cognitive regime. By contrast, D2 receptors respond only to high concentrations of dopamine and their activation produces a destabilizing, "rapid updating" change in the organisms's cognitive regime.[96] If this is true, then it is particularly interesting that D2 receptor distribution appears to be somewhat lateralized, favoring the right hemisphere.[97] This may be at least part of the explanation behind the preferential relationship between cognitive novelty and the right hemisphere.

While the phenomenal distinctness, even oppositeness, of perseveration and field-dependent behavior is not in question, the distinctness of the underlying mechanisms is far from settled. In *Computational Explorations in Cognitive Neuroscience*, Randall O'Reilly and Yuko Munakata[98] have articulated a very important insight that goes against the grain of the intuitions prompted by clinical observations. The gist of this insight is that perseveration and field-dependent behavior do not reflect the breakdown of two different mechanisms within the frontal lobes. Instead, they are viewed as the consequence of the breakdown of a certain unitary frontally mediated regulation acting (or rather failing to act) on the posterior neural networks, presumably in the posterior portions of the hemispheres, which are organized in two different ways. In other words, the key to the dual nature of frontal symptomatology is found not only in the frontal lobes themselves but also in the diversity of neural organization landscapes in the posterior networks upon which the frontal lobes act. If these posterior networks are organized as a collection of subnetwoks strongly interconnected within but poorly interconnected across, then the failure of frontal regulation will result in the patterns of activation getting "stuck" within one such subnetwork unable to get out, hence perseveration. On the other hand, if these posterior networks are relatively homogeneous, then the failure of frontal regulation will result in an excessive diffusion of activation, hence field-dependent behavior.

The description of the two kinds of neural architectures, broken up into a distinctive subnetwork vs. a relatively homogeneous one, sounds very much like the organization of the two hemispheres proposed earlier in this chapter: the left hemisphere consisting of relatively distinctive subnetworks and the right hemisphere being a relatively homogeneous master network. We then arrive at an interesting syllogism. If O'Reilly's and Munataka's hypothesis and the account of the hemispheric differences articulated here (and earlier in *The Wisdom Paradox*[99]) are both valid, then damage to the left frontal lobe should produce mostly perseveration, and damage to the right frontal lobe should produce mostly field-dependent behavior. Do we have any data to test this prediction? They answer is, yes.

For better or worse, my mentor Alexandr Luria eschewed standard psychometric tests. Instead, he had a collection of bedside procedures—some of his own design, others adapted from the writings of an earlier generation of great European neurologists—which he administered in an improvisational, fluid way, depending on the diagnostic questions at hand. Most of these procedures were designed to elicit positive rather than negative symptomatology, that is, manifestations produced by disease and not part of normal behavior, as opposed to decrements in behavior. Almost without exception, by virtue of its uniqueness, positive symptomatology is much more informative than negative symptomatology, so in experienced hands, Luria's bedside procedures amounted to an impressively powerful diagnostic arsenal. Today this approach to neuropsychological diagnosis is sometimes bombastically and with various emphases referred to as "process oriented," "qualitative," "hypothesis testing" as distinct from a "fixed battery" approach. All the members of Luria's clinical entourage, myself included, learned from him in an apprenticeship kind of way and usually acquired considerable facility in this brand of fluid, Socratic diagnosis. Among Luria's bedside probe collection, there were a few ingenious procedures designed to elicit "frontal" symptoms (or rather signs), including perseveration and echo behaviors.

Many years later, already in the United States, I decided to formalize these procedures, wedding Luria's ingenuity with the common expectations of standartization. This effort resulted in *The Executive Control Battery (ECB)* which I co-authored with my former students and associates Bob Bilder, Judy Jaeger, and Ken Podell.[100] It consists of four brief subtests, two of which are designed to elicit various types of graphomotor and motor perseveration, and two others to elicit various types of echopraxic responses. In addition to a normative sample of neurologically healthy individuals, we administered ECB to various clinical samples, including patients with lateralized prefrontal lesions.

The findings were quite dramatic. Perseveration was almost twice as severe following left frontal lesions than following right frontal lesions. By contrast, echopraxia was twice as severe following right frontal lesions than following left frontal lesions.[101] These findings confirmed informal observations that I had made many years earlier, while still working in Luria's laboratory at the Bourdenko Institute of Neurosurgery in Moscow, that perseveration and field-dependent behavior are often caused by oppositely lateralized frontal lesions. Assuming the O'Reily's and Munakata's hypothesis is correct, this is precisely what one would predict based on the differences in the left- and right-hemispheric neural net organization proposeded earlier in this chapter. While these findings do not prove the contrasting nature of the left- and right-hemispheric neural landscapes, one broken up into distinctive subnets, the other one more homegeneous and smooth, they are certainly very consistent with this model. Likewise, assuming that the hypothesis about the hemispheric differences in neural organization articulated here is correct, then the ECB findings lend strong support to the hypothesis by O'Reilly and Munakata about the single mechanism underlyng perseveration and field-dependent behavior but playing itself out differently on different landscapes of the posterior parts of the two hemispheres.

This is not the whole story, however. The double dissociation between perseveration and echopraxia and the left and right frontal lesions was present only in males. In females no such dissociation was evident, and the effects of left and right frontal lesions were much more alike. Does this suggest, in keeping with our line of reasoning, that the neural organization of the two hemispheres is more similar in females than in males? We will examine this issue more closely in Chapter 9.

7

The Conductor:

A Closer Look at the Frontal Lobes

Novelty and the Frontal Lobes

The repertoire of every orchestra or troupe consists of pieces that have been its mainstay for years as well as relatively new additions. Likewise, the products manufactured by a company consist of older lines of products and relatively new ones. Which pieces (or products) require closer ongoing attention by the conductor/director (or the CEO)? Common sense suggests that the less streamlined or rehearsed the activities, the less likely they are to be successfully accomplished "on autopilot." Therefore, the less rehearsed, more novel activities require closer direction from the leader.

Functional neuroimaging experiments by Raichle and his colleagues highlight the relationship between the frontal lobes and novelty quite dramatically.[1] These researchers used positron emission tomography (PET) to study the relationship between regional cerebral blood flow levels and task novelty. When the task (saying an appropriate verb to a visually presented noun) was first introduced, the blood flow level in the frontal lobes reached its highest level. As the subjects' familiarization with the task increased, frontal lobe involvement all but disappeared. When a new task was introduced that generally resembled the first task but was not exactly like it, frontal blood flow increased somewhat but did not quite reach its initial level (Fig. 7.1). There appears to be a strong relationship between the task novelty and blood flow level in the frontal lobes: it is highest when the task is novel, lowest when the task is familiar, and intermediate when the task is partly novel. To the extent that blood flow levels are correlated with neural activity (which most scientists believe to be the case), these experiments provide strong and direct evidence about the role of the frontal lobes in dealing with cognitive novelty.

Of course, the distinction between cognitive novelty and cognitive routines is not a binary one but, rather, a matter of degree. Likewise, the relative role of the prefrontal cortex in novel in contrast to familiar cognitive situations is not characterized by a precipitous discontinuity—it is also a matter of degree. Jordan Grafman and his colleagues at the National Institutes of Health have shown that the anterior prefrontal cortex is particularly active during novel tasks, but medial and more posterior prefrontal regions are active during familiar tasks.[2] This finding would be consistent with the hierarchical nature of action representation in the prefrontal cortex. According to this view, more posterior prefrontal regions are involved in the representation of specific actions, "tagging" specific neural circuits in the posterior cortex, whose activation is necessary to complete the action. By contrast, a novel task is approached by activating more widely distributed regions, which contain the circuits representing somewhat similar familiar tasks.

You may recall that novelty is associated with the right hemisphere. Does this mean that the frontal lobes are more intimately involved with the workings of the right hemisphere than of the left hemisphere? It just may. The right frontal lobe is larger in the

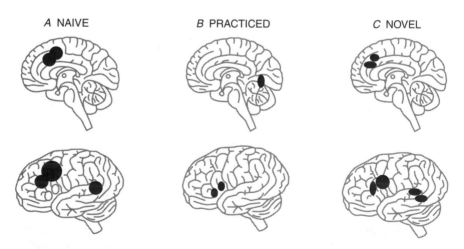

Figure 7.1 Frontal lobes and novelty. (A) Prefrontal cortex is active when the cognitive task is novel. (B) Frontal activation drops with task familiarization. (C) Prefrontal cortex becomes partially activated again when a somewhat different task is introduced, similar but not identical to the first one. [Adapted from Raichle et al. (1994).[1] Reprinted with permission.]

right hemisphere than in the left hemisphere. And while it is specious to draw overly direct parallels between structure and function, most scientists believe that more neural tissue implies greater computational capacity. It may also be the case that the pathway connectivity in the right hemisphere (including the right prefrontal cortex) is conducive toward the activation spread within a larger region than in the left hemisphere, due to a greater representation of long pathways, for example, axons emanating from the spindle cells known to be more numerous in the right than in the left prefrontal regions (see discussion in Chapter 6). The special role played by the frontal lobes and the right hemisphere in dealing with novelty and by the left hemisphere in implementing routines suggests that the dynamic changes associated with learning are at least twofold. With learning, the locus of cognitive control shifts from the right hemisphere to the left hemisphere, and from the frontal to the posterior parts of the cortex.

This dual phenomenon, which I had described earlier, was demonstrated by Jim Gold and his colleagues at The National Institute of Mental Health.[3] Using PET, they studied changes in blood flow patterns in the course of performing a complex "delayed alternating response" task. Frontal lobe activation was very strong at the early (naive) stage and subsided considerably at the late (practiced) stage of learning the task. Its regional pattern had also changed. At the early learning stage the activation was greater in the right prefrontal regions than that in the left. At the late stage the pattern was reversed: there was more activation in the left than right prefrontal regions. This is depicted in Figure 7.2.

In another PET study, Anthony McIntosh and his colleagues at the Rothman Research Institute in Toronto demonstrated particular changes in the left but not

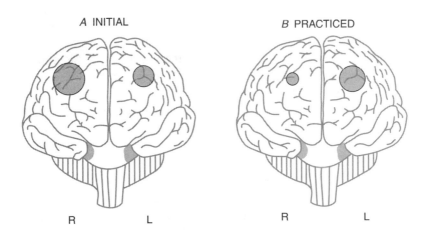

Figure 7.2 Frontal lobes, hemispheres and novelty. (*A*) A novel task activates predominantly the right prefrontal cortex. (*B*) As the task becomes familiar, the overall level of activation drops and shifts from the right to the left prefrontal cortex. [Adapted from Gold et al. (1996).[3] Reprinted with permission.]

right prefrontal cortex with learning with awareness.[4] As discussed in Chapter 6, a gradual transition from right prefrontal to left posterior activation was demonstrated by a group of Japanese scientists in a study of gamma EEG changes with increased task familiarity.[5] A right–left/prefrontal–fusiform interaction was also apparent in a study of priming effects by Ian Dobbins and colleagues.[6] Thus, there is a growing body of evidence of a complex, at least two-dimensional right-frontal to left-posterior spatiotemporal dynamics of learning.

To my knowledge, no data have been reported demonstrating the presence or absence of such an effect in primates, even though single-neuron activity in the course of learning a new task has been recorded in the monkey prefrontal cortex.[7] But absence of evidence is no evidence of absence, and it may be necessary to look for such effects in animals in order to see them.

In the old literature the right hemisphere was referred to as the "minor hemisphere" and the frontal lobes as the "silent lobes." Today we know that these structures are neither minor nor silent, although their functions may be elusive. The functions of the right hemisphere are less transparent than those of the left hemisphere, and the functions of the frontal lobes are less transparent than those of the posterior cortex, precisely because they deal with situations defying easy codification and reduction to an algorithm. So much for the minor hemisphere and the silent lobe! It has taken a longer time to appreciate their functions, but we are beginning to understand their true complexity and the central role they play in our mental processes.

Working Memory—or Working with Memory?

Memory does not sound like a mysterious concept to most people. In fact, the general public is so conditioned to the term that it is often used inclusively, and thus meaninglessly, to refer indiscriminately to every aspect of the mind. Ask 10 people what memory does, and the answers will be pretty uniform: learning names, telephone numbers, and the multiplication table, and recalling for the final exam the dates of historical events one could do without. Memory is also among the most heavily studied aspects of the mind. In a typical memory study a subject is asked to memorize a list of words or a series of pictures of faces, and then to recall or recognize the material under various conditions.

Unfortunately, both the general-public preconceptions about memory and the traditional ways of conducting memory research have very little to do with the way memory operates in real life. In a typical study of memory, a subject is asked to memorize information and then recall it. The subject memorizes certain information because the examiner instructs the subject to do so. Memorization and recall are the end unto themselves, and the decision about what to recall rests with the examiner, not with the subject.

In most real-life situations we store and recall information not for the sake of recall itself but as a prerequisite for solving a problem at hand. Here recall is a means to an end, not the end. Furthermore, certain memories are accessed and retrieved not in response to an external command coming from someone else but in response to an internally generated need. Instead of being told what to recall, I have to decide which information is useful to me in the context of my ongoing activities at the moment.

All of us know all kinds of things. I know the location of barbershops on the West Side of Manhattan, the names of major Russian composers, the multiplication table, the main airports in Australia, the ages of my distant cousins, and on and on. How is it, then, that as I am sitting in front of my computer writing this book, I promptly access my knowledge about the frontal lobes and write about them, and not about the French Revolution or my favorite restaurants in New York? Furthermore, how is it that, having developed an appetite after a few hours of strenuous typing, I equally promptly access my knowledge of neighborhood restaurants instead of that about the frontal lobes, this transition being seamless and instantaneous?

Most real-life acts of memory recall involve deciding what type of information is useful to us at the moment, and then selecting this information out of the huge totality of all the knowledge available. Furthermore, as the nature of our activities changes, we make a smooth, instantaneous switch from one selection to another, and then do this again and again. We make such decisions, selections, and transitions virtually every moment of our waking lives, most of the time automatically and effortlessly. But given the total amount of diverse information available to us at any given time, these decisions are anything but trivial. They require intricate neural computations, which are carried out by the frontal lobes. Memory based on such ever-changing, fluid decision making, selection, and switches is guided by the frontal lobes and is called *working memory*. At every point of the process we need to access a particular type of information that represents but a tiny fraction of our total knowledge. Our ability to access it is like an instantaneous finding of a needle in a haystack—it is nothing short of astounding.

Therein lies a crucial difference between a typical memory experiment and the way memory is used in real life. In real life, I have to make the decision what to remember. In a typical memory experiment the decision is made for me by the examiner: "Listen to these words and remember them." By shifting the decision-making process from the individual to the examiner, we remove the role of the frontal lobes and the memory task is no longer a working memory task. Most real-life acts of recall involve working memory and the frontal lobes, but most procedures used in memory research and to examine patients with memory disorders do not.

The disparity between the way memory is used in real life and the way it is studied in the laboratory helps explain the confusion about the role of the frontal lobes in memory. An inconclusive debate on the subject has been going on for years, since the subject was first raised by Jacobsen[8] and Luria.[9] Recently, in large measure due to the work of the neuroscientists Patricia Goldman-Rakic[10] and Joaquin Fuster,[11] the role of the frontal lobes in memory has been reasserted and the concept of working memory has gained prominence. Much has been written on the subject of working memory over the last few years. A book by the Swedish cognitive neuroscientist Torkel Klingberg, *The Overflowing Brain*,[12] stands out as a particularly lucid rendition of the subject. Working memory is closely linked to the critical role that the frontal lobes play in the temporal organization of behavior and in controlling the proper sequence in which various mental operations are enacted to meet the organism's objective.[13] Pharmacological disruption of the prefrontal cortex results in working memory impairment,[14] particularly when D1 or D2 receptors are affected.[15] Today the concept of working memory is among the trendiest in cognitive neuroscience. As is the case with trendy concepts, it is often used arbitrarily and loosely, at times being rendered meaningless. This is why it is particularly important to discuss this concept carefully and rigorously. It is often said that "working memory is like short-term memory." Well, if it is so much like short-term memory, then why do we need a new term? Creating duplicate terminology without new meaning obfuscates things rather than clarifying them.

Somewhat in the minority among fellow neuroscientists, I define working memory as *the selection of task-relevant information.* To fully appreciate the centrality of the selection process to working memory, it is important to remember that the first evidence of the role of the frontal lobes in memory came from animal experiments. It was precisely that aspect of memory which appeared to depend on the frontal lobes that was termed working memory. At the time, human research did not support the role of the frontal lobes in memory—hippocampi, diencephalon, yes, but not the frontal lobes. What was the reason for this chasm between animal and human memory research?

To answer this question, put yourself first in the position of a researcher designing an animal experiment, and then in the position of an experimental rat, or a monkey. To the experimenter the task is to memorize a maze, or a sequence of alternating responses; it is a memory task. But the rat or the monkey doesn't care about the experiment's objective as seen through the eyes of the researcher. To the experimental animal the task is to get the bait by whatever means it takes; it is a foraging task. The animal then discovers that in order to get the bait, it has to remember the maze rather than the color of the experimenter's eyes or the brilliance of his or her smile. More than anything else, it is this act of selection of task-appropriate information that draws the frontal lobes into the process, and this is the essence of working memory.

The selection aspect is absent in most memory paradigms used in human research—subjects are explicitly told what it is that they need to memorize, which is both antithetical to the assessment of working memory and unrealistic in terms of everyday uses of memory. As discussed earlier, this is precisely what accounts for the disparity between human and animal literature on the role of the frontal lobes in memory. When a selection requirement is incorporated into a memory task, the prefrontal cortex becomes engaged, as the functional magnetic resonance imaging (fMRI) study by Rowe and colleagues from the Wellcome Department of Cognitive Neurology of London's Institute of Neurology has shown.[16] Likewise, prefrontal (dorsolateral, ventrolateral, and anterior cingulate) activation decreases as the forgetting of memories selected for their "unworthiness to be remembered" takes place. Suppression of memories represents the ultimate form of "negative" selectivity of long-term storage.[17] Depue and colleagues at the University of Colorado have demonstrated a combined involvement of the right inferior, right medial frontal gyri, and frontopolar regions in memory suppression.[18]

To the extent that a selection component is present in a neuropsychological memory test, the test can be shown to engage the frontal lobes. This is precisely what makes The California Verbal Learning Test (CVLT)[19] such a good test of verbal memory. It is up to the subject to discover (or fail to discover) and then to choose to use (or fail to choose) the tacit option of semantic clustering that facilitates recall. This tacit option introduces a genuine element of selection, which in turn engages the frontal lobes, as the work of Monti Buchsbaum and colleagues using PET has shown.[20] I would imagine that the extent of frontal activation on the CVLT is directly proportionate to the extent to which the subject relies on semantic clustering while performing the task. Unfortunately, very few of the procedures touted in neuropsychological test catalogues as tests of working memory have a strong selection component, and one can only hope that this admonition will get the attention of the editors from Psychological Corporation, Psychological Assessment Resources, and other major test publishers. What we really need is a new generation of memory tests with an explicit selection component. They will be the real "working memory tests."

Since the selection of the information required to solve the problem at hand is made in the frontal lobes, they must "know," at least roughly, where in the brain this information is stored. This requirement suggests that all the cortical regions are somehow represented in the frontal lobes, an assertion first made by Hughlings Jackson at the end of the nineteenth century.[21] Such representation is probably coarse, rather than specific, enabling the frontal lobes to know what type of information is stored where, but not the specific information itself. The frontal lobes then contact the appropriate parts of the brain and bring the memory (or, as scientists say, the "engram") "on-line," by activating the circuitry that embodies the engram. The analogy between the frontal lobes and the corporate chief executive officer comes in handy again. Having signed a new contract, the CEO may have none of the technical skills required to do the project, but he or she knows who on the staff does, and the CEO has the ability to correctly select the employees for the project on the basis of their particular expertise.

Since different stages of solving a problem may require different types of information, the frontal lobes must constantly, and rapidly, bring new engrams on-line, while letting go of the old ones. Furthermore, we must often make rapid transitions from one cognitive task to another. To make things even more challenging, we frequently deal with several problems in parallel. This activity highlights a very peculiar feature of working memory: its constantly and rapidly changing content. Imagine that you have five bank accounts with activities (deposits and withdrawals) taking place simultaneously and frequently. Imagine further that you have to keep track of the five balances in your head, without the benefit of a notebook or a computer, in order to run your business. Instead of memorizing a body of static information, you must be able to rapidly update the content of your memory all the time.

The five-account banking situation sounds pretty fantastic. But how different is it from the challenge facing a corporate executive, entrepreneur, mutual fund manager, or political or military leader who must monitor and act on a number of situations rapidly unfolding in parallel? Imagine a juggler with five balls in the air who has to keep track of all five balls constantly in motion. Now imagine mental juggling, which is what running a corporation, a business, or a scientific lab amounts to. This is analogous to what working memory does. With malfunctioning working memory, all the balls will soon be on the ground.

To return to the corporate executive, suppose this person needs to assemble a team of experts for a complex, long-term project with unforeseeable contingencies. At every stage of the project he or she must identify the required expertise; decide how to locate the experts' names; actually find them; remember their names and telephone numbers or know how to access them at least for the duration of the project; identify the needs dictated by the next stage of the project; and so on. Imagine, further, that at every stage of the project the CEO needs more than one type of expert, so that several parallel searches take place. This would be a reasonably accurate description of working memory. Working memory is very different from the activities we traditionally associate with the word *memory*— learning a fixed body of information and hanging on to it.

But the role of working memory is not restricted to large-scale decision making. We depend on working memory even in the most mundane situations. In your memory you have the telephone numbers of your favorite restaurant and of your dentist. You know where you keep your shoes and your vacuum cleaner. Even though this information is in your memory at all times, it is not the focus of your attention all the time. When you need to entertain your friends, you call your restaurant and not your dentist. When you are getting dressed in the morning, you go to the closet containing the shoes and not to the closet containing the vacuum cleaner. These seemingly trivial and effortless decisions also require working memory.

We have the ability to bring task-relevant information into focus as needed and then go on to the next bit of relevant information. The selection of task-appropriate information occurs automatically and effortlessly, and the smoothness of this selection is ensured by the frontal lobes. But patients at early stages of dementia often report "inane" actions. They may take dirty dishes to the bedroom instead of the kitchen, or open the refrigerator looking for gloves. This is an early breakdown of the frontal lobes' ability to select and bring on-line task-appropriate information. Working memory frequently suffers in early dementias. People with severely impaired working memory will rapidly find themselves in a state of hopeless confusion.

The paradox of working memory is that even though the frontal lobes are critical for accessing and activating task-relevant information, they do not themselves contain this information—other parts of the brain do. To demonstrate this relationship, Patricia Goldman-Rakic and her colleagues at Yale studied delayed responses in the monkey.[22] They recorded neurons in the monkey frontal lobes, which fire as long as an engram (memory trace) must be "held on" to but stop firing once the response has been initiated. These neurons are involved in keeping the engram on-line, but not in the storage of the engram.

Different parts of the prefrontal cortex are involved in different aspects of working memory, and a peculiar parallelism exists between the functional organization of the frontal lobes and the posterior cortical regions. It has been known for years that the primate (including human) visual system consists of two distinct components. The "what" system, extending along the occipitotemporal gradient, processes information about object identity. The "where" system, extending along the occipitoparietal gradient, processes information about object location. Presumably, visual spatial knowledge is also distributed. The memories for "what" are formed within the occipitotemporal system, and the memories for "where" are within the occipitoparietal system.

Is *access* to these two types of visual memory controlled by the same frontal regions or by different ones? Susan Courtney and her colleagues at the National Institute of Mental Health answered the question in a PET experiment with an ingenious activation task.[23] A set of faces appeared in a 4 × 6 grid, followed by another set of faces. The subjects were asked to answer the "what" question ("Are the faces the same?") or the "where" question ("Did they appear in the same positions within the grid?"). The two tasks produced two distinct patterns of activation within the frontal lobes, in the inferior portions for "what" and the superior portions for "where." Similar findings were obtained using single-cell recordings in monkeys by Patricia Goldman-Rakic and her colleagues at Yale.[24]

Apparently, different aspects of working memory are under the control of different regions within the frontal lobes. Does this mean that every part of the prefrontal cortex is linked to a particular system outside the frontal lobes? What happened to the conductor at large? Is there a part of the frontal lobes whose contribution is truly integral? We are only beginning to understand the functions of the areas around the frontal poles, the furthest forward extension of the frontal lobe (consisting mostly but not exclusively of Brodmann area 10). I would not be surprised if future research were to show that the areas immediately surrounding the frontal poles serve a particularly synthetic function and superimpose an additional level of neural hierarchy over the dorsolateral and orbitofrontal cortical regions. This assertion is supported by the ingenious studies by Jordan Grafman and his colleagues at the National Institutes of Health,[25] Joshua Hoffman and his colleagues at the University of California,[26] Berkeley, and Koechlin and colleagues,[27] reviewed earlier in Chapter 5. Certain additional aspects of the synthetic functions probably played by this part of the brain are discussed in the next section.

The neural circuitry of working memory is the focus of intense research with both experimental and computational methods.[28] It is aimed at understanding the mechanisms of keeping information "on-line" for the duration of its utility to the task at hand. Both electrophysiological (persistent reverberations within neuronal groupings) and biochemical (calcium-mediated synaptic facilitation) mechanisms have been proposed.[29] These are important and interesting studies. In my opinion, however, they address the second question while ignoring the first one that needs to be answered in order to understand the mechanisms of working memory: How does the organism decide which information is important for solving the task at hand? In most experimental paradigms used to study working memory, both in humans and in animal models, the task is constrained in such a way that the demands on the selection process are negligible. In my opinion, this design removes working memory from the equation, instead of highlighting it, and reduces the frontal lobe participation in the process. Any cogent research into the mechanisms of working memory will have to put the selection process at the front of the line.

Freedom of Choice, Ambiguity, and the Frontal Lobes

Consider the following everyday problems: *(1)* My checking account had a balance of $1000 and I withdrew $300. How much do I have left? *(2)* What shall I put on today: a blue jacket, a black jacket, or a gray jacket? *(3)* What is my dentist's telephone number? *(4)* Shall I go on vacation to the Caribbean, Hawaii, or Greece? *(5)* What is my boss's secretary's name? *(6)* Shall I order lobster fra diavolo, lamb chops, or chicken Kiev for dinner? (My doctor says none of the above.)

Situations 1, 3, and 5 are deterministic. Each of them has a single correct solution intrinsic in the situation, all the other responses being false. By finding the correct solution—the "truth"—I engage in *veridical decision making*. Situations 2, 4, and 6 are inherently ambiguous. Neither has an intrinsically correct solution. I choose the lamb chops not because they are "intrinsically correct" but because I like them. By making my choice, I engage in *adaptive decision making* (my doctor says maladaptive).

In school we are given a problem and must find the correct answer. Only one correct answer usually exists. The answer is hidden. The question is clear-cut.

But most real-life situations, outside of the realm of narrow technical problems, are inherently ambiguous. The answer is hidden, and so is the question. Our purposes in life are general and vague. The "pursuit of happiness" is an amorphous notion meaning different things to different people, or even to the same person under different circumstances. At any given time, each of us must decide what the pursuit of happiness means here and now for me. In her famous retort to the question: "What is the answer?" Gertrude Stein captured this very well: "What is the question?"

We live in an ambiguous world. Aside from high school exams, college tests, and factual and computational trivia, most decisions we make in our everyday lives do not have intrinsically correct solutions. The choices we make are not inherent in the situations at hand. They are a complex interplay between the properties of the situations and our own properties, our aspirations, our doubts, and our histories. It is only logical to expect that the prefrontal cortex is central to such decision making, since it is the only part of the brain where the inputs from within the organism converge with the inputs from the outside world.

Finding solutions for deterministic situations is often accomplished algorithmically. It is increasingly delegated to various devices: calculators, computers, directories of all kinds. But making choices in the absence of inherently correct solutions remains, at least for now, a uniquely human territory. In a sense, freedom of choice is possible only when ambiguity is present.

The absence of absolute algorithmically computable truths is precisely what sets leadership decisions apart from technical decisions. A conductor's or stage director's foremost responsibility is to provide an interpretation of a musical or theatrical piece—an intrinsically subjective proposition. A corporate CEO makes strategic decisions in an ambiguous, fluid environment. Military genius is still regarded as the purview of art more than science.

Resolving ambiguity, or "disambiguating the situation" in scientific parlance, often means choosing the question first, that is, reducing the situation to a question that has a single correct answer. In choosing the clothes to wear, there are many questions I may decide to ask: *(1)* Which jacket best matches the weather? (and choose the warmest jacket); *(2)* Which one is more fashionable? (and choose the newest jacket); *(3)* Which one is my favorite? (and choose the gray jacket). Precisely how I disambiguate the situation depends on my priorities at the moment, which themselves may change depending on the context. An inability to reduce ambiguity leads to vacillating, uncertain, inconsistent behavior. One is reminded of Buridan's jackass, standing in front of two haystacks and starving, unable to choose. Even the ancient Romans understood the perils of persistent ambiguity and coined the saying "dura lex sed lex" ("hard law is better than no law").

At the same time, an individual must have the flexibility to adopt different perspectives on the same situation at different times. The organism must be able to disambiguate the same situation in multiple ways and have the capacity to switch between them at will. Dealing with inherent ambiguity is among the foremost functions of the frontal lobes. In a sense, whether you are decisive or wishy-washy depends on how well your frontal lobes work. Studies have shown that patients with frontal lobe damage approach inherently ambiguous situations differently from the way healthy people do. The loss of the ability to make decisions is among the most common signs of early dementia. Damage to other parts of the brain does not seem to affect these processes.

In a nutshell, veridical decisions deal with "finding the truth," and adaptive, actor-centered decisions involve choosing "what is good for me." Most "executive leadership" decisions are priority based, made in ambiguous environments, and adaptive, rather than veridical, in nature. The cognitive processes involved in resolving ambiguous situations through priorities are very different from those involved in solving strictly deterministic situations. Ironically, cognitive ambiguity and priority-based decision making have been all but ignored in cognitive neuropsychology. This is not to say that other branches of psychology have ignored them. Projective tests like the Rorschach Inkblots have always been accorded a respected role in the psychodynamic tradition. But in its quest for precision and measurement, cognitive science has rejected such procedures as too vague, too subjective. Yet the lack of satisfactory scientific methods does not change the fact that priority-based, adaptive decision-making in ambiguous situations is central to our lives, and that the frontal lobes are particularly important in such decision making. So rather than brushing the problem aside as "unworthy," the appropriate scientific methods must be found.

With my former graduate student Ken Podell, I tried to remedy the shortcoming with a simple experiment, using an original procedure called the Cognitive Bias Task (CBT).[30] Subjects were shown a geometric design (target), then two other designs appeared (choices), and were asked to "look at the target and select the choice you like the most." (The CBT card is shown in Fig. 7.3.) We made it clear to subjects that there were no intrinsically correct or incorrect responses, and that the choice was up to them. The experiment consisted of a large number of such trials, no two of them being completely identical.

So the subjects were encouraged to do what they pleased. In reality, however, the designs were arranged in such a way that the subjects had two options: to base their response on either the properties of the targets (which changed from trial to trial) or some stable preference unrelated to the target (e.g., favorite color or shape). As is often the case in life, "freedom of choice" was an illusion and the subjects' responses were tacitly constrained by the experimental design. Despite the seemingly loose nature of our experiment, the subjects' responses could be clearly quantified and were highly replicable. Our cognitive projective paradigm proved to be very informative, and we will return to it in several parts of this book.

We conducted our experiment with healthy individuals and with patients with various types of brain damage. Damage to the frontal lobes dramatically changed the nature of responses. Damage to other parts of the brain had very little or

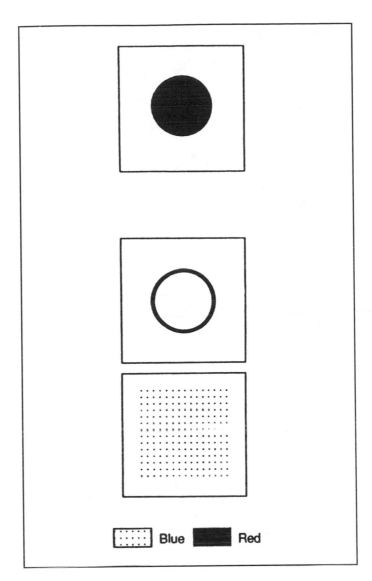

Figure 7.3 The Cognitive Bias Task (CBT). In the actor-centered condition of CBT a subject is asked to look at the top form and then choose one of the two bottom forms that he or she likes most. In the veridical conditions of CBT the subject is asked to look at the top form and then choose the bottom form more similar to it (or more different from it). Unbeknownst to the subject, one of the two bottom choices is always more similar to the target than the other one. [After Goldberg et al. (1994).[30] Copyright 1994 by Massachusetts Institute of Technology. Reprinted with permission.]

no effect. We repeated the experiment, but this time disambiguated the task in two different ways. Instead of instructing the subjects to "make the choice you like the best," we asked them to "make the choice most similar to the target," and then to do it again, this time making the choice "most different from the target." In disambiguated conditions the effects of frontal lesions disappeared and the subjects with brain lesions were able to perform the task as well as the healthy controls (see Fig. 7.4).

The effect can also be demonstrated in normal subjects through fMRI. In an experiment conducted in collaboration with Kai Vogeley and his colleagues, prefrontal activation was evident in the actor-centered CBT condition, but it disappeared in the veridical CBT condition[31] (see Fig. 7.5).

Our experiments show that the frontal lobes are critical in a free-choice situation, when *it is up to the subject to decide how to interpret an ambiguous situation.* Once the situation has been disambiguated for the subject and the task has been reduced to the computation of the only correct response possible, the input of the frontal lobes is no longer critical, even though all the other aspects of the task remain the same. Bijan Pesaran and colleagues from New York University have demonstrated that an interaction between the monkey's frontal cortex and the posterior cortical regions is particularly great during free-choice behavior compared to that in an instruction-driven behavior.[32] So the role of the frontal lobes in guiding inherently ambiguous, preference-based behaviors is not unique to humans; it appears to be critical across a range of simian species.

Of all the aspects of the human mind, none are more intriguing than intentionality, volition, and free will. These attributes of the human mind are fully at play, however, only in situations affording multiple choices. We humans tend to claim the mental abilities that we perceive as the most advanced to be uniquely ours. Numerous assertions have been made by philosophers and scientists that volition and intentionality are uniquely human traits. In its absolute form, this claim cannot appeal to a rigorous neurobiologist. It is more likely that these properties of the mind have developed gradually through evolution, possibly following an exponential course. Indeed, it has been shown by Justin Wood and colleagues that the perception of intentionality is possible already in various nonhuman primate species. Interestingly, this ability appears to be more developed in chimpanzees and old-world rhesus macaque monkeys, and less developed in the more primitive new-world tamarin monkeys.[33] Without claiming any scientific rigor, I believe that my bullmastiff dog Brit is also capable of perceiving intentionality to a modest degree. On the other hand, neither chimpanzees nor orangutans approach 2.5-year-old human children in their performance on tests of social cognition, even though they can match them on tests dealing with the physical world.[34] An argument can be made that development of the ability to perceive intentionality, and particularly social cognition, parallels development of the frontal lobes. Just to belabor the canine theme in a comparative-neurobiological context, a study of

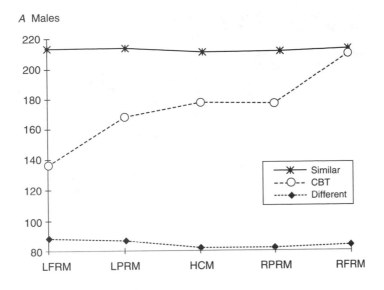

A Males

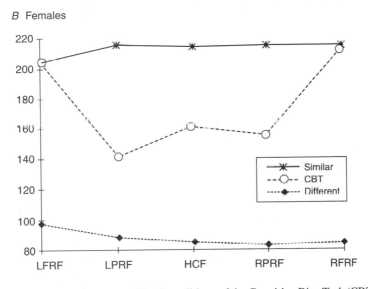

B Females

Figure 7.4 Actor-centered versus veridical conditions of the Cognitive Bias Task (CBT). In the actor-centered condition, frontal lesions produce dramatic changes in performance on CBT. The effects of lesions disappear in the two veridical conditions of CBT. This is true both for right-handed males (A) and for right-handed females (B). Key: LFRM, left-frontal male lesion group; LPRM, left-posterior male lesion group; HCM, healthy control male group; RPRM, right-posterior male lesion group; RFRM, right-frontal male lesion group; LFRF, left-frontal female lesion group; LPRF, left-posterior female lesion group; HCF, healthy control female group; RPRF, right-posterior female lesion group; RFRF, right-frontal female lesion group. [After Goldberg et al. (1994).[30] Copyright 1994 by Massachusetts Institute of technology. Reprinted with permission.]

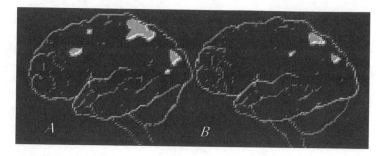

Figure 7.5 Brain activation in actor-centered (*A*) and veridical (*B*) tasks on fMRI. (*A*) Choosing geometric forms on the basis of preference results in combined prefrontal and occipitoparietal activation. (*B*) Choosing geometric forms on the basis of perceptual mismatch produces only occipitoparietal activation whereas prefrontal activation disappears. [Adapted with permission from Vogeley et al. (2003).][31]

spotted hyenas revealed their particularly social nature. It also turns out that they possess the largest frontal lobes among all (four of) the hyena species.[35]

Cognitive neuroscientists are not the only ones who ignore actor-centered, adaptive decision-making at their peril. Far worse, actor-centered decision making has also been ignored by educators. Our entire educational system is based on teaching veridical decision making. This is true not just in the United States but everywhere, at least within the Western cultural tradition. Strategies of actor-centered, adaptive decision-making are simply not taught. Instead, they are acquired by each individual idiosyncratically, as a personal cognitive discovery, through trial and error. Designing ways of explicitly teaching the principles of actor-centered problem solving is among the most worthy challenges for educators and school psychologists. Developmental psychology also focuses on veridical decision making; the chronology and staging of actor-centered adaptive decision making are virtually unknown.

We do know, however, that adaptive decision-making declines before veridical decision-making at early stages of dementia. My former postdoctoral student Allan Kluger and I conducted a study at the Millhauser Dementia Research Center of New York University School of Medicine.[36] We compared the decline of perfor-mance on the Cognitive Bias Task and on its disambiguated, veridical analogue in patients at different stages of Alzheimer's-type dementia. Performance on the actor-centered, preference-based version of the task declined much earlier in the disease process than did performance on the veridical, "match-to-similarity" version. This is reflected in Figures 7.6A and 7.6B.

This finding is important in more ways than one. It challenges the prevailing notion that the frontal lobes are relatively invulnerable in Alzheimer's-type dementia. Most research suggests that Alzheimer's disease affects particularly the hippocam-pus and the neocortex.[37] Traditionally it has been assumed that at the neocortical

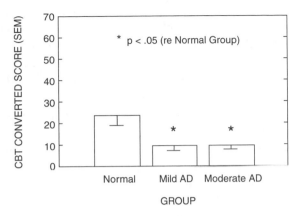

A   PERFORMANCE LEVEL ON THE COGNITIVE BIAS TASK (CBT)

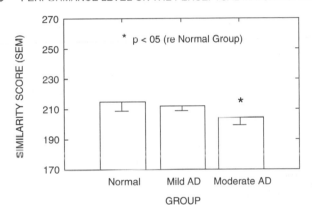

B   PERFORMANCE LEVEL ON THE PERCEPTUAL MATCHING TASK

Figure 7.6 Actor-centered versus veridical decision-making decline in dementia of Alzheimer's type (AD). Actor-centered decision-making declines already at an earlier stage of disease process (*A*). Veridical decision making begins to decline only at a later stage (*B*). [After Goldberg et al. (1997).[36]]

level the parietal lobes are especially vulnerable in Alzheimer's disease, and the frontal lobes less so. This well-entrenched assumption is probably a misconception caused by the systematic failure to recognize early cognitive symptoms of frontal lobe dysfunction as early signs of dementia. In fact, if you listen carefully to dementia patients and their family members, it becomes obvious that indecision, hesitation, and an increasing reliance on others for making choices are easily as common as memory impairment or word-finding difficulties at early stages of cognitive decline in the elderly. Unfortunately, the breakdown in actor-centered decision making is often misdiagnosed as depression or something else, often remaining completely unrecognized as a clinically significant symptom, an early symptom of frontal lobe dysfunction. This is likely to result in a systematic sampling bias in the selection of brains for the brain banks serving as the databases for neuropatological studies, which in turn results in lopsided conclusions regarding the relative vulnerability of various brain structures to disease.

The search for highly sensitive cognitive signs of early dementia is a major challenge for clinicians, dementia researchers, and pharmaceutical companies. With the advent of new drugs for the treatment of dementia, a welcome and increasingly realistic prospect, it will become particularly important to have sensitive cognitive tools to measure the therapeutic effects of the new "cognotropic" drugs. The exceptional vulnerability of actor-centered decision making in brain disease offers an innovative strategy for developing cognitive markers of very early stages of dementia and highly sensitive tools for the assessment of cognotropic drug effects.

The simultaneous breakdown of actor-centered decision making along with the sparing of veridical decision making has been documented in other disorders as well. Using the Cognitive Bias Task and The Iowa Gambling Test, Antonio Verdejo and his colleagues demonstrated this combination in a group of substance abusers in a large-scale study conducted in Spain.[38] So the superior diagnostic utility of actor-centered tasks is evident across several clinical populations.

In my book *The Wisdom Paradox*[39] I refer to veridical cognition as *descriptive* and to actor-centered cognition as *prescriptive*. I believe this to be a very important distinction, easily on a par with the distinction between semantic and episodic knowledge, or procedural and declarative knowledge. To the extent that complex cognitive constructs can be mapped on neuroanatomical structure, descriptive cognition relies mostly on the posterior parts of the hemispheres and prescriptive cognition relies mostly on the frontal lobes (see Fig. 7.7). In order to fully understand the functions of the frontal lobes, a new generation of cognitive paradigms must be created, designed to investigate nonveridical prescriptive cognition. Such paradigms are increasingly used in cognitive neuroscience research, but they have yet to percolate into the world of diagnostic neuropsychological tests.

The difference between descriptive and prescriptive cognition and their respective links to the posterior or frontal cortex finds an interesting parallel in

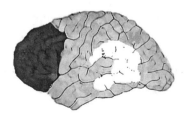

Figure 7.7 Cortical territory of actor-centered (prescriptive) cognition—dark shading. Cortical territory of veridical (descriptive) cognition—light shading.

computational neuroscience. In an attempt to capture the differences between the frontal lobes and posterior cortex in neural-net models, Randall O'Reilly has proposed that the prefrontal cortex has certain features of digital computation, whereas the posterior cortex has certain features of analogue computation.[40] He has also proposed that the posterior cortex operates mostly on the basis of Hebbian learning (driven by the features of the outside world), whereas the frontal lobes operate mostly on the basis of backprop-like mechanisms (driven by the internal representation of a goal).[41] It is unclear how far and how literally this analogy can be taken, but it is certainly an appealing metaphor and perhaps even a useful heuristic. Hebbian associative learning is driven by the properties of the environment surrounding the learner and it captures the properties of the world as it presents itself to the person. By contrast, back-propagation learning is driven by a task and an active process.

The issue of actor-centered decision making is closely linked to the issue of intentionality. The body of rigorous neuroscientific work on intentionality still remains sparse. Among the recent studies, an experiment by Haqwan Lau and his colleagues stands out.[42] They attempted to capture the dynamic neuroanatomy of bringing intention into conscious focus (paying "attention to intention") in an fMRI study of voluntary action. Because of the specific nature of the action (hand movement), the supplementary and parietal regions were unsurprisingly activated. But in addition to this, there was also activation of the right dorsal prefrontal region. It would be particularly interesting to find out whether the prefrontal activation would be present across different tasks involving intentionality, thus representing an invariant component linked to intentionality itself rather than to specific task demands. It would also be interesting to see if its lateralization to the right hemisphere is invariant across time, or whether it is a function of task familiarity and would eventually shift to the left.

At the time of this writing, the concept of working memory has been embraced by most cognitive neuroscientists as key to the understanding of frontal lobe function. But considered in isolation from actor-centered decision making and other issues discussed in this chapter, the cognitive definition of working memory has proved to be disquietingly opaque. Some researchers try to circumvent this opaqueness by defining working memory as that form of memory that depends on the frontal lobes. But this is circular logic. Many aspects of cognition depend on the frontal lobes. Unless you have a definition of working memory that is independent of neuroanatomy, how do you know which of the frontal lobe–dependent mental operations is "working memory"?

In clinical neurosciences there is growing appreciation of the centrality of executive deficit in a wide range of disorders, including dementias, traumatic brain injury, and others. Consequently, there has been more interest in developing intervention tools (in the forms of cognitive-exercise software and pharmacology) to address the issue. But to treat a disorder one needs to know exactly which variable is to be measured and affected. Contrary to what research literature on the executive functions would lead one to believe, anyone working with brain-damaged patients who are suffering from an "executive deficit" knows that the main problem facing these patients is not "working memory" in its standard opaque definition, but poor judgment and decision making in underconstrained situations. It is not commonly evaluated in clinical practice or measured in clinical research, not because it is deemed unimportant but because we simply do not have sound instruments to accomplish this goal.

I strongly believe that clinically meaningful effectiveness of any diagnosis of or therapies for executive deficit will depend overwhelmingly on the ability to document and impact patients' capacity for sound actor-centered decision making. For this to happen, neuropsychology will have to come up with rigorous ways of measuring such capacities. Until this happen we will continue to bark up the wrong tree in our attempts to both help our patients and understand the underlying basic neurocognitive processes.

As already discussed, frontal lobe damage is particularly likely to affect prescriptive decision making. The disparity between the relatively spared perfunctory, rhetorical knowledge of the expected behavior and the severely impaired ability to parlay this knowledge into actual behavior is quite common in patients with frontal lobe damage regardless of its etiology. Alexandr Luria is credited with introducing simple bedside procedures for eliciting this disparity in patients: the patient is asked to do the opposite of what you are doing: "When I raise my finger please raise your fist; and when I raise my fist please raise your finger." It is not uncommon for a "frontal" patient to lapse into imitative echopractic behavior while reciting the correct instruction all the while. These procedures have been formalized in *The Executive Control Battery*,[43] which we designed and published a number of years ago. It is precisely this disparity between perfunctory knowledge and the ability to guide behavior by such knowledge that limits the utility of the hypothetical "moral dilemma" scenarios in studying meta-cognition in patients with frontal lobe dysfunction. While very few standard clinical diagnostic procedures exist designed to examine the relationship between knowledge and action, every seasoned clinician knows that the capacity of self-initiated choice making is particularly fragile in a wide range of conditions including dementias.

Further understanding and appreciation of the difference between descriptive and prescriptive cognition have far-reaching societal implications above and beyond the narrowly defined clinical neuropsychology. The legal ramifications of this distinction were recognized in the 2002 opinion of the U.S. Supreme Court regarding capital punishment for the mentally retarded.[44] Ruling against such punishment reflected the High Court's recognition of the fact that a cognitively impaired individual may have the necessary perfunctory knowledge of what constitutes socially acceptable behavior, yet may lack the ability to parlay this knowledge into actual behavior.

Neuroeverything

Whereas clinical neuropsychology has been remiss in developing cogent tools for assessing decision making in ambiguous situations, we have witnessed a surge of interest in such processes in a range of new applications of cognitive neuroscience.

Sometime in the mid-1980s I used the then freshly minted term *cognitive neuroscience* in the company of respectable molecular neuroscientists, which triggered a barrage of dismissive looks and disparaging grunts. Today, of course, cognitive neuroscience is all the rage and nobody questions the legitimacy of this designation. Well past that point, we are witnessing the advent of new terminology that even a decade ago would have struck the reader as outlandish: social neuroscience, neuroeconomics, neuromarketing, neuroethics, neurolaw, and even neuropolitics. Each of these terms reflects a growing confidence that the field is ready to proceed with a rigorous examination of the biological mechanisms of complex decision-making inherent in various social, economic, and political situations. Even morality and ethical behavior have become the subjects of neurobiological exploration, which we will address in some detail in Chapter 11.

Neuroeconomics and social neuroscience in particular are developing so rapidly that doing them justice would require separate books. In fact, such books exist, notably *Decisions, Uncertainty, and the Brain*, by Paul Glimcher.[45] At the time of this writing, several laboratories have been especially prolific in researching these topics, notably those at New York University and Princeton University. Most of the research in these new areas of inquiry involves experimental methods, particularly functional neuroimaging. Analytic, modeling, and computer simulation methods have also been used.[46]

What sets these new applications apart from the more traditional areas of cognitive neuroscience is the focus on the decision making and action selection in underconstrained, ambiguous situations and on the mechanisms of making decisions guided to a large extent by subjective choices rather than by transparent true–false criteria. These researchers are concerned with an agenda broadly similar to the one I have been trying to inject into the assessment of patients with frontal lobe dysfunction and other forms of brain damage. Most of these fledgling extensions of cognitive neuroscience implicate the prefrontal cortex and related structures of the anterior cingulate cortex and the striatum, which is why I felt that at least a cursory mention of these assorted "neuro's" belongs in the book.

One should think of these new areas of study as applications, because the basic mechanisms of decision making deployed by the brain in the economic, moral, or legal contexts under study are the same ones that operate in other cognitive contexts. There are no thematically specialized modules with distinct neuroanatomic characteristics in the brain. For instance, there is no reason to believe that the decision-making processes underlying marketplace interactions are mediated by a special-purpose neural circuitry that is separate from the circuitry involved in various other forms of "executive" decision making. "Neuroeconomics" and other recent-coinage "neuro's" are justified mostly as areas of application but not as areas of inquiry into the fundamental aspects of brain function. While neuroscientists and neuropsychologists understand this very well, the general public, deluged by popular media accounts about "specific brain centers lighting up" when a subject in an MRI scanner is told to think about money, love, or the next political elections, may not.

Thus I learned from CNN (on March 21, 2008)[47] that people generous in giving had their striatum (reported as "stiratum") light up in a neuroimaging study; this is so because the striatum is the "happiness center" of the brain. "To give or not to give" is, of course, a decision shrouded in ambiguity in a number of contexts, but it is precisely this kind of "neurophrenology" that compelled an acquaintance of mine, a highly intelligent man and a generous philanthropist with a long-standing history of supporting neuroscience, to stop giving money to the field. Presumably, fed up with this kind of opportunistic but cute and media-genic sound bite, his striatum went blank, at least as far as brain research is concerned, and I am now in the process of trying to convince him that not all neuroscience is that shallow.

The truly unfortunate thing is that the advent of functional neuroimaging has spawned a whole wave of such studies—flashy, engaging, sometimes even dramatic, creating the illusion of clarity, but devoid of theoretical cohesion and, ultimately, relatively useless in advancing our knowledge of the brain or of anything else. Such studies are often even misleading. Unlike the low-tech methods dominating much of twentieth-century psychology, the tools of new-wave neurophrenology are very expensive. Because of their high-tech glitter they create the illusion of understanding where often little or none is gained.

Fortunately, a growing body of serious, principled work in neuroeconomics exists, and more broadly on the subject of decision making in ambiguous environments. There is plenty of genuinely good work under way, which will be the focus of my brief review here.

As stated earlier, studies on the brain mechanisms of decision making in the market place, in neuroeconomics, has stimulated interest in cognitive ambiguity and in decision making that occurs in cognitively ambiguous environments. In such studies, one must pay attention to how the term *cognitive ambiguity* is used, since its use is itself infused with ambiguity. Sometimes it is used in reference to conflicting situations, for example, when the correct choice of action is opposite to the most habitual action and thus requires the overcoming of a cognitive "knee-jerk" response, as in the Stroop Test. On other occasions *cognitive ambiguity* refers to probabilistic environments. Sometimes it refers to situations in which critical information about the environment is unavailable to the subject. But most of these definitions still imply the existence of one "objectively" correct choice, albeit a hidden one. By contrast, when I use the term *cognitive ambiguity* I am likely to refer to choices based on truly subjective preference rather than on the uncovering of hidden truths ("Shall I order steak or fish?" as opposed to "Which action is likely to bring the greatest monetary reward?") So in reading scientific reports it is important to begin by "disambiguating the ambiguity" by grasping exactly which aspect of cognitive ambiguity is being studied.

As we already know, the prefrontal cortex consists of several neuroanatomically distinct regions. Two such regions have been closely linked to intentionality in ambiguous situations: dorsolateral prefrontal cortex (DLPF) and the anterior cingulate cortex (ACC). These two regions are closely interconnected neuroanatomically and functionally, as revealed by a variety of mapping techniques. They also exhibit a remarkable pattern of co-activation, revealed by neuroimaging techniques such as PET, which may be a result of direct pathway connectivity between the DLPF and ACC, or of both structures receiving projections from the ventral tegmental area via the mesocortical dopamine pathway. The ACC has been implicated in conflict resolution;[48] in error monitoring, in which the prediction of action is compared with its outcome; in assessing error likelihood in a given context;[49] in resolving cognitive ambiguity;[50] and in assessing task difficulty due to lack of familiarity.[51] Still, the exact role of ACC remains somewhat obscure, as is the division of labor between ACC and the DLPF in conflict resolution and adjustment.[52]

This is not to detract from the diverse and on the whole very interesting neuroimaging studies of ACC. But most of these studies, while attempting to investigate the role of ACC and the DLPF in conflict resolution or conflict monitoring, still employ veridical paradigms like the Flanker test (indicating the direction of an arrow often in conflict with the surrounding error direction)[53] or the Stroop Test (naming print color conflicting with color name),[54] both of which have intrinsically correct and intrinsically false choices. As is the case with the prefrontal cortex, it will remain impossible to understand the functions of the anterior cingulate cortex as long as we cling to the cognitive probes based on the veridical paradigms. I strongly believe that our understanding of the role of the anterior cingulate cortex in human cognition will be greatly enhanced by the introduction of a new generation of cognitive and neuropsychological paradigms based on the actor-centered principle. Until this happens, our attempts to understand the function of the prefrontal cortex and the anterior cingulate cortex will continue to miss the point, at least to a degree. The distinction between cognitive novelty and cognitive familiarity developed earlier in this book may also prove to be central in elucidating the role of the anterior cingulate cortex in assessing task difficulty, in error detection, and in predicting error likelihood in a given cognitive context. This approach implies paying closer attention to the expression of lateralized differences in the anterior cingulate cortex.

The relationship between the prefrontal cortex and the striatum in decision making in probabilistically ambiguous situations has been another focus of interest,[55] as has that in probabilistic situations with critical information missing.[56] Sabrina Tom and her colleagues at the University of California Los Angeles have studied the neural mechanisms of "risk aversion,"[57] a well-known phenomenon in which most people are more sensitive to loss than to gain, so that a disproportionately large gain is required to offset the fear of loss in financial-choice strategies. They found that the prefrontal cortex and striatum are involved in this process. So it appears that these two structures are closely linked across a wide range of situations involving decision making in probabilistically ambiguous situations.

When it comes to truly subjective aspects of quazi-economic decision making, the study by Joseph Kable and Paul Glimcher stands out.[58] They examined the neural mechanisms of assigning subjective value to the delays of monetary rewards. Immediate monetary reward is often perceived by individuals as more "valuable" than a delayed reward of the same monetary quantity. This devaluation is truly subjective, and the curves characterizing the extent of subjective "devaluation" as the function of the delay length is highly idiosyncratic. One might argue that this function can be "objectively" computed by somehow entering into the consideration the interest accrued or the return on investment likely to accumulate over the elapsed delay time, but this is not how people seem to assign this value. Kable and Glimcher have shown that individual subjective value calculation appears to involve three regions: ventral striatum, medial prefrontal cortex, and the posterior cingulate cortex.

Samuel McClure and colleagues have demonstrated the difference between neural substrates mediating decisions concerning immediate vs. delayed monetary rewards. Decisions concerning immediately available monetary rewards activate mostly the brain stem and limbic structures. By contrast, decisions concerning rewards potentially available in the future activate mostly the neocortical structures, particularly the prefrontal cortical regions—both those found on the frontal convexity (dorsolateral and ventrolateral) and the orbitofrontal cortex.[59]

In a somewhat related study, Mathias Pessiglione and colleagues have shown that certain basal forebrain structures, including ventral striatum and the amygdala, are critical for energizing behavior in response to anticipated rewards, even at an unconscious level.[60] Other structures have also been implicated in assigning value to various stimuli. Neurons in the monkey orbitofrontal cortex are particularly likely to fire in response to "valuable" rewards—a banana or an apple. Some of these neurons exhibit sensitivity to relative value: the same neuron may fire more vigorously in response to the more attractive item in a pair, depending on the cognitive context. It will fire more vigorously in response to an apple if it is paired with a piece of lettuce (a relatively less attractive item), but not if it is paired with a banana (a relatively more attractive item).[61]

Since the classic work by Kahnemann and Tversky it has been shown that economic decisions are not made in antiseptically rational, dispassionate ways;[62]

both moral considerations of fairness and emotion play a role. The emotional contribution to decision making can be demonstrated with the so-called framing effect. The same set of conditions can be presented ("framed") in terms of gains or in terms of losses ("You stand to keep 60% of the money" vs. "You stand to lose 40% of the money"). Even though the two statements are equivalent, experiments have shown that they impact economic decision-making in different ways. Interestingly, the "framing" effect was particularly associated with amygdala activity, whereas the frame-independent, "rational" decision-making pattern was associated with activation in the orbitofrontal and anterior cingulate regions.[63] Thus one can surmise that the framing effect is essentially due to the impact of emotions.

The role of moral considerations of fairness was demonstrated by Alan Sanfey and colleagues at Princeton University in a study of the neural mechanisms of decision making in the Ultimatum Game, where one player proposes how to split a sum of money and the other player accepts or rejects the proposal.[64] Unfair offers elicited activity in the dorsolateral prefrontal cortex (particularly on the right side) and the anterior insula, the implication being that both rational and emotional factors played a role.

Interestingly, chimpanzees' behavior in an Ultimatum Game is driven strictly by self-interest in maximizing their own gain; the righteous indignation about other players' unfairness does not seem to play a role in their decision making. Under certain conditions this is also true for humans. Daria Knoch and her colleagues from the University Hospital in Zurich and Harvard Medical School reported that when the right (but not left) dorsolateral prefrontal cortex is temporarily disabled by low-frequency transcranial magnetic stimulation (TMS), subjects lose their capacity for righteous dismay at other players' greed and do what is best for them regardless of the abstract considerations of fairness.[65] This finding is particularly interesting in light of the lateralization of emotions, discussed later in Chapter 8 of this book. The fronto-amygdaloid system in the right hemisphere appears to mediate negative affect, whereas the left fronto-amygdaloid system mediates positive affect. So perhaps temporary disabling of the negative-affect loop with TMS reduces a subject's capacity for dwelling on the situation's downside, and the gleeful anticipation of personal gain takes over.

In "altruistic punishment," the upright members of a group are prepared to punish their social norm-violating peer even if they incur some costs as a result of their actions. Such behavior represents another interesting model of economic decision making colored by emotion. A multidisciplinary team of Swiss scientists led by Dominique de Quervain have demonstrated increased right caudate activation in people experiencing a strong desire to inflict "effective" (economically consequential instead of symbolic) punishment on their transgressing peers.[66]

In a somewhat similar vein, Brooks King-Kasas and colleagues studied reciprocity and mutual trust in two-person simulation of economic exchanges, in which the reciprocity relationship could be "benevolent," "malevolent," or "neutral."[67] Vast regions of the brain were activated in non-neutral situations, including the frontal lobes, the thalamus, and the brain stem, and the head of the caudate nucleus appeared to be critical for "fairness computation" and response selection based on this computation. A complex relationship between perceived fairness in other people, empathy toward them, and desire for revenge in response to perceived unfairness was studied by Tania Singer and colleagues.[68] Fronto-insular and anterior cingulate activation was associated with empathy toward fair players suffering from experimentally inflicted pain. This response was attenuated in males, but not in females, in response to unfair players experiencing pain. In males, but not in females, increased activity in the nucleus accumbens, perhaps reflecting desire for revenge, was associated with the perception of unfair players suffering from pain.

So it appears that quasi-economic decision making involves a complex neural machinery irreducible to a single structure. It is centered on the greater frontal lobes involving various subdivisions of the prefrontal cortex, cingulate cortex, and the basal ganglia, but it also involves the "emotional" structures such as the amygdala. The picture of a vast network of general-purpose structures emerges, each involved in a wide range of other activities, rather than anything approaching dedicated, narrowly specialized circuitry. This conclusion is in keeping with animal studies examining what might be regarded as "proto-economic" decision making. Choice making by *Macaca mulatta* monkeys between different juices involves neuronal firing in the orbitofrontal cortex.[69]

But more important than these neuroanatomic findings, the new field of neuroeconomics has introduced a new generation of inventive, even if at times excessively convoluted, paradigms of much greater complexity than that of the diagnostic tools traditionally used in clinical neuropsychology. Clinical neuropsychologists need to adapt some of the paradigms developed in neuroeconomics and in other explorations of cognitive ambiguity in functional neuroimaging studies of normal subjects as the basis for clinical neuropsychological test design.

8

Emotion and Cognition

The Emotional Frontal Lobes

Rigorous neuroscientific exploration of emotions was slow in coming, but owing to the work by Joseph LeDoux and others we now know that the amygdala plays a critical role in how with think and what we feel.[1] From the work of LeDoux and colleagues we also know that a direct pathway exists between the thalamus and the amygdala, ensuring a preconscious, very rapid, and very coarse emotional appraisal of the environment. Presumably, this phylogenetically old mechanism of emotional appraisal is not just subcortical but also precortical. The thalamo-amygdaloid interface is often thought of as the most rudimentary mechanism of emotions, even though in evolutionary terms it makes sense to think of it as a middling one, the tectal–tegmental interface of the midbrain being the truly most ancient precursor of emotional regulation.

For years, a misconception was prominent, particularly in popular science and among the general public, that rational thought processes are controlled exclusively by the neocortex and emotions, by subcortical structures. But just as the thalamus can be thought of as the evolutionarily early functional antecedent of the posterior cortex, the basal ganglia and the amygdala can be viewed as the functional antecedent of the frontal lobes. In this vein, if the thalamo-amygdaloid interface serves as the phylogenetically old, coarse mechanism of emotion, then a younger interface should also exist that provides the mechanism for more refined and more conscious emotional regulation. This mechanism should be cortico-cortical in nature and involve appraisal by the frontal lobes of the inputs from the posterior cortex.

Our emotional reactions to things are not really part of the veridical account of the world but are about the relationship of these things to us, to our needs, and to our well-being. Emotions do not capture the intrinsic properties of the individuals, objects, or events that trigger them; instead, they instruct us about how to act with respect to these individuals and objects (to approach, to avoid, to fight, to flee), or what to expect from them—good or bad, both being transitive notions. One can think of emotions as pattern recognition, but of a prescriptive, actor-centered pattern recognition rather than a descriptive kind. Emotional reactions to novel situations and things, or to strangers, have the same instantaneous quality as that of our ability to recognize unfamiliar things as members of familiar categories and as meaningful objects.

To extend the analogy, it may be of heuristic value to think of the breakdown of emotional processing as parallel to the associative agnosias discussed earlier in the book. If the ability to recognize new items as members of familiar generic categories (that the item is a table, a chair, or a pen) depends on the association cortex of the posterior parts of the hemispheres (occipital, parietal, and temporal), the ability to recognize new situations as representing familiar threats or rewards depends on the prefrontal cortex. This stands to reason, since we already know that the prefrontal cortex is in charge of actor-centered, prescriptive cognition. Just as damage to the posterior association cortex may result in agnosias, damage to the prefrontal cortex may result in emotional dysregulation.

In retrospect, the notion that the prefrontal cortex plays a role in emotional control should have come as no surprise. The effects of prefrontal lesions on emotional dysregulation were apparent already to early students of the frontal lobes, such as Kurt Goldstein and Alexandr Luria.[2] As we already know, damage to the frontal lobes often produces profound emotional dysregulation: extreme emotional flattening in the dorsolateral frontal syndrome, and extreme emotional disinhibition (sometimes referred to as *Witzelsucht*) in the orbitofrontal syndrome.[3] The similarities between certain frontal lobe syndromes and some aberrant emotional states have been described in numerous sources, including the earlier chapters of this book. These similarities were reflected in the classic neurological nomenclature, where the dorsolateral prefrontal syndrome was commonly referred to as "pseudodepressed." It was understood, however, that the aspontaneity so common in the dorsolateral syndrome was more akin to the lack of affect than to negative affect, and that the disinhibition common in the orbitofrontal (ventromedial) syndrome was more akin to poor impulse control than to euphoria. The emphasis in the classic studies of frontal lobe syndromes was on cognition rather than on affect. Even though these syndromes have been known since the turn of the twentieth century, they were first systematically described by my mentor, Alexandr Luria.[4]

The systematic examination of the role of the frontal lobes in emotional control began much more recently and has blossomed over the last few decades. Nonetheless, to this day, exploration of the frontal lobe's role in cognition and its role in emotions is generally conducted by two different scientific groups, with astoundingly little overlap. Very few attempts have been made to interweave the cognitive and emotional aspects of frontal lobe dysfunction into a coherent narrative, the work by Antonio Damasio representing a notable exception.[5]

Several methodologies have been employed, including studies of the effects of focal lesions in neurological patients, spearheaded by Robert Robinson at the University of Iowa,[6] and electrophysiological and functional neuroimaging studies in normal subjects, led by Richard Davidson at the University of Wisconsin.[7] Their work has helped dispel a second misconception prominent among the general public and pop-science media: that the left hemisphere is the seat of rationality, whereas the right hemisphere is the seat of emotions. With impressive consistency, these studies have demonstrated that not only are the frontal lobes central to emotional control, but their contribution is lateralized. Focal lesions of the left hemisphere tend to produce negative affect, and the strength of this effect is directly proportional to the lesion proximity to the left frontal pole. This finding was confirmed by further studies of depression in traumatic brain injury associated with left dorsolateral frontal and left basal ganglia lesions.[8]

By contrast, lesions of the right hemisphere tend to produce euphoria—the closer to the right frontal pole, the stronger the effect is. Through research conducted over the last few decades, it has become increasingly clear that emotions are complex, multilayered processes under the combined control of subcortical structures, particularly the amygdala, and of the neocortex, particularly the prefrontal cortex. Research has also shown that both the left and the right amygdalae and prefrontal cortices play a role in emotional control. Furthermore, the role played by the left and right amygdalae in emotional control exhibits a certain degree of sexual dimorphism.[9]

Robert Robinson and his colleagues, who studied the effects of stroke on emotional regulation, were probably the first to systematically examine a peculiar division of labor between the left and right prefrontal regions. Left prefrontal stroke often produces a depression-like condition, and right prefrontal stroke produces nonchalance (sometimes referred as *belle indifference*) bordering on euphoria. The affective changes caused by the lateralized stroke can be quite extreme; patients with left-hemispheric stroke can engage in pathological crying and patients with right-hemispheric stroke, in pathological laughter.[10] The often extreme nature of these phenomena makes it highly unlikely that the difference in affective changes, caused by a lateralized stroke, is a mere consequence of different degrees of awareness of deficit (right-hemispheric stroke often causing anosognosia, which is usually less pronounced or entirely absent following a left-hemispheric stroke). This difference in the impact of lateralized lesions on affect clearly suggests that the neocortex plays an important role in emotional regulation, and that the notion of a dispassionate left hemisphere is a fallacy.

Furthermore, the closer the stroke is to one or the other frontal poles along the posterior–anterior axis, the stronger the respective effect. This pattern clearly suggests that the prefrontal cortex plays a particularly critical role in affective regulation. Later, in Chapter 11, we will discuss how patients with ventromedial prefrontal lesions are incapable of using emotional input in moral judgement[11] and how frontal lobotomy results in the elimination, or at least attenuation, of the emotional aspects of physical pain.[12] So it appears that the prefrontal cortex is critical for mediating emotion on several levels: for the experience of emotion, and for the use of emotional information for interpretative purposes in various aspects of cognition, including social cognition.

The role of the frontal lobes in emotions, as well as its lateralized nature, has been further elucidated in functional neuroimaging studies of neurologically intact people. Much of this work was pioneered by Richard Davidson and colleagues. Studies of normal subjects, conducted with EEG and subsequently with PET and fMRI, provided convergent evidence.[13] Presented with pleasant stimuli (e.g., viewing pleasant movie clips), the subjects exhibited left prefrontal activation, but presented with unpleasant or sad stimuli (e.g., sad movie clips), they exhibited right prefrontal activation. Experiments with built-in financial gains or financial losses in a video game resulted in similar findings: left frontal activation was associated with financial gains and right frontal activation with financial losses.

In a study of subjects playing the Ultimatum Game, when one player accepted or rejected the proposal by the other player on how to split a sum of money, the right dorsolateral prefrontal cortex was shown to be active much more in response to unfair than to fair offers,[14] a neural substrate of "moral indignation." As we already know, temporary disabling of the right dorsolateral prefrontal cortex by low-frequency transcranial magnetic stimulation (TMS) leads to a change of subjective "weights" of conflicting motives of personal gain (positive) and recognition of the other player's unfairness (negative) in favor of the former.[15] "Altruistic punishment," which can also be construed as a morally indignant desire to punish a social-norm violator even at a cost to the punisher, is also associated with the punisher's right caudate pattern of activation.

Suppression of memories (presumably because of their negative valence) occurs under the control of the right prefrontal (inferior and medial) cortex[16] or under the dorsolateral prefrontal control bilaterally.[17,18] Interestingly, such prefrontal activation in the suppression of unwanted memories was also associated with modulation of right hippocampal activation, further implicating the right hemisphere in negative affect. Studies of meditation provide a particularly impressive, if somewhat unconventional, source of evidence in the same direction: immersion into states of pleasant, soothing relaxation triggers activation in the left prefrontal cortex and deactivation in the right prefrontal cortex.[19]

By contrast, vicarious experience of pain, which informs our social cognition when we observe another person suffer, is associated with right frontal activation, as demonstrated by Naomi Eisenberger in a study of social exclusion.[20] This study complements Antonio Damasio's findings of the emotional obtuseness that derails social cognition in patients with ventromedial frontal damage when they are faced with hypothetical moral dilemmas.[21] So a robust division of labor is apparently present between the two frontal lobes in the control of affective states across a wide range of contexts: the left prefrontal regions are linked to positive affect, and the right prefrontal regions are linked to negative affect.

A similar dichotomy is evident when the individual differences in emotional traits are examined. According to Davidson and colleagues, patterns of lateralized prefrontal activation provide an interesting basis for the typology of emotional styles. People with an optimistic, sunny disposition consistently exhibit the preponderance of activation in the left prefrontal regions. By contrast, gloomy, habitually dysphoric and brooding types given to depression consistently exhibit a preponderance of activation in the right prefrontal regions.[22] These findings are so stable in given individuals that it is possible to talk about electrophysiological traits corresponding to emotional traits.

The electrophysiological signatures of different emotional styles become apparent already in early infancy. This finding suggests their hereditary basis and perhaps even reflects innate emotional traits: cheerful 10-month olds exhibit the preponderance of left frontal activation, and whining 10 month olds exhibit the preponderance of right frontal activation.[23] Remarkable consistency exists across lesion studies and studies of normal states and of normal traits in both children and adults, all pointing toward a profound and dichotomously specialized role of the frontal lobes in emotional control.

What is the relationship between the prefrontal cortex and the amygdala, the subcortical structure most often implicated in emotional control? The vertical integration across different phylogenetic layers characteristic of most functional systems in the brain appears to be at work as well in the mechanisms of emotions. At a minimum, one must consider a two-by-two circuitry design in trying to map the functional neuroanatomy of emotions: the left and right prefrontal cortex, and the left and right amygdala. In this circuit, the prefrontal cortex, most likely the orbitofrontal cortex, is likely to exert a certain "editorial" function over the amygdala, by modulating, modifying, and even suppressing the outputs from the amygdala.[24] Indeed, Richard Davidson and colleagues have shown that people with a greater baseline prefrontal activity were better able to modulate their emotions in certain experimental situations. Conversely, in people who committed affectively charged, impulsive violent crimes, a reduction of baseline prefrontal metabolism was noted, as well as exaggerated metabolism in several subcortical structures, including the amygdala.[25]

The amygdala has been traditionally associated with negative emotions, fear response, and memory for aversive stimuli; this is particularly true for the lateral amygdala.[26] But recent research suggests that the amygdala is instrumental in mediating a wide range of emotional states, both negative and positive.[27] The amygdalae exhibit functional lateralization that parallels that of the frontal lobes (although for evolutionary reasons it may be more appropriate to reverse the statement).

Like the left prefrontal cortex, the left amygdala is more active in response to pleasant stimuli, but its activity is reduced in depressed states. Furthermore, the ability to suppress negative emotions is associated with greater baseline activation in the left prefrontal regions.[28] Fear-engendering stimuli produce an exaggerated activation in the right amygdala, and damage to the right amygdala leads to an impaired ability to appreciate fear. Findings of brain pathology concur with this pattern. It has been suggested that certain forms of anxiety disorder are associated with an increased activation of the right amygdala, or even with a morphologically abnormally large right amygdala. Criminals who committed affectively charged, impulsive crimes showed exaggerated metabolic activation rates in subcortical structures of the right hemisphere, including the right amygdala.[29] On the other hand, removal of the right amygdala (usually in the context of surgical treatment of temporal-lobe seizure disorder) results in a decreased ability to recognize and appreciate the facial expressions of fear. Interestingly, lateralization of several important neuromodulators was found in anxious rats: greater concentrations of serotonin were found in the right than the left amygdala, as well as (somewhat surprisingly to those who believe in evolutionary continuities) increased concentration of dopamine in the right frontal cortex.[30]

This discussion leads to an intriguing question, although tangential to the main theme of the book. What, if any, relationship exists between the personalities and dominant affective tone of various historical figures (as conveyed in their writings and in accounts provided by their contemporaries) with presumed temporal-lobe seizure disorder and the side of their seizure focus? If several neurohistorical reconstructions are to be believed, both Martin Luther and Joan d'Arc suffered from temporal-lobe seizures. According to most historical accounts, Joan d'Arc's dominant affective state was one of exaltation and bliss. By contrast, Martin Luther is usually described as a brooding and hostile individual. Is it possible that the Maiden of Orleans had her seizure focus close to the left amygdala, and the founder of Protestantism, close to his right amygdala? We will never know, nor will we ever know how the course of civilization would have turned had these and other remarkable historical personalities had the benefit of anticonvulsant pharmacology.

So, a distinct parallel exists between the functional lateralization in the prefrontal cortex and that in the amygdalae, and it is possible to talk about two lateralized, integrated fronto-amygdaloid circuits of emotional control, operating in a synergistic fashion. One can envision two vertically integrated emotional-control circuits: left for positive emotions and right for the negative emotions. In each of these two circuits the amygdala contributes an automatic component not under conscious control, and the prefrontal cortex contributes a more reasoned and consciously controlled "oversight" over our emotional world. In most real-life situations these two levels of control are well integrated and blend into a seamless emotional whole. But these two levels of emotional control may become dissociated in various neurological and neuropsychiatric conditions, the previously described effects of lateralized frontal stroke or of the orbitofrontal "pseudopsychopathic" syndrome serving as examples.

The differences between ventromedial prefrontal and amygdaloid contributions to the appraisal of emotionally charged situations are reflected in corresponding lesion effects. Both types of lesions interfered with decision making in a simulated gambling experiment, but only the amygdaloid lesions resulted in the failure to generate a skin-conductance response (change in electric skin conductivity) commonly associated with emotional states.[31] A somewhat similar division of roles between the ventromedial prefrontal cortex and the amygdala was demonstrated by Mobbs and colleagues in a study of "threats" by predators in a virtual reality environments. Distant threats were associated with ventromedial prefrontal activation, but as the threat was getting closer the central amygdaloid activation began to predominate.[32] Presumably, the appreciation of a distant threat is mediated mostly by the cognitive mechanisms of the prefrontal cortex, whereas a more immediate threat engages the more automatic amygdala-mediated response.

Under certain circumstances, the dissociation between the "cognitive" neocortical and "automatic" amygdaloid contributions may occur even in the daily experiences of healthy individuals. In my book *The Wisdom Paradox*,[33] I describe a scene during a visit to Kenya many years ago in which was I was invited to take in my hands a just-hatched baby crocodile, a tiny and obviously harmless creature. To my own utter disbelief, I could not prevail upon myself to touch the skinny hatchling. A peculiar tug-of-war ensued between me and something inside me that I didn't even recognize as being part of my conscious self. As *I* (my frontal lobes) was commanding me to extend my hand toward the baby crocodile, *it* (my amygdala) was pulling it back. This neural tug-of-war between my frontal lobes and amygdala was not accompanied by a familiar feeling of fear in the usual sense; in fact I was quite relaxed and even amused by my internal goings on at a conscious level. But it was accompanied by a visceral revulsion and resistance of the sort that I had very rarely, if ever, experienced before. The frontally and amygdala-generated inputs appeared to result in qualitatively different kinds of subjective experiences. To my total astonishment and amusement, the amygdala prevailed and I was unable to touch the skinny reptile.

Other neural structures may also be part of the vertically integrated circuits of emotional control. In all likelihood, the contribution of these additional structures is similarly lateralized. More recently, the role of the anterior cingulate cortex (ACC) in emotional control has drawn considerable attention. Elizabeth Phelps and her colleagues at New York University's Center for Neural Studies have shown that individuals with a consistently optimistic personality exhibit the pattern of activation in the amygdala and the rostral ACC.[34] Evidence thus exists supporting the notion of a unified "emotional learning" circuitry, which includes the amygdale, dorsomedial prefrontal cortex, and the anterior cingulate cortex.[35]

Emotions, Novelty, and Cerebral Hemispheres

Earlier in the book we discussed hemispheric specialization and interaction as a fundamental aspect of cognition. Now, in considering the role of the frontal lobes in emotion, the hemispheric theme has resurfaced again, but in a very different context.

What is the relationship between the cognitive and the emotional aspects of functional lateralization of the frontal lobes and other structures? How can they be integrated into a coherently unified theory of hemispheric specialization and integration? Is there an intrinsic relationship between the cognitive and emotional hemispheric dichotomies, or do these two aspects of hemispheric specialization cohabit in a merely coincidental way? As long as our understanding of hemispheric specialization was dominated by the language–visuospatial dichotomy, the answer had to be the latter. One would be very hard pressed to argue the existence of an intrinsic link between language and positive emotion, or between visuospatial processes and negative emotion. So it is not surprising that traditionally the cognitive and emotional aspects of hemispheric specialization have been regarded separately, almost orthogonally, without any attempts to interweave them into a unified, coherent theory. Such a theory simply could not have been formulated within the framework of the verbal–nonverbal dichotomy of hemispheric specialization. This was a highly unsatisfactory state of affairs, since both intellectual and aesthetic considerations expect a scientific narrative to be parsimonious and not just a laundry list of disjointed propositions. By contrast, the novelty–routinization theory of hemispheric specialization allows one to integrate the cognitive and emotional themes into a coherent understanding of hemispheric specialization.

Indeed, one can argue that an intrinsic relationship exists between novelty seeking and negative affect. Novelty seeking implies dissatisfaction with the status quo. In my earlier book *The Wisdom Paradox*,[36] I argued, half in jest, that the great globe-trotting, path-breaking mariners, like Christopher Columbus and Magellan, would have never embarked on their great voyages had they not been temperamentally dysphoric and had Prozac been available in those days. Considered in this light, the widely reported prevalence of bipolar disorder among creative individuals comes as no surprise. One has to be dissatisfied with that which *is*, in order to embark on the attainment of that which *should be*. So the seat of novelty and the seat of negative affect are logically linked together in a shared neural territory of the right hemisphere, as the negative affect drives novelty seeking.

By contrast, the left hemisphere is the repository of long-term, generic knowledge and cognitive routines. But the brain is highly selective about what is "permitted" into the long-term store. Most of the information we acquire is forgotten and never makes it into long-term memory. With few exceptions, only information recognized by the brain as highly important makes it into long-term memory. What are the biologically plausible mechanisms of rating information in terms of its importance? Both bottom-up and top-down mechanisms may be in existence. The bottom-up mechanism is based on the frequency of use, since frequently needed information is by definition important; and this is the likely mechanism of forming and storing generic knowledge. The top-down mechanism is based on the assignation of importance value by the prefrontal cortex. In some sense, information contained in the left hemisphere's long-term store is "good" by virtue of being recognized and reinforced as "useful".

Dopamine is likely to play an important role in both mechanisms. As we already know, dopamine is more prevalent in the left hemisphere than in the right hemisphere. We also know that positive affect is mediated predominantly by the left hemisphere and negative affect by the right hemisphere. Dopamine is often referred to as the "reward" neuromodulator,[37] and it appears to play a particularly important role in positive reward. Michael Frank and colleagues have demonstrated that patients with Parkinson's disease, suffering from the depletion of the dopamine system, tend to learn how to avoid choices leading to negative outcomes more readily than learning how to select choices leading to positive outcomes. This negative-response learning bias is reversed with the administration of dopamine agonists.[38]

This discussion of the novelty–routinization principle of hemispheric integration emphasizes mostly the neocortical structures. But the same principle may play itself out in the subcortical structures usually associated with affective control. So-called crossed-disconnection lesions in monkeys, involving the amygdala in one hemisphere and the orbitofrontal cortex in the other hemisphere, result in an inability to update the reward value of significant stimuli.[39] This response can be construed as a breakdown of learning a new, changing relationship between a stimulus and a reward.

9

Different Lobes for Different Folks:

Decision-Making Styles and the Frontal Lobes

The Neuropsychology of Individual Differences

Comparing the function of the normal and abnormal brain has been the mainstay of neuropsychology. It is understood that brain disease may take many forms, each corresponding to its own neurological or psychiatric condition: dementia, head injury, stroke, and so on. On the other hand, traditional neuropsychology and cognitive neuroscience have adopted an abstraction, the "normal brain," envisioned as a grand average of all individual brains. This simplistic notion has been frequently taken to an absurd extreme in many areas of cognitive neuroscience, including functional neuroimaging, the increasingly dominant methodology allowing scientists and clinicians to examine brain physiology and not just brain structure. The imaging data were fitted onto "Talairach space" (named after its inventor),[1] which is basically the brain of a single French woman, presumably selected on the assumption that it serves as a good approximation of all the other brains. To make matters worse, only one hemisphere was selected and mirrored, ignoring all we know about hemispheric differences.

Neuroscientists are not unique in recognizing and appreciating the diversity of human minds, talents, and personalities as variations of normality.

The world would indeed be a boring place were everyone the same and, therefore, to a large extent predictable. By noting that Joe Doe is mathematically gifted, musically inept, and short-tempered while Jane Blane is musically gifted, mathematically inept, and sweet, we do not automatically conclude that one is normal and the other abnormal. In most instances we assume that both are normal, but different. A whole field of psychology has emerged to study the *individual differences as multiple expressions of normality.*

But does the brain have anything to do with these differences, or are they entirely a reflection of our different surroundings, upbringings, and experiences? Neuroanatomists have known for a long time that individual "normal" brains differ profoundly in overall size, relative sizes of different parts, and proportions. More recent findings suggest that individual brain biochemistry is also highly variable. These differences are particularly pronounced in the frontal lobes.[2]

Is there a relationship between the variability of human brains and the variability of human minds? In particular, are the differences in decision-making styles related to the differences in the anatomy and chemistry of the frontal lobes? We are only beginning to ask these questions, and in doing so, we are laying the ground for a new discipline, the *neuropsychology of individual and group differences.* In due time, we may be able to understand the contribution of individual *neural* differences to individual *cognitive* differences. In fact, there has been a growing number of studies attempting to use the methods of neuroscience in identifying individual differences in risk taking (discussed later in this chapter), economic decision-making patterns, and even political preferences, as in liberals vs. conservatives.[3]

This inquiry will proceed in steps, first by establishing this relationship with respect to groups rather than individuals.

Male and Female Cognitive Styles

Intuitively, we understand that no individual cognitive landscape is a flat line. Instead, it consists of peaks and valleys, the peaks corresponding to individual strengths and the valleys to individual weaknesses. The quest for understanding the relationship between individual cognitive landscapes and individual brains drove the earliest attempts at mapping cortical functions, giving rise to Gall's phrenology. In this tradition, individual cognitive differences have been understood in terms of who is better at what ("better" presumably corresponding to "bigger" in terms of regional cortical space).

Individual differences can also be approached in terms of cognitive *styles*, rather than cognitive *abilities*. Particularly, we can ask questions about the individual differences in decision-making styles. This brings us back to the distinction between adaptive and veridical decision making made earlier in the book (see Chapter 7).

If cognitive abilities influence the ease with which we acquire cognitive skills, then decision-making styles influence the ways in which we deal with life situations as individuals. Most real-life situations of any degree of complexity do not contain a tacit unequivocal, single solution (the way the statement "2 + 2 = . . ." does). Placed into the same situation, different people will act in different ways; one is not unequivocally right and all the rest unequivocally wrong. How do we make our choices and what accounts for the differences in the ways we make them? Finally, what are the brain mechanisms responsible for the differences in decision-making styles?

My colleagues and I approached these questions by giving our deliberately loosely designed Cognitive Bias Task (CBT) to neurologically healthy subjects.[4] The subjects were shown three geometric forms (one target and two choices) and asked to look at the target and make the choice that they "liked the most" (see Fig. 7.3). It was clear that different subjects exhibited different response patterns. These response patterns gravitated toward one of two distinct strategies. Some subjects matched their choice to the target, and as the targets changed, so did their choices. We called this decision-making strategy *context-dependent*. Other subjects made their choices based on stable preferences, regardless of the target. They always picked blue, or red, or circle, or square. We called this decision-making strategy *context-independent*. To our surprise, males and females made their choices in strikingly different ways: males were more context-dependent and females were more context-independent (see Fig. 9.1). Although there was an overlap between the two curves, the gender differences were both robust and significant.

Gender differences in cognition is a relatively new and increasingly hot topic. For decades, neuroscientists treated humanity as a homogeneous mass, ignoring the self-evident truth apparent to every man and woman in the street: that males and females are different. But we are finding out increasingly that one ignores gender differences in cognition at one's own peril. Early work on cognitive gender differences focused on specific cognitive skills, on who is better in what. This inquiry focused on *veridical* decision making. Some of the most quoted research suggests, for instance, that males are better at mathematics and spatial relationships, and females are better at languages. But very little, if anything, has been said about gender differences in general cognitive styles. In particular, next to nothing has been said in the cognitive literature about gender differences in the general approach to decision making, about *adaptive* decision making. Our work with CBT is among the first such accounts.

Could the gender differences observed in our esoteric experiment correspond to some real-life traits? Common sense suggests that they could. Imagine two approaches to personal finances. Jane Blane and Joe Blow are self-employed consultants whose incomes fluctuate from month to month. Jane Blane practices a context-independent approach to life. She always saves 5% of her income, never buys clothes costing more than $500 per item, and always takes her vacation

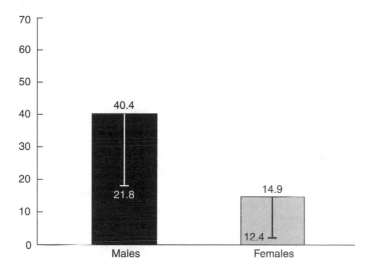

Figure 9.1 Gender differences in actor-centered decision making. Males exhibit a more context-dependent response selection preference on the Cognitive Bias Task (higher score). Females exhibit a more context-independent response selection preference (lower score). [After Goldberg et al. (1994).[4] Copyright by Massachusetts Institute of Technology. Reprinted with permission.]

in August. By contrast, Joe Blow's approach to life is context-dependent. When his monthly income is below $5000 he saves nothing, when it is between $5000 and $7000 he saves 5%, and he saves 10% when his monthly income exceeds $7000. He tends not to buy clothes costing more than $500, except when his monthly income is particularly high. He takes a vacation whenever his workload permits. This is just an example, but it models basic lifelong individual differences in actor-centered decision making.

In a very broad sense, the context-independent strategy can be thought of as a "universal default strategy." It represents an attempt by the organism to formulate all-purpose "best" responses averaged, in some sense, across all the possible life situations. The organism will accumulate a repertoire of such responses as a concise sum total of lifelong experiences. The "all-purpose" repertoire will be updated with new experiences, but very slowly and gradually, since it is the conservator of the individual's "universal wisdom."

The problem with such a strategy is that real-life situations are often so different from one another that any attempt at "averaging" becomes meaningless. In statistics, drawing a mean value across exemplars makes sense only if all the exemplars represent the same population. If the exemplars are drawn from different populations, then the mean will be misleading. Nonetheless, such a "default" strategy may be your best bet when faced with a totally novel situation, for which you have no specific experience or knowledge.

By contrast, a context-dependent strategy reflects an attempt to capture the unique, or at least specific, properties of the situation at hand and to custom tailor the organism's response. Having encountered a new situation, the organism attempts to recognize it as a familiar pattern representing a familiar *narrow class* of situation, a "known quantity." This accomplished, the organism applies the specific experience of dealing with such familiar situations. But faced with a radically new situation, the organism's attempt at pattern recognition will fail. In that case, an organism guided by a context-dependent strategy, a no-default option, will attempt to capture the unique properties of the situation at hand right away, even though the available information may be woefully insufficient. This will produce a "bouncy" behavior with precipitous changes at every transition to a new situation.

The optimal decision-making strategy is probably achieved through a dynamic balance between the context-dependent and context-independent approaches. Indeed, very few people adhere to one or the other strategy in its pure form; most people are able to switch between them at will, or to adopt mixed strategies, depending on the situation. But in subtle ways individuals tend to gravitate toward one or the other approach to life. Likewise, our research shows that females as a group have a subtle preference toward context-independence and males toward context-dependence.

Neither strategy is better than the other in an absolute sense. Their relative advantages depend on how stationary the environment is. In a relatively stationary environment a context-independent approach to decision making is probably the sounder one. In a highly unstable environment a context-dependent approach is preferable. The choice of strategy also depends on how good a grasp the individual has on the specific situations at hand. If his or her grasp on the particular situation is good, then a context-dependent strategy is probably better. But if an individual's grasp on a situation is shaky because the individual lacks familiarity with the situation or it is inherently complex, then it may be more prudent to rely on a compact set of tried and true default principles.

Evolution seems to value both decision-making strategies, as both are represented in our species. Do they work better synergistically than either one by itself? How do they complement each other? Which one is better suited for which type of cognitive challenges? What evolutionary pressures resulted in their slight divergence by sex? Do the two decision-making strategies adaptively suit the distinct male and female roles in our success as a species? Do these differences correspond to the different roles played by females and males at early stages of human evolution? Are the gender differences in decision-making styles biologically or culturally determined to begin with? Are these differences found in other primates? Or are they found in most mammalian species? Are people born with them, or do boys and girls diverge in their decision-making styles only as they approach sexual maturity? Does the decision-making style change in females with menopause?

Do the gender differences in decision-making styles recede as the societal roles of males and females continue to converge? These fascinating questions await their answers through future research.

Research into cognitive gender differences, although increasingly prominent, is sometimes assaulted when a statement of gender *difference* is misconstrued as a statement of gender *inferiority*. I was once a target of such misguided political correctness while giving a guest lecture at a prominent medical center in New York City in the mid-1990s. A young postdoctoral fellow interrupted my presentation and stridently accused me of male chauvinism as I was presenting the findings described in this chapter. I responded by saying that not having been particularly concerned about political correctness in my old country, the Soviet Union, where the consequences of political incorrectness could be quite dire, I saw no reason to worry about it in the United States, where the worst that could happen was wasting my time on a stupid argument. To their credit, the audience of doctors and medical students reacted with a round of applause.

It may be interesting to create a taxonomy of activities that lend themselves better to context-dependent and to context-independent decision making. To a degree, this can be accomplished empirically. But the distinction between the context-dependent and context-independent strategies also lends itself to relatively straightforward computational modeling with neural nets and other methods. In addition to modeling individual organisms, a collective behavior of such organisms can be examined, when some of them are context-dependent and some are context independent. Furthermore, the relative prevalence of these two decision-making biases can be varied in different environments. By examining such group behaviors of neural nets, it may be possible to begin to understand the adaptive value of having different decision-making strategies combined in a population. In the long run, such theoretical computational models may provide particularly important insights into the individual differences and the adaptive value of having several decision-making types represented in society.

Frontal Lobes, Hemispheres, and Cognitive Styles

What are the brain mechanisms of different cognitive styles? Do different decision-making strategies depend on different parts of the brain? Are these mechanisms different in males and females? Decision-making styles seem to depend on the frontal lobes. They also exhibit gender differences and are lateralized. This brings us to the issue of the lateralization of frontal lobe functions.

Hemispheric specialization has always been a central topic in neuropsychology. However, the frontal lobes have traditionally been on the periphery of such inquiry, an afterthought. This was an understandable consequence of the prevailing belief that the functional differences between the two hemispheres revolved around the verbal–visuospatial distinction. Since the prefrontal cortex has not been tradition-ally regarded as the seat of either language or visual–spatial processes, it was not regarded particularly pertinent to this distinction.

But this flies in the face of common sense, if we believe that brain structure and brain biochemistry have more than a passing relationship to brain function. The frontal lobes exhibit morphological gender differences and asymmetries, which humans share with several nonhuman species. The protrusion of the right frontal pole over the left frontal pole, known as the *Yakovlevian torque* (the other half of the torque includes a protrusion of the left occipital lobe over the right occipital lobe), is conspicuous in male humans and less pronounced in female humans. But it is also present in fossil humans.[5] The cortical thickness of the left and right fron-tal lobes is similar in female humans but different in male humans (right thicker than left). Humans share the gender difference in frontal cortical thickness with several mammalian species. Humans also share the differences in left and right frontal cortical thickness in males with several other species.[6] Spindle cells, with their long axons, are more prolific in the right than in the left frontal lobes of several species.[7]

Biochemical differences found in the frontal lobes are also shared by humans with other species. Estrogen receptors are symmetrically distributed across the frontal lobes in female humans and asymmetrically distributed in male humans—and in several nonhuman mammalian species.[8] Some of the major neurotransmit-ters also exhibit hemispheric asymmetry. Dopamine pathways tend to be more prevalent in the left than right frontal lobe, and noradrenergic pathways tend to be more prevalent in the right than left frontal lobe. This dual asymmetry is found in humans, the monkey, and the rat.[9]

With this background, it is highly probable that the frontal lobes are function-ally different in males and females. It is also probable that the left and right frontal lobes are functionally different in males but less so in females. By the same token, it is highly *improbable* that these functional differences are restricted to the differ-ence between language and nonverbal processes—for the simple reason that this distinction has no meaning in monkeys, rats, and such.

On the basis of our earlier work with the Executive Control Battery, we already knew that lateralized frontal lesions produce different effects in males and in females.[10] Nonetheless, we wanted to clarify these differences further. As before, my colleagues and I felt that we stood the best chance of cracking the problem by applying our nonveridical, actor-centered tasks. For this study we chose patients with isolated lesions in the left frontal lobe or the right frontal lobe, males and females. We first limited our study to right-handed patients. When we gave the Cognitive Bias Task to the patients, a rather striking picture emerged.[11]

Males with a damaged right frontal lobe behaved in an extremely context-depen-dent manner and males with a damaged left frontal lobe behaved in an extremely context-independent manner. Neurologically intact normal controls were somewhere in the middle of the range. So it appears that in males the two frontal lobes make their choices in very different, opposite, ways. In a normal brain these two decision-making strategies coexist in dynamic balance, with one or the other assuming the leading role depending on the situation. But this flexibility of decision making is lost in brain damage, and behavior deteriorates toward one or the other maladaptive extreme. In females the picture was entirely different. Both left and right frontal lesions produced extremely context-dependent behavior, whereas neurologically healthy normal females exhibited, as we already know, relatively context-independent behavior (see Fig. 9.2).

These findings of functional lateralization and gender differences in the frontal lobes are among the most robust findings in the literature. Why have the numerous other studies asking similar questions failed to turn up anything nearly as robust? I think the answer to this question lies in the power of the actor-centered paradigm. To make this point, we compared two tasks in their ability to discriminate between the effects of left and right frontal lesions in males. The first task was our Cognitive

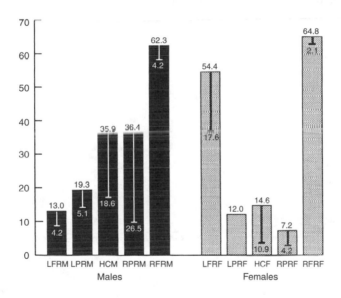

Figure 9.2 Gender differences in lateralized lesion effects. In males left frontal lesions produce extreme context-independent response selection preference (low score) and right frontal lesions produce extreme context-dependent response selection preference (high score) on the Cognitive Bias Task (CBT). In females both left and right frontal lesions produce extreme context-dependent response selection preference on the CBT (high score). Key: LFRM, left-frontal male lesion group; LPRM, left-posterior male lesion group; HCM, healthy control male group; RPRM, right-posterior male lesion group; RFRM, right-frontal male lesion group; LFRF, left-frontal female lesion group; LPRF, left-posterior female lesion group; HCF, healthy control female group; RPRF, right-posterior female lesion group; RFRF, right-frontal female lesion group. [After Goldberg et al. (1994).[4] Copyright by Massachusetts Institute of Technology. Reprinted with permission.]

Bias Task (CBT), which is actor centered in nature (Fig. 9.3). The second task was the Wisconsin Card Sorting Test (WCST),[12] regarded by many as the gold standard of neuropsychological frontal-lobe assessment, which is veridical in nature (Fig. 9.4). As Figures 9.3 and 9.4 show, despite its exhalted status, the WCST fails to differentiate between the lateralized frontal lesion effects, whereas the CBT does a perfect job. This is yet further evidence that neuropsychologists and the neuropsychological test publishers need to invest their time and energies in the design of a new generation of actor-centered procedures.

Of course, the next logical step is to study normal subjects with functional neuroimaging, which is what we are doing as of this writing. The expectation is that healthy right-handed males with the preference for context-dependent decision making will show a particular activation of the left prefrontal cortex while doing the task. By contrast, healthy right-handed males with the preference for context-independent decision making will show a particular activation of the right prefrontal cortex. In females a totally different picture can be expected. Healthy right-handed females with the preference toward context-independent decision making will show a particular activation of the prefrontal cortex bilaterally, and females with the preference for context-dependent decision making will show a particular activation of the posterior cortex bilaterally.

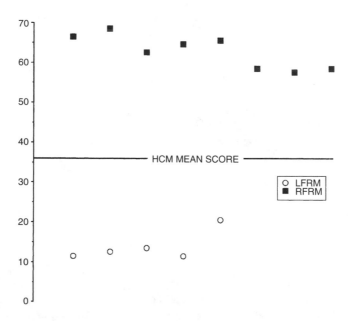

Figure 9.3 Cognitive Bias Task (CBT) individual score distribution in right-handed males with lateralized frontal lesions. Key: LFRM, left-frontal male lesion group; RFRM, right-frontal male lesion group; HCM, healthy control males. [After Podell et al. (1995). Copyright by American Psychiatric Press, Inc.]

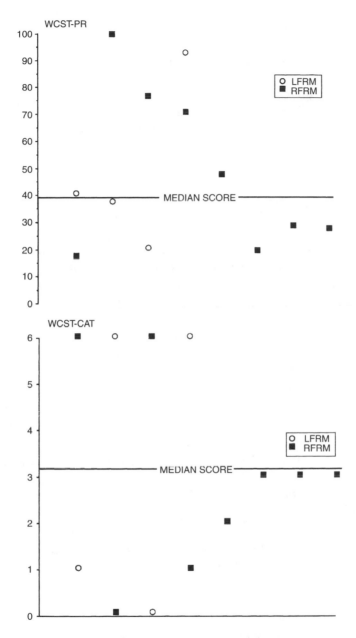

Figure 9.4 Wisconsin Card Sorting Test individual score distribution in right-handed males with lateralized frontal lesions. Top: Number of perseverative responses (WCST-PR). Bottom: Number of categories achieved (WCST-CAT). Key: LFRM, left-frontal male lesion group; RFRM, right-frontal male lesion group; IICM, healthy control males. [After Podell et al. (1995). Copyright by American Psychiatric Press, Inc.]

Cognitive Styles and Brain Wiring

The male and female cognitive decision-making strategies are different, as are the patterns of lateralization of their frontal lobe functions. It has been known for some time that structural, biochemical, and functional differences between the hemispheres are greater in males than in females.[13] So it should come as no surprise that the functional differences are greater between the two male frontal lobes than between the two female frontal lobes.

Among many possible ramifications of these differences, one is particularly interesting: the fact that various diseases of the brain afflict males and females at different rates. Schizophrenia,[14] Tourette's syndrome,[15] and attention deficit hyperactivity disorder (ADHD)[16] are all more common in men than in women. As we will find out later in this book, all three disorders are understood today as dysfunction of the frontal lobes, or of structures closely linked to the frontal lobes. Could it be that males are more vulnerable than females to any disorder affecting predominantly the frontal lobes? The two female frontal lobes are functionally more alike and thus each of them is more capable of taking over the functions of the other in the case of lateralized frontal lobe dysfunction. Indeed, a suggestion of lateralized, rather than completely bilateral, brain dysfunction is present in schizophrenia,[17] Tourette's syndrome,[18] and possibly even in ADHD.[19]

Does all this mean that female cortex is generally less functionally differentiated than male cortex? Traditionally this question was asked narrowly, only with respect to the cerebral hemispheres, thus the answer had to be yes. But recent research suggests that in certain respects the female cortex is *more* functionally differentiated than the male cortex. Our own work also pointed in this direction when we compared the effects of posterior (parietal and temporal) lesions on the response selection strategies.[20]

The effects of posterior (parietal and temporal) lesions in males and females on CBT performance were considerably less significant than the effects of frontal lesions. This was to be expected if actor-centered decision making is primarily under the control of the frontal lobes. Nonetheless, the effects of posterior brain lesions were also gender dimorphic. In males the direction of posterior-lesion effects was the same as the frontal-lesion effects, albeit much weaker: left-sided lesions made behavior more context-independent, and right-sided lesions made behavior more context-dependent. But in females the effects of posterior lesions were opposite those of the frontal lesions: they made performance less context-dependent rather than more context-dependent.

Taken together, the male and female findings lead to a provocative conclusion. These findings challenge the established belief that the same pattern of functional cortical differentiation is present in both sexes, but expressed more strongly in males than in females. Our findings suggest that the difference is not merely in degree but in kind, that a qualitative difference is present. The female cortex is no less functionally differentiated than the male cortex—and no more. The two sexes emphasize different aspects of functional cortical differentiation. In the male brain the left–right differences are better articulated than in the female brain. But in the female brain the front–back differences are better articulated than in the male brain.

This conclusion is supported by earlier research studying the effects of lesions[21] and examining the patterns of regional cerebral blood flow[22] and functional magnetic resonance imaging (fMRI) activation in males and females.[23] When the task was to process verbal information, coactivation of the frontal and posterior regions within the same hemisphere, the left hemisphere, was seen in males. By contrast, in females the coactivation was symmetric (*homologous*), that is, coactivation of the two opposite hemispheres was recorded.

What could be the mechanism of these two alternative emphases in the male and female functional cortical organization? This question may be best dealt with if instead of functional *differentiation* we consider functional *integration*. The degree of functional integration as opposed to differentiation between brain structures depends, in turn, on the degree of interaction among them. The greater the interaction between two brain structures, the greater their functional integration. The more limited the interaction between these structures, the greater their functional differentiation.

With this reasoning in mind, let us consider what is known about the main connections within the brain. The corpus callosum is the structure that, together with the anterior and posterior comissures, connects the two cortical hemispheres. Certain aspects of the corpus callosum are thicker in females than in males.[24] To the extent that we believe in a more or less direct relationship between structure and function (a tempting, albeit precarious proposition), this may account for greater functional interaction, hence greater functional integration and lesser functional differentiation, between the cortical hemispheres in females.

Next let us consider the main connecting structures between the front (anterior) and back (posterior) aspects of the *same* hemisphere, the longitudinal fasciculi and other long white-matter bundles connecting distant cortical regions *within* a hemisphere. Recent studies have shown that these structures are somewhat larger in males than in females.[25] Following the logic of analysis adopted in this section, this may account for greater functional interaction, hence a greater degree of functional integration and less of functional differentiation, between the frontal and posterior portions of a hemisphere in males.

A rather elegant, equitable picture of two complementary neuroanatomical connection emphases in males and females emerges, which may account for some of the fundamental cognitive differences between the two sexes. How exactly do these two patterns of connectivity affect cognition? Which pattern of connectivity is "better" for what cognitive task? What is the adaptive evolutionary value of having these two complementary patterns of neural organization represented within the species in roughly equal proportions (a teleological question that I keep asking and that would have incurred the wrath of Stephen Jay Gould)?

These are all fascinating, and fundamental, questions. In trying to answer them it is tempting to capitalize on the relatively straightforward way in which the neuroanatomical gender differences described here lend themselves to formalization in a computational model. These questions are best answered, in my opinion, through experimentation with computational models, perhaps formal neural nets, comparing the emergent properties of enhanced connections *within* layers with the emergent properties of enhanced connections *between* layers in a bicameral model. Among the many challenges of cognitive neuroscience, those that allow natural (as opposed to contrived) theoretical models are particularly attractive, since they help move the field of neuropsychology out of the purely empirical domain into the domain of developed theoretical disciplines. The puzzle of cognitive differences between the sexes may prove to be among these challenges.

Rebels in Small Proportion: Handedness and Novelty Seeking

It would appear that novelty seeking should be the cardinal attribute of our restless species, but it is not. Humans tend to be conservative, gravitating toward the familiar. During my presentations for the general public I am always amused by how people want to hear what they already know and not what is truly novel. Journalists, including those who occasionally interview me about the brain for various features in the lay press, have the same inclination.

In fact, it can be argued that monkeys tend to be attracted to novelty much more than humans are. In an experiment that Mortimer Mishkin and Karl Pribram conducted in the 1950s, a monkey had to choose between an object identical to one previously shown and a different object.[26] The monkey saw an object. Then the monkey saw another object, which was either identical to the baited object or different from it. Two conditions were compared: when the identical (familiar) object was reinforced and when the different (novel) object was reinforced. On the whole, the monkeys learned to respond to novel stimuli faster than to the familiar ones, which suggests that they tend to be more attracted to the novel than to the familiar.

In a comparable situation, humans act in a very different manner. The preferences exhibited by our subjects on the Cognitive Bias Task (when they were asked to look at the target and make one of the two choices that they "liked the best") were very different from those of the monkeys. Humans almost invariably chose the items more similar to the target instead of the more different ones. This was true both for the right-handed healthy subjects and brain-damaged patients.

Such an emphasis on the familiar is understandable, since humans, at least adult humans, are guided by previously accumulated knowledge to a much larger extent than any other species. To put it in different terms, the ratio of de novo discovery to the previously accumulated body of knowledge is relatively low in adult humans compared to other species. This is because no other species has the mechanism of storing and transmitting the collective knowledge of the species accumulated over many generations in external cultural devices, such as books, films, and the like. Therefore, our bias toward the familiar serves an adaptive function. By contrast, the assimilation of previously accumulated knowledge in a monkey is limited to imitation of other monkeys' behavior. By and large, a young animal embarks on a cognitive voyage, discovering its world on its own.

Human predisposition toward familiarity may change, as new knowledge accumulates at an exponential rate. A sociologist of science may someday devise a formula relating the amount of knowledge acquired within a generation to the amount of knowledge inherited from previous generations. The paradox is that this ratio changes in a nonmonotonic way. The ratio is high in nonhuman primates and probably during the prehistoric stages of human civilization, low through ancient history and dark middle ages, and picks up the speed through recent history, reaching exponential growth in modern times. The first peak of this ratio reflects an absence of effective cultural devices for information storage and transmission. By contrast, the second peak reflects the power of such devices, which permits an increasingly rapid accumulation of information. In human societies a low acquired-to-inherited knowledge ratio found in traditional cultures is associated with the cult of the elders as the repositories of accumulated wisdom. By contrast, a high acquired-to-inherited knowledge ratio found in modern societies is associated with the cult of the young as the vehicle of discovery and progress.

But a society cannot thrive on conservatism alone. For progress to occur, a mechanism must exist balancing conservatism and innovation. An excessively conservative society will be stagnant. A society too ready to give up established principles and concepts and rush headlong toward the new and untested ones will be dangerously flimsy and unstable. This delicate balance is maintained in every society through tacit conventions and explicit rules that determine the height of the hurdle that a new idea must clear to gain acceptance. Different societies set these hurdles at different levels for different situations. In science, for instance, the more radical a new idea, the higher the threshold for acceptance. An increasingly more rapid rate of knowledge accumulation through history is accompanied by the society's increasing willingness to revise the prevailing established assumptions. Yet it can be argued that even modern societies put a premium on preservation over modification.

Is there a mechanism operating at the biological, possibly genetic, level that regulates the balance between conservatism and innovation in human population? Merely phrasing a question in these terms has an outlandish, provocative ring. Yet our work has not only led me to suspect that such a mechanism exists, it suggests what the mechanism may be.

Earlier I mentioned that the overwhelming majority of our subjects showed preference for similarity on the Cognitive Bias Task—as long as they were right-handed. Among the left-handers the response pattern was distinctly different, and many of them exhibited a preference for the choice that *differed* from the target rather than resembled it.[27] This was particularly true for the left-handed males. To the extent that our experiment elicits the preference toward the familiar versus the novel, it appears that left-handers, particularly left-handed males, are the novelty seekers.

Folkloric claims about the high prevalence of left-handedness among creative individuals have been around for many years. I have heard them repeated in different cultures on both sides of the Atlantic and have always dismissed them as gratuitous—until seeing our own findings. Now I cannot help but entertain the intriguing possibility that different types of handedness may be associated with different biases toward the routine or the novel.

Handedness is not unique to humans. In many simian species, both apes and monkeys, one hand plays the leading role and the other hand plays a subordinate role consistently throughout the animal's lifetime.[28] This is also true for rodents. Furthemore, a relationship exists between the lateralization of hippocampal dopamine concentration and lateralized preferences in T-shaped bifurcating mazes in individual rats.[29] The difference between us and them is that in simians no consistent preference is exhibited *within the population* and the handedness split across the members of the species is roughly even. In humans, by contrast, approximately 90% of the population exhibits various degrees of right-handedness, and only about 10% gravitates toward left-handedness.[30] Among all the species exhibiting *individual* handedness, humans exhibit the most strong and consistent *population* trend in handedness.

Numerous attempts to find cognitive correlates of handedness have basically failed.[31] What sets our study apart from most of the earlier research is our emphasis on actor-centered, rather than veridical, aspects of decision making. We are looking at cognitive *styles* rather than cognitive *abilities*. Once the question is phrased in this manner, an intriguing possibility emerges: left-handers are neither like right-handers nor the neuropsychological inverse of right-handers; they represent a distinctly different cognitive style.

If handedness is correlated with bias toward familiarity or toward novelty, then the roughly 9:1 ratio (at least according to traditional statistics) of right-handers to left-handers in the human population merits further examination. Could it be that this ratio reflects adaptive balance between conservation and innovation tendencies in the population, and that the population handedness bias serves as the mechanism to control this balance? In this scenario left-handers would be the innovation seekers, cultural rebels whose presence is necessary for societal ferment, but their proportion would be kept relatively low, lest society lose its broad cultural mooring.

To be viable, such a mechanism would have to allow some variation to regulate the conservation-to-innovation ratio in an adaptive manner. We do not know how variable the "true" biological handedness ratio is in different cultures at different historical stages. We do know, however, that cultural–anthropological factors affect this ratio in many societies. On the whole it seems that traditional societies, committed to the preservation of tradition more than innovation, tend to ostracize left-handedness and enforce right-handedness. Educational doctrines based on this tradition, perceived as misguided by modern Western society, persisted in most European and Asian societies well into the second half of twentieth century and continue to persist in many cultures even now. Born and schooled in Eastern Europe, I am myself a product of this educational atavism and a converted left-hander. By contrast, the more dynamic North American society, which is less affected by cultural "baggage," has been less bent on policing handedness, thus allowing a greater proportion of left-handers. While the enforced left- to right-handedness switch is very unlikely to change the underlying neurobiology and cognitive styles in any real sense, the policing of handedness may have been traditional societies' naive reaction to the observations that iconoclastic behavior is often associated with left-handedness.

An even broader question can be asked: Is it possible that in other, nonhuman primates, handedness serves as a mechanism for regulating the conservation-versus-innovation population balance? Let's return to Mishkin's experiment. Could it be that in his sample the familiarity-seeking monkeys were right-handed, and the novelty-seeking monkeys were left-handed? Unfortunately, no handedness data from this study are available.[32] Using a somewhat similar paradigm, Jonathan Wallis and colleagues at the Massachusetts Institute of Technology recorded neurons in the monkey's prefrontal cortex, whose firing pattern suggested their involvement in the encoding of abstract rules.[33] Two rules were used: responding to sameness and responding to difference. It would be very interesting to see if an interaction existed between the type of rule, the side of firing neurons, and monkey handedness.

What are the mechanisms relating handedness to the conservation–innovation bias? In our earlier discussion we linked the left hemisphere with cognitive routines and the right hemisphere with cognitive novelty. By virtue of the contralaterality of motor control, right-handedness tends to preferentially engage the left hemisphere and left-handedness tends to preferentially engage the right hemisphere. This reasoning implies that the roles of the two hemispheres with respect to the novelty–routinization distinction are unchanged in right-handers and left-handers. However, our own research using actor-centered cognitive tasks has shown that the functional roles of the two frontal lobes are reversed in left-handers compared to those in right-handers.[34] This further highlights the complex relationship between handedness and hemispheric specialization. It could be, for instance, that certain aspects of hemispheric specialization are reversed in left-handers, while certain others remain unchanged.

Another possibility is prompted by studies relating personality traits to brain biochemistry. Here dopamine receptors have been implicated in several species. People conspicuous in their predilection to risk taking seem to have an exceptionally high representation of a certain type of dopamine receptors.[35] Dopamine, of course, is a neurotransmitter that is very closely linked to the frontal lobes. Is it possible that this receptor type, an allele of D4 receptors, is particularly common among left-handers? Is it especially common among people exhibiting novelty seeking on cognitive tasks such as the Cognitive Bias Task? In Lister hooded rats, trait impulsivity was found to be linked to the reduction of dopamine D2/3 receptors in the nucleus accumbens.[36] The relevance of this finding to human personality typology is unclear at this time and should be examined further.

Until these questions are rigorously answered, the thesis developed in this chapter will remain speculative. Still, the intriguing possibility exists that the left-handers in our midst represent the restless, creative, novelty-seeking ferment in history—a catalyst indispensable for progress, yet best kept in check, lest it upset our societal apple cart. In the book *The Thirteenth Tribe*, Arthur Koestler quotes a tenth-century Arabic traveler writing about a Volga Bulgar tribe: "When they observe a man who excels through quickwittedness and knowledge, they say: 'for this one it is more befitting to serve our Lord.' They seize him, put a rope round his neck and hang him on a tree where he is left until he rots away."[37] One wonders how many among the unfortunate Bulgars were left-handed.

Whatever the underlying neurobiology, on a phenomenal level we know that some people are better at innovation and others, at following routines. Indeed, these different gifts are often incompatible. Visionaries who develop new trends in science, culture, or business often fail at implementing their own ideas in a sustained and systematic way; and other people, incapable of developing new trends but necessary to sustain them, have to take over to make things happen. Does this mean that trail-blazing visionaries have a particularly well-developed right hemisphere and cautious conventional types have a more developed left hemisphere? This is a fascinating proposition to examine concerning the neuropsychology of individual differences.

Like creativity, mental illness and neurodevelopmental disorders have also been linked to left-handedness. Schizophrenia, autism, dyslexia, and attention deficit disorder (ADD) are all characterized by an unusually high proportion of left-handers. While many cases of left-handedness are "pathological" (acquired due to early brain damage),[38] many others are hereditary, or genetically determined. The parallels between creativity and madness have fascinated both scientists and poets. Particularly interesting are cases of fluid boundaries, of geniuses gone mad, such as van Gogh and Nijinsky. Both genius and madness are deviations from the statistical norm. The romantic view holds that creative insights too far ahead of their time are often denounced by contemporaries as madness. The cynical view suggests that some of the more enduring cultural beliefs were a result of psychosis. Although the relationship between creativity and mental illness is well outside the scope of this book, their shared relationship to left-handedness is highly provocative.

Executive Talents: The *S* Factor and the Theory of Mind

Human brains are as variable in their individual features as any other part of the body. Weight, relative sizes of different lobes, the articulation of gyri and sulci— all are highly variable. Although the cognitive neuroscience of individual differences has yet to come together, it makes intuitive sense that the individual cognitive traits and talents have something to do with the individual variation in brain organization. Notably, the individual variation of human brain morphology is particularly pronounced in the frontal lobes.[39]

We tend to define people by their talents and shortcomings. Someone is musically gifted but has no spatial sense; someone else has a way with words but has a deaf ear. Such descriptions capture the person's special traits but not the person's essence. But when we call someone "smart" or "shrewd" and someone else "dumb" or "obtuse," we are no longer talking about narrow special traits. We are alluding to something both more elusive and more profound. We come much closer to defining the person's essence, to defining the person him- or herself, rather than the person's attributes. Being "smart" (or "dumb") is not an attribute of you; it *is* you. Peculiarly, a certain degree of independence exists between this global dimension of human mind and the more narrow special traits. An individual may be devoid of any special talents, musical, literary, or athletic, yet be considered by others to be very "smart." The opposite is also possible, when a uniquely gifted individual is nonetheless perceived as "dumb." At the risk of committing cultural sacrilege, I will suggest that, on the basis of biographic accounts, Mozart was probably somewhat a "dumb" genius. Lack of everyday wisdom could probably also be imputed in the case of one of my intellectual heroes, Alan Turing. Of course, the examples of the opposite, the "ordinary smart," are numerous and, by definition, anonymous. Many readers of this book will probably qualify.

But what do we mean by the terms *shrewd* and *obtuse*? And what are the brain structures whose individual variations determine these global traits? This question is directly related to the search for general intelligence—the "G factor"—and for measures of it, which are outside the scope of this book. The issue remains a matter of heated scientific debate. The last few decades have witnessed a departure from the notion of a single *G* factor in favor of "multiple intelligences." Introduced by Gardner[40] and Goleman,[41] these domain-specific "intelligences" broadly correspond to the cognitive variables systematically studied by cognitive neuroscientists and tested by clinical neuropsychologists and known to be dissociable in both neurological health and neurological illness.

Regardless of how the cognitive construct of general intelligence is defined, I am not aware of the existence of any distinct, single brain characteristic shown to account for such a G factor. The few available studies of genius brains failed to turn up compelling findings, and some of them are outright counterintuitive (which goes to show how flawed our intuitions are on the subject). For example, the brain of author Anatole France was known for its small size.[42] Einstein's brain reveals a peculiar lack of differentiation between the temporal and parietal lobes, as if a portion of the temporal lobe was "appropriated" by the parietal lobe.[43] This may possibly account for his self-reported preference for visualization over formalisms in developing his ideas (as well as for his reported dyslexia). But unless we believe in a homunculus inhabiting the general region of the angular/supramarginal gyrus, the finding is too local, too regional to account for an all-encompassing G. This leads us to the conclusion that many forms of "genius" reflect local properties of the mind (and, by inference, of the brain) and may have little to do with our intuitive sense of "being smart" as a global, central, defining personal attribute. The local nature of genius is suggested by the biographic accounts of Mozart and Turing. Based on what we know of their lives, neither would have been regarded as smart by most people.

But what about the S factor (S for "smart")? I believe that, unlike the G factor, the S factor does exist. In this, I enjoy the tacit support of scores of ordinary people totally oblivious to G but acutely sensitive to S. Lay people, unencumbered by any particular psychological preconceptions but endowed with common sense, are amazingly confident, effortlessly and consistently judging who is smart—and who is not. What are they responding to in fellow human beings? What is the basis of their intuition? I have always thought this question worth asking but have been unable to find an answer in the literature. The underpinnings of everyday perception of intelligence are a fascinating subject on the interface of neuropsychology and social psychology.

The study that I envision should be as naturalistic as possible. It would start with assembling a panel of lay "judges" who are unencumbered by any psychological preconceptions and unconstrained by excessive instructions from the researcher, then recruiting a sample of equally lay subjects. The judges would have to rate the subjects on a 10-point scale of "smartness," based on a sample of live one-on-one freewheeling 1-hour-long interactions or (less desirable) on a prerecorded tape of the subjects interacting with someone else or among themselves. The situation (live or taped) should be as naturalistic and unconstrained as possible. After the experiment all the subjects would be put through an extensive battery of neuropsychological tests. What are your predictions? Do you expect the S ratings to be culture-dependent or culture-invariant?

I predict that the judges' ratings, or at least rankings, of the subjects would be highly consistent. Although cultural and professional factors undoubtedly play a role in judging smartness, I believe that fundamental cultural invariants of smartness exist which are perceived similarly in every society, just as they have been suggested to exist for physical beauty. I predict further that of all the neuropsychological tests, the smartness ratings would be best correlated with the tests of executive functions. In the multiple-intelligence scheme of things, it is the executive intelligence that we intuitively recognize as "being smart," the S factor. And of all the aspects of intelligence, the S factor—the "executive talent"—shapes our perception of a person as a persona, and not just as a carrier of a certain cognitive trait.

But every scale has its range defined by two extreme points. Therefore, rating people on the S factor is tantamount to also rating them on a D factor (D for "dumb"). This would turn the proposed experiment into a highly inflammatory enterprise, which might never see the light of day in our correctness-preoccupied culture. That would be a shame.

To a large extent, the trait in question refers to our ability to form insight into other people and to anticipate their behavior, motives, and intentions. Given the communal nature of our lives, this ability is of paramount importance to our success in the broadest possible sense. Whether you want to cooperate with someone's intentions or thwart them (and particularly in the latter case), you must first understand and anticipate the other person's intentions.

In my description in Chapter 3 of the essential executive functions, I emphasized their sequential, planning, temporal ordering aspect. Now imagine that you have to plan and sequentially organize *your* actions in coordination with a group of other individuals and institutions engaged in the planning and sequential organization of *their* actions. Your relationship with these other individuals and institutions may be cooperative, adversarial, or both. Furthermore, the nature of this relationship may change over time. To succeed in this interaction, you must be able to have not only an action plan of your own but also an insight into the nature of the other person's plan. You must be able to foresee not only the consequences of your own actions but also those of the other person's actions. To do that, you must have the capacity to form an internal representation of the other person's mental life or to use the high language of cognitive neuropsychology to form the "theory of mind" of the other person. Your own actions will then be chosen under the influence of your theory of the next person's mind formulated in your own mind. And the next person presumably will have a theory of *your* mind formulated in *his or her* head. The relative success of each of you will depend largely on the accuracy and degree of precision of your relative abilities to form the internal representation of the other. This makes the executive processes required for success in an interactive social (or rather *societal*) environment much more complex than the executive processes required in a solitary situation, such as solving a puzzle. This is true for competitive, cooperative, or mixed interactive situations.

Chess or checkers represents a formalized, highly distilled example of such "social" executive functions. The activities of business, political, or military leaders are also fundamentally based on their abilities to form the theory of mind of their opposite number, or very often their opposite numbers. In all such environments the essential questions are, "What will he do next?" and "What should I do if he does this?" In my own experience, the game I had to play against the institutions of the state to extricate myself from the Soviet Union was the most extreme and demanding instance of a real-life high-stake chess game I have ever encountered. My capacity for insight into, and anticipation of, the other side's moves and intentions made all the difference between success and failure of my audacious enterprise.

The capacity for insight into other people's mental states is fundamental to social interactions. It finds very few prototypes in the animal world, if any. One of the most refined forms this capacity may take is deception, since deception requires manipulating the adversary into acquiring certain mental states, which the deceiver can then exploit. Frith and Frith argue that even apes lack this ability to any appreciable degree and that it is a uniquely human attribute.[44] The ironic corollary of this conclusion is that just as developed social interactions are uniquely human, so is sociopathy.

Someone with an insight into other people's minds is intuitively perceived as "smart" or "shrewd," and someone without this ability as "dumb" or "obtuse." We use these descriptions to capture the individual's cognitive essence, not his or her narrow cognitive traits. While it may be possible to respect a "dumb" person's special gift, we find it very difficult to respect the person as an individual. Based on everything we know about the brain, this elusive but fundamental ability rests with the frontal lobes. In a number of studies normal subjects were asked to imagine the mental states of other people while their brains were being scanned with PET or fMRI. Invariably, particular activation was found in the medial and lateral inferior prefrontal cortex.[45]

We encounter enhanced capacity for insight into other people's inner worlds in successful corporate, political, and military leaders. But just as often, or more, we encounter this capacity diminished. Poor ability to form the theory of mind may be an expression of the normal variability in frontal lobe function without necessarily implying outright frontal lobe pathology, just as most everyday instances of inarticulate language do not imply outright damage to the temporal lobe.

As a clinician, I encounter this "benign" nonpathological diminution of the ability to form a theory of mind and presumably a subtle functional weakness of the frontal lobes quite frequently. I used to find it annoying but have come to enjoy it, as a cognitive voyeur of sorts and a casual student of the individual variation of frontal lobe function in everyday life.

A patient walks into my office and I begin to inquire into the circumstances of his car accident. The response goes roughly as follows. "Last night I opened the fridge and saw that we are running out of milk. My wife always has cereal for breakfast and how is she going to have it without milk! So the next morning I had to go to the grocery to buy some milk. We have three groceries in the neighbor-hood but I always buy from Joe because he is a nice guy and we served in the Navy together. So I get into my green station wagon, but then it occurs to me that I need to go the bank first . . ." and on and on, until, with any luck, we get to the street intersection where the collision happened.

My good patient clearly failed to form an accurate theory of my mind, or else he would have spared me (and himself) all the details that have no relevance what-soever to anything I need to know as a neuropsychologist about his problem. Was his rambling an expression of the good man's frontal lobe damage suffered in the accident? I doubt it. The odds are that he has always been like that: a bit, well, "dumb." He is allowed: we recognize individual differences in everything and respect the normal curve. Besides, it turns out that my patient is an excellent amateur musician and I am not—individual differences again.

A case of a much more extreme incapacity to form the theory of my mind forces me to conclude the presence of frank frontal lobe pathology. A man in his early 40s was referred for a neuropsychological evaluation. He was suffering from a myste-rious neurodegenerative disease, probably hereditary, unnamed, and malignant. He strode vigorously into my office, neatly dressed and well put together, without any discernible stigmata of a neurological patient. I put him through my standard history-taking interview: age, education, marital status, handedness. His responses were to the point, in well-formed language.

Then I asked about his favorite pastimes. "Movies!"—came the response with the exhilaration of an adolescent reliving his first trip to Disneyland. And before I could put in a word or ask my next question, a rapid-fire account of all the recently seen movies came out, one after another, with colorful detail, delivered in an excited language, impatient to get it all out at once. My first impulse was to move things along, but then I decided to let the patient carry on and see what hap-pened. The movie accounts kept coming out exuberantly and endlessly, dozens of them. The man *was* into movies and had watched them *all*—and now I, his doctor, was being made privy to this unforgettable and joyful personal experience. The movie plots kept spilling out for about 40 minutes and would have continued to spill out had I not interrupted my patient finally and moved things along.

The "movie man" is etched in my memory as a case of a patient without a clue about his doctor's informational needs. The deficit in this patient's ability to form the theory of my mind was more profound than that in the earlier case of the milk-fetching car accident victim, and I strongly suspected the presence of frontal lobe damage. Indeed, the results of the subsequent neuropsychological testing were suggestive of particularly severe frontal lobe dysfunction. My patient's inability to monitor and control his own output is common in frontal lobe disease and is often considered one of its central features. As we will see later in the cases of the injured student Vladimir and the horse-riding accident victim Kevin, it may take many forms (see Chapters 10 and 12). This consequence of frontal lobe dysfunction is particularly damaging to the individual's societal interactions both in overtly clinical forms and in more subtle, relatively benign everyday forms.

Clearly, the ability to form an internal representation of a different person's mind is linked to another fundamental cognitive ability: the concept of *mental self and mental self–nonself differentiation*. The sense of self is fundamental to our mental life, and it would appear that no complex cognition can exist without it. Yet scientific evidence suggests that the sense of self emerges late in evolution and is linked to the development of the frontal lobes.

Experimental studies of the evolution of the "self" concept use the method of self–nonself (or self–other) differentiation.[46] Suppose you put an animal in front of a mirror. Will it relate to its own image as to self or as to a different animal? Dogs relate to their own image as they would to a different animal. They bark, growl, and engage in dominance displays. Only great apes and, to a lesser extent, monkeys relate to their mirror image as their own self.[47] They use the mirror as an opportunity to groom hard-to-reach body parts and to erase marks painted on their foreheads by experimenters.

From these humble evolutionary beginnings, we humans have developed elaborate mental machinery for representing our own internal states. And again, the prefrontal cortex is implicated in this process. When subjects are asked to focus on their own mental states, and not on external reality, medial prefrontal cortex lights up.[48] Both the internal representation of one's own mental states and the internal representations of the mental states of others rely on the frontal lobes. And so the complex, coordinated neural computations integrate and interweave the mental representations of "self" and "others." Truly, the prefrontal cortex is the closest there is to the neural substrate of social being.

That the capacity for self–nonself differentiation should depend on the frontal lobes comes as no surprise. As we have established before, the prefrontal cortex is the only part of the brain, and certainly of the neocortex, where information about the organism's internal environment converges with information about the world outside. The prefrontal cortex is the only part of the brain with the neural machinery capable of integrating the two sources of data.

But how capable is it? How precisely does the emergence of this ability parallel the development of the frontal lobes? How closely does the development of this cognitive capability follow the emergence of its putative neural substrate? Is the development of self–nonself differentiation solely a function of frontal lobe emergence in evolution, or did it also require the emergence of certain conceptual structures incrementally externalized in the culture? In *The Origins of Consciousness and the Breakdown of the Bicameral Brain*, Julian Jaynes proposed that self-consciousness emerged rather late in human cultural evolution, possibly as late as in the second millennium B.C.E.[49]

I also suspect that many enduring cultural beliefs (which, as a scientist, I tend to regard as supernatural), including religious beliefs, are vestiges of early humans' inability to recognize their own internal representations of other people as part of "self" rather than of "nonself." Rich sensory images of other persons, and even one's own thought processes, would be interpreted as "spirits." A rich sensory memory of a deceased tribesman would be interpreted as the tribesman's "ghost" or as evidence of the tribesman's "life after death." According to this scenario, some of the more literal religious and magical beliefs, which persisted for millennia, are vestiges of early humans' inability to distinguish between one's own memories of other people (internal representations, parts of "self") and those actual people themselves ("nonselves," others). This may have been precisely what Jaynes[50] refers to as the "hallucinatory experiences" of ancient humans. A careful cross-cultural investigation of cognitive self–nonself differentiation involving the few remaining relatively "primitive" cultures (e.g., Indian tribes of the Amazon, and Papua-New Guinea and Irian Jaya highlanders) could be particularly illuminating in this regard.

According to Jaynes, the self–nonself confusion was not confined to prehistoric times. It extended well into the early history populated by individuals we assume to be neurobiologically "modern." If this is so, then one of two possibilities (or a combination of the two) must be considered. The first is that the biological evolution of the frontal lobes is not in and of itself sufficient for the completion of cognitive self–nonself differentiation and some additional, cumulative cultural effect is required, as Jaynes suggests. The second possibility is that the biological evolution of the frontal lobes extended later into history than our established evolutionary assumptions would have it. The humanization of the great ape may have taken even longer than we thought.

10

When the Leader Is Wounded

The Fragile Frontal Lobes

The definition of disease changes over time. Classic neuropsychology was concerned with the effects of brain lesions (bullet wounds, strokes, and tumors) on cognition. This was the knowledge base on which our understanding of brain function was built. Gradually, the scope of neuropsychology has expanded, and today there are more neuropsychologists employed in psychiatric and geriatric settings than on traditional neurology services.

The expansion of neuropsychology reflects the expansion of the definition of brain disease. This, in turn, is a consequence of our society becoming more enlightened, more affluent, and, our occasional misgivings notwithstanding, on the whole more humane. In the old days, it was considered normal that by a certain age people would start "losing their marbles." Today we know that this is not part of normal aging but rather a consequence of distinct brain disorders, such as Alzheimer's disease. In the old days, a poor learner was scolded by his parents, and an unruly pupil was flogged. Today we know about learning disabilities and attention deficit disorder.

I recall my first faculty position in the United States in the late 1970s at one of the most prestigious Ivy League departments of psychiatry. Clinical conferences were replete with endless debates over whether a particular patient was "schizophrenic" or "organic," *organic* meaning suffering a dysfunction of the brain. The old Cartesian distinction between the body and the soul, which had fooled the general public for so many years, had permeated psychiatry as well.

Today we know that schizophrenia is organic, since both biochemical and structural abnormalities have been discovered in the patients' brains. This is also true for depression, obsessive-compulsive disorder, attention deficit disorder, Tourette's syndrome, and other conditions. The distinction between "diseases of the brain" and "diseases of the soul" is becoming increasingly blurred. The ailments of the "soul" are understood increasingly as diseases of the brain. "Descartes' error," to use Antonio Damasio's elegant phrase,[1] is finally being corrected.

As we continue to discover the neural basis of diseases previously thought to be in the soul department, the extreme degree of frontal lobe involvement in virtually all of these conditions becomes increasingly apparent. This involvement speaks to a particular biological vulnerability of the frontal lobes. Indeed, frontal lobe dysfunction often reflects more than direct damage to the frontal lobes.[2]

The frontal lobes appear to be the bottleneck, the point of convergence of the effects of damage virtually anywhere in the brain.[3] Considering the military analogy, this should not come as a surprise. Injury to the leader will disrupt the activities of many units in the field, producing remote effects. Equally, the functions of leadership will be disrupted if the lines of communication from the front to the leader are cut off.

Damage to the frontal lobes produces wide ripple effects through the whole brain. At the same time, damage anywhere in the brain sets off ripple effects interfering with frontal lobe function. This unique feature reflects the role of the frontal lobes as the "nerve center" of the nervous system, with a singularly rich set of connections to and from other brain structures.

The unique sensitivity of the frontal lobes to brain disease can be demonstrated in a number of ways. Swedish neuroscientists Asa Lilja and Jarl Risberg studied the patterns of regional cerebral blood flow (rCBF) disruption caused by brain tumors.[4] To their surprise, they found the blood flow particularly disrupted in the frontal lobes regardless of tumor location. This was true even if the tumor itself was as far away from the frontal lobes as possible without leaving the cranium, so to speak.

Scientists at the New York State Psychiatric Institute studied regional blood flow patterns in patients with depression.[5] Disruption of blood flow was most pronounced in the frontal lobes, despite the fact that serotonin (a major neurotransmitter whose deficiency is presumed to be responsible for depression) is ubiquitous in the brain, without showing any particular frontal lobe preponderance. In Sweden, Risberg studied the transient effects of electroconvulsive therapy (ECT) on regional cerebral blood flow.[6] Again, most disruption was found in the frontal lobes even though the electrodes through which the current was delivered to the brain were applied to the temporal lobes.

In another study conducted at the New York State Psychiatric Institute, healthy volunteers were given scopolamine, a chemical substance interfering with the action of acetylcholine, one of the main neurotransmitters in the brain.[7] Scopolamine was given to create an experimental simulation of memory disorders in Alzheimer's disease. (The rationale for the experiment was based on the assumption that cholinergic transmission is particularly affected in Alzheimer's disease.) Again, the greatest disruption of regional cerebral blood flow was observed in the frontal lobes—despite the fact that unlike some other neurotransmitters, acetylcholine is not exceptionally prevalent in the frontal lobes.

Working at the New York University Aging and Dementia Center, my colleagues and I have shown that frontal lobes become dysfunctional at a very early stage of Alzheimer's type dementia.[8] This is expressed as an inability to make decisions in ambiguous situations. Given the ambiguous nature of most real-life situations, the loss of this ability is fraught with particularly devastating consequences.

But cognitive changes occur in normal aging as well. It is not uncommon for people in their 60s and 70s to notice that their memory is not quite as sharp as it used to be. What most people fail to realize is that the so-called normal age-related changes affect the functions of the frontal lobes as much as they affect memory.

To conclude, the frontal lobes are more vulnerable and are affected in a broader range of brain disorders—neurodevelopmental, neuropsychiatric, neurogeriatric, and so on—than any other part of the brain. The frontal lobes have an exceptionally low "functional breakdown threshold." This led me many years ago to conclude that frontal lobe dysfunction is to brain disease what fever is to bacterial infection; it is both highly predictable and often nonspecific.[9] Hughlings Jackson understood this very well when he introduced his law of "evolution and dissolution."[10] According to this law, the phylogenetically youngest brain structures are the first to succumb to brain disease. But I believe that the frontal lobes' unique vulnerability is the price they pay for the exceptional richness of their connections. The "noise summation" effect, the aggregation of faulty signals that probably take place in the prefrontal cortex following diffuse brain damage, can be demonstrated computationally. In fact, I designed a mathematical demonstration of this effect in collaboration with Yelena Artemyeva at the University of Moscow in the late 1960s using John von Neumann's parallel low-reliability automata as the model. The clinical corollary of this conclusion is that frontal lobe dysfunction does not always signify a frontal lobe lesion—in most instances it probably does not. Instead, it is a remote effect of a diffuse, distributed, or distant lesion.

Frontal Lobe Syndromes

Consider the sequence of events required for every purposeful behavior. First, behavior must be initiated. Second, the objective must be identified, the goal of action formulated. Third, a plan of action must be forged according to the goal. Fourth, the means by which the plan can be accomplished must be selected in a proper temporal sequence. Fifth, the various steps of the plan must be executed in an appropriate order with a smooth transition from step to step. Finally, a comparison must be made between the objective and the outcome of the action: does the outcome correspond to the objective? Is it "mission accomplished" or "mission failed"? If "failed," then by how much and in which aspect of the task? In a nutshell, these are the functions of the executive in charge of the workings of an organization. These are also the functions of the frontal lobes. This is why the frontal lobe functions are often called "executive functions."

The importance of executive functions can be best appreciated through analysis of their disintegration following brain damage. A patient with damaged frontal lobes retains, at least to a certain degree, the ability to exercise most cognitive skills in isolation.[11] The basic abilities, such as reading, writing, simple computations, verbal expression, and movements, remain largely unimpaired. Deceptively, the patient will perform well on the psychological tests measuring these functions in isolation. However, any synthetic activity requiring the coordination of many cognitive skills into a coherent, goal-directed process will become severely impaired.

But even a cursory review of frontal lobe neuroanatomy suggests their tremendous complexity, which in turn suggests a functional diversity of each distinct part. And indeed, damage to different parts of the frontal lobes produces distinct, clinically rather different syndromes. The most common among them are the *dorsolateral* and *orbitofrontal* syndromes.[12]

In early neurological literature the dorsolateral syndrome was known as "pseudodepression," alluding to the similarity of some frontal lobe patients to depressed patients. In both conditions extreme inertia and inability to initiate behaviors is present, sometimes to a high degree. A patient with a severe dorsolateral frontal syndrome will lie passively in bed, not eating, drinking, or attending to any other needs. He will fail to respond readily to any attempt to engage him in any activity. He will look somewhat like a patient with severe depression. But the similarity ends here. A depressed patient has a sad mood and a sense of pervasive misery, but a dorsolateral frontal patient has a flat affect and sense of indifference. The patient with dorsolateral frontal lesion is neither sad nor happy; in a sense, he has no mood. No matter what happens to the patient, good things or bad things, this state of indifference will persist.

The indifference of dorsolateral frontal patients is sometimes so extreme that it reduces their response to pain. Most people have heard about frontal lobotomy, a neurosurgical procedure severing the connections between the frontal lobes and the rest of the brain.[13] Introduced in 1935 by a Portuguese physician, Egas Moniz,[14] frontal lobotomy had its heyday in the United States in the 1940s and 1950s and has since been discredited and largely abandoned. For better or worse, it was used most often to treat psychosis. It was also used, however, to treat intractable pain, a rare condition of extreme suffering unresponsive to medications.

Frontal lobotomy, or a related procedure called *cingulotomy*, "cured" such patients, permanently or temporarily, from the subjective feeling of suffering, but not from the physical sensation of pain.[15] Bizarrely, they continued to report their sensation in terms virtually identical to those used before the surgery. But what was once the source of unbearable suffering was now met with utter indifference. The patients were no longer bothered by pain, despite its persistent presence.

Robert Iacono, a neurosurgeon from southern California, brought to my attention the case of a patient suffering from excruciating and debilitating rectal pain along with depression, sleep disturbance, and morphine addiction. Following cingulotomy, the patient no longer initiated complaints about pain, even though she continued to complain about pain when asked. For the first time in many months she appeared relaxed. The family was astonished at her personality change from extremely demanding to eerily compliant. During the next few weeks the patient's sleep notably improved and she voiced considerably fewer spontaneous complaints. She also became highly suggestible.[16]

The observation is extremely interesting, since it informs us both about the frontal lobes and about the mechanisms of pain. The sensory experience alone is not sufficient to produce the subjective feeling of suffering. A higher-order interpretative process is required, which appears to be somehow linked to the frontal lobes and the anterior cingulate cortex. Frontal lobotomy "cured" pain by producing the dorsolateral frontal lobe syndrome in the patient. As will be made clear by the following discussion, the price of such a cure is very high.

Recent functional neuroimaging studies have shown, for instance, that the expectation of pain activates the medial frontal lobe regions.[17,18] When the signal about the aversive sensory experience fails to reach the frontal lobes, the experience fails to cause the subjective, affective sense of suffering. The role of the frontal lobes in modifying the sensory experience of pain was further studied by Tor Wager and his colleagues, who examined the mechanisms of placebo.[19] With the introduction of effective placebo, activation in the regions comprising the so-called pain matrix (the thalamus, insula, and the cingulate cortex) was reduced, and activation in the prefrontal cortex (both dorsolateral and orbital) was increased. Interestingly, activation was also increased in the periaqueductal gray of the brain stem. This finding suggests a tripartite process: the prefrontal cortex impacting the brain stem regions linked to the opiate release, which in turn act on the "pain matrix," dulling it.[20]

As already mentioned, the role of the prefrontal cortex and cingulate cortex in the higher-order interpretative aspect of pain was demonstrated in two ingenious studies of suffering that was social, rather than physical, in nature. Tania Singer and her colleagues examined the mechanisms of empathy in someone observing pain inflicted on another person. They found that the rostral parts of the anterior cingulate, as well as the anterior insula, were activated in observing pain even in the absence of the sensory experience itself.[21] Naomi Eisenberg and her colleagues studied the effects of social exclusion in a computer videogame. The extent of distress caused by exclusion from the game was positively correlated with the extent of anterior cingulate activation and negatively correlated with the right ventral preforntal cortex. The study implicates both structures in the mediation of social distress and points to their respective roles. It appears that the right ventral prefrontal cortex moderates social distress by controlling the anterior cingulate cortex.[22]

Drive and Newtonian Bodies: A Dorsolateral Case Study

Vladimir was a promising engineering student in Moscow in his mid-20s. One day, he was standing on the platform of the Moscow subway, the famous, bombastically imposing "metro," Stalin's great pyramid built with the labor of Gulag slaves. When the soccer ball Vladimir was tossing around fell on the rails, he jumped down to get it. He was hit by an approaching train, suffered severe head injury, and was rushed to the Bourdenko Institute of Neurosurgery, where I did my research at the time under Luria's supervision. I first encountered Vladimir 2 or 3 months after his injury. By that time, Vladimir was medically stable, his life no longer in danger.

Vladimir was particularly interesting because, as a result of his injury, he had to undergo surgical resection of both frontal poles. At the time, Luria was becoming increasingly interested in the frontal lobes and I, the youngest among his immediate entourage, was unattached to any particular project. So the frontal lobes became my project and Vladimir became "my" patient. Conveniently, I was one of the few males on Luria's largely female staff and thus could be relied on to deal with Vladimir's clinical antics.

The career of every clinician is punctuated by a few formative cases. Vladimir was my first such case. Unwittingly, through his tragedy, he introduced me to the rich phenomena of frontal lobe disease, triggered my interest in the frontal lobes, and thus helped shape my career. We were roughly the same age, in our 20s; he was a few years older.

Vladimir spent most of his time in bed staring blankly into space. He ignored most attempts to engage him in any kind of activity. Persistent attempts could provoke a trickle of profanities, and a particularly vigorous intruder ran the risk of being hit with a chamber pot. Occasionally attracted by something in his environment, Vladimir attempted to get out of bed, but the bed was surrounded with a protective net.

The nurses would call on me to help coax Vladimir out of bed to go for a medical procedure or to give him an injection (the surest way to encounter

Vladimir's chamber pot). I reasoned with Vladimir in a casually profane, locker room–style banter, and it usually had a calming effect. A friendship of sorts developed between a brain-damaged student and a student of brain damage. As a result, I was able to engage Vladimir in all kinds of little bedside experiments with relative ease, despite his general inertia. He would follow my instructions in a detached, stone-faced, zombie-like fashion.

To most of us the word *drive* connotes a certain personality trait, one particularly valued in our achievement-oriented society. We associate drive with accomplishment, competition, success, winning spirit. A person without drive is perceived as a loser unworthy of respect, almost an anomaly in our competitive culture. To most people, drive is a highly desirable social trait, a virtual sine qua non.

Like most human traits, drive has a biological basis. The frontal lobes are central to the maintenance of drive. I like to compare patients with dorsolateral frontal lobe disease to bodies in Newtonian physics. To set in motion a body in classical Newtonian mechanics, an application of external force is required. Likewise, external force is required to terminate motion or to set it on a new course. In an odd way, patients with dorsolateral frontal damage behave like Newtonian objects. The most conspicuous feature of their behavior is an inability to initiate any behavior. Once engaged in a behavior, however, the patient is equally unable to terminate or change it on his own.

Vladimir's inertia, so striking in his everyday behavior (or lack thereof), could also be elicited experimentally. Asked to draw a cross, he would first ignore the instruction. I had to lift his hand with mine, place it on the page, and give it a little push, and only then would he start drawing. But having started, he could not stop and continued to draw little crosses until I took his hand in mine and lifted it off the page (Fig. 10.1). Such combined inertia of initiation and termination is seen in various disorders affecting the frontal lobes, including chronic schizophrenia.

I was first struck by the combined presentation of the inertia of initiation and inertia of termination while studying patients with frontal lobe damage under Luria's tutelage in Moscow in the late 1960s. Their similarity and near-perfect correlation in patients suggested shared mechanisms, even though no direct evidence of the existence of such shared mechanisms was available at the time. More recently,

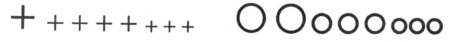

"draw a cross"   "draw a circle"

Figure 10.1 Frontal-lobe patient as a Newtonian body. A patient is asked to draw a cross. It takes a long time to entice him to do so, but once started he is unable to terminate his activity and keeps drawing crosses. At a later point he is asked to draw a circle and the cycle repeats itself. [Adapted from Goldberg and Costa (1985).[12] Reprinted with permission.]

Fujii and Graybiel discovered "sequence-bounding" bursts of spiking activity in the macaque's prefrontal neurons.[23] These neurons burst into action in the beginning and in the end of a motor sequence, thus delineating its proper initiation and termination. The breakdown of this frontal lobe machinery, which in all probability exists in humans as well, is likely to be responsible both for the initiation and termination difficulties and for perseveration.

But back to Vladimir. When the task was to listen to a story and then recall it, Vladimir would start slowly and then carry on in a monotonous voice. He would go on and on and when asked to finish, he would say, "Not yet." The never-ending monologue was an expression of "reverse inertia," an inability to terminate activity.

I asked Vladimir to listen to a simple children's story, "A Lion and a Mouse," and then recall it. The story goes as follows:

A lion was asleep and a mouse was running around him making noises. The lion woke up, caught the mouse, and was about to eat him up, but then decided to show mercy and let the mouse go. A few days later, hunters caught the lion and tied him to a tree with ropes. The mouse learned about it, ran down, gnawed the ropes and set the lion free.

This is how Vladimir recalled the story:

So the lion made friends with the mouse. The mouse was caught by the lion. He wanted to strangle him but then let him go. The mouse started dancing around him, singing songs, and was released. After that the mouse was accepted in his house by . . . lions, various animals. After that he was released, so to speak, he hadn't been captured, he was still free. But after that he was completely released and was walking free.

At this point I asked: "Are you finished?" But Vladimir said, "Not yet," and carried on:

So, he was released by the lion completely, after the lion listened to him, and he was released to go to all the four directions. He didn't run away and remained to live in his cave. Then the lion caught him again, some time later. . . . I don't remember it exactly. So he caught him and released him again. Now the mouse got out of there and went to his hangout, to his pad. The mouse goes on and on and talks about his pad. And there is another mouse there. So the mouse opens the door to this . . . what do you call it? Hi! Hi! How are you doing! OK, more or less. I am all set. Glad to see you. I have an apartment . . . and a house . . . and a room. The bigger mouse asks the smaller one: How are you doing? How is it coming along?

I say: "You better finish." But Vladimir again says, "Not yet!" and continues:

So it was all right. I had a lot of friends. They often get together . . . but the friendship broke up, so tell him that I miss these brief get-togethers.

Vladimir continued his monologue until I turned off the tape-recorder and left.

Vladimir's inertia, both the inertia of initiation and that of termination, was pervasive. It was evident both in his drawings and in his verbal output. The pervasive nature of inertia is typical in dorsolateral frontal lobe syndrome.

Vladimir's case was extreme. But following even mild head trauma, it is common for the patient to become indifferent and devoid of initiative and drive. The change may be subtle, and it is not always apparent to family members or even doctors that the change is neurological in nature, that it is a mild form of the frontal lobe syndrome. These symptoms are often called "personality change," but "personality" is not an extracranial attribute of a person, carried on our skin. Our personality is determined to a large extent by our neurobiology, and personality disorders, unlike skin disease, are caused by changes in the brain. The frontal lobes have more to do with our "personalities" than any other part of the brain, and frontal lobe damage produces profound personality change.

A subtle decrease in drive, initiative, and interest in the world around is also a common early sign of dementia. In popular folklore, early signs of dementia are associated with memory loss first and foremost. In reality, however, subtle frontal lobe dysfunction is as common. As I point out in Chapter 7, the tendency to misdiagnose the symptoms of frontal lobe dysfunction as "depression" has very likely resulted in the underestimation of the degree of frontal lobe involvement in dementias and to a skewed epidemiological picture. In reality, just as depression may masquerade as dementia producing so-called pseudodementia, so, too, is the opposite possible: dementia with frontal lobe involvement may masquerade as depression producing "pseudodepression." While the mental health and gerontological communities are very familiar with the concept of "pseudodementia," the concept of "pseudodepression" is not nearly as widely known, this resulting in a systematic diagnostic bias.[24]

The degree to which frontal lobe symptoms can be elusive to the uninitiated eye becomes clear from the example of Jane, a woman in her late 50s, referred to me for a second opinion. A few years earlier, Jane had developed tremors and was promptly referred to one of the best movement disorders clinics in town. The diagnosis of Parkinson's disease was promptly made and Jane was put on Sinemet, a dopamine-enhancing medication commonly used in these circumstances. But gradually a cognitive impairment became noticeable, affecting her memory, attention, and judgment. When her family members brought this to the doctors' attention, they were not particularly concerned and changed the Sinemet dosage. Contrary to their expectations, Jane's cognition did not improve; it continued to deteriorate. She then lapsed into a psychotic episode, running up and down the block undressed, screaming that her neighbors were setting the building on fire. Other psychotic episodes followed, mostly with paranoid overtones. There was also some suggestion of hallucinations.

At this point, Jane's tremors were the least of her family's concerns, and they kept pleading with the doctors to do something about the cognitive impairment and psychosis. But the doctors just continued to adjust the Sinemet doses. They obviously assumed that the psychosis and the memory loss were side effects of the medication. But there was no improvement and things were getting out of hand. Finally, the exasperated family decided to seek another opinion, as it happened, from me.

The history of Jane's illness was recounted to me by her husband, a lucid, educated, and caring man in his early 60s, a senior executive. The story had the telltale ring of Lewy body disease, a lesser-known dementia with a clinical course often actually more malignant than in Alzheimer's disease. Jane was taken off Sinemet and put on Cognex, a cholinergic enhancer, and a slight improvement was noted.

Becoming increasingly convinced that Jane indeed suffered from Lewy body disease, I decided to probe her husband a little more about the very early disease stage. As a result, a strikingly different clinical picture emerged. As it turned out, Jane's husband had left out a very significant feature of Jane's condition. At least a year prior to the first appearance of the tremors and possibly even earlier, a subtle change in Jane's personality had become increasingly apparent. Always vivacious and sociable, a great entertainer who put a lot of energy and gusto into her social life, Jane began to withdraw.

Uncharacteristically, she began to refuse to go out, preferring to stay at home. She stopped entertaining, saying that she had no energy or interest. Jane's husband had noticed the change and responded with a mixture of concern and annoyance. But it simply did not occur to this highly intelligent and devoted man that the changes in his wife's personality signaled a clinical disorder. Had this thought crossed his mind, the whole process of Jane's treatment would have taken a different course from the beginning. It was obvious to me that Jane's "personality change" reflected the involvement of her frontal lobes at the earliest stage of the disease, well before the tremors or anything else.

Plans and "Memories of the Future"

In 1985 David Ingvar, a Swedish psychiatrist and neuroscientist, coined a phrase both poetic and implausible: "memory of the future."[25] What is a memory of the future? Memories are supposed to be about the past.

The confusion is resolved when we consider one of the most important functions of advanced organisms: making plans and then following the plans to guide behavior. Unlike primitive organisms, humans are active, rather than reactive, beings. The transition from mostly reactive to mostly proactive behavior is probably the central theme of the evolution of the nervous system. We are able to form goals, our visions of the future. Then we act according to our goals. But to guide our behavior in a sustained fashion, these mental images of the future must become the content of our memory; thus the memories of the future are formed.

The role of the prefrontal cortex in forming predictions about the future appears to be ubiquitous across tasks and time scales. On one end of this continuum are the "top-down" expectations that guide our visual perception in real time.[26] On the other end are projections into the future inherent in complex economic decisions. As already discussed, the brain mechanisms of planning and of the ability to project into the future are of great interest in the context of several new applications of neuroscience, including neuroeconomics. How do humans make complex decisions, about their personal finances and of strategic importance to national and global economic systems? Here, the role of the frontal lobes has been highlighted in several studies. Samuel McClure and colleagues demonstrated the difference between neural substrates mediating decisions concerning immediate vs. delayed monetary rewards (see Chapter 7). Decisions concerning immediately available monetary rewards activate mostly the brain stem and limbic structures. By contrast, decisions about rewards potentially available in the future activate mostly the neocortical structures, particularly the prefrontal cortical regions, those found on both the frontal convexity (dorsolateral and ventrolateral) and the orbitofrontal cortex.[27]

Interestingly, a vaguely comparable study in the rat has yielded very different results: impulsive choice of a poor immediate reward over a larger but delayed reward was caused by damage to the subcortical, limbic nucleus accumbens, whereas damage to the anterior cingulate and medial prefrontal cortex did not produce such impulsivity.[28] Further research may clarify whether the differences between the results of these two studies reflect certain profound changes in the mechanisms of executive control in the course of mammalian evolution or whether they simply reflect some differences in the two experimental paradigms.

We anticipate the future on the basis of our past experiences and act according to our anticipations. The ability to organize behavior in time and to extrapolate in time is also the responsibility of the frontal lobes. Whether you have good foresight and planning ability or fly by the seat of your pants depends on how well your frontal lobes work. Patients with frontal lobe damage are notorious for their inability to plan and to anticipate the consequences of their actions. Damage to other parts of the brain does not seem to affect these abilities. One of the first signs of dementia, a subtle impairment of planning and foresight, is also present in other conditions, usually reflecting frontal lobe dysfunction.

A simple experiment illustrates Vladimir's severely impaired ability to follow plans. I asked Vladimir to listen to a story, "A Hen and Golden Eggs," and then recite it from memory. The story goes as follows:

> A man owned a hen that was laying golden eggs. The man was greedy and wanted to get more gold at once. He killed the hen and cut it open hoping to find a lot of gold inside, but there was none.

Vladimir repeated the story as follows:

> A man was living with a hen . . . or rather the man was the hen's owner. She was producing gold. . . . The man . . . the owner wanted more gold at once . . . so he cut the hen into pieces but there was no gold. . . . No gold at all . . . he cuts the hen more . . . no gold . . . the hen remains empty. . . . So he searches again and again. . . . No gold . . . he searches all around in all places. . . . The search is going on with a tape-recorder . . . they are looking here and there, nothing new around. They leave the tape-recorder turned on, something is spinning there. . . . What the hell are they recording there . . . some digits . . . 0, 2, 3, 0 . . .

so they are recording all these digits . . . not very many of them. . . . That's why all the other digits were recorded . . . turned out to be not very many of them either . . . so, everything was recorded [monologue continues].[29]

The sheer length of Vladimir's monologue is out of proportion to the original story, showing his inability to terminate an activity—the inertia in reverse. He also perseverates, as he continues to rehash the phrases and themes of the story. But at a certain point new content is introduced, a spinning tape-recorder. All of a sudden, Vladimir's story is a complete non sequitur: it is no longer about the golden eggs, but about a tape-recorder.

The explanation for this strange behavior lies in the environment. I am sitting in front of Vladimir with a portable tape-recorder on my lap, taping the very monologue that we are discussing here. Vladimir's task is to recall the story. The tape-recorder is completely incidental to this task. But its mere presence in the environment is sufficient to derail Vladimir's ability to follow the task at hand. Instead of being guided by the plan of action, Vladimir merely recites what he sees in front of him: the spinning and blinking of the tape-recorder. His train of thought is hopelessly lost and no longer bears any relation to the task at hand. He is unable to recapture the lost train of thought and continues to engage in his "field-dependent" digression.

Being at the mercy of incidental distractions and displaying an inability to follow plans are common features of frontal lobe disease. This is known as *field-dependent behavior*. A frontal lobe patient will drink from an empty cup, put on a jacket belonging to someone else, or scribble with a pencil on the table surface, merely because the cup, the jacket, and the pencil are there, even though these actions make no sense. This phenomenon was studied extensively by the French neurologist François Lhermitte, who called it "utilization behavior."[30]

I recall the indignation of the nurses on the university hospital neurology service where I used to consult many years ago. A few patients on the unit invariably kept wandering into the other patients' rooms, inciting the wrath of the nurses, who accused the patients of every conceivable malicious intent. The reality was much simpler and sadder. The wandering patients were entering through the doors just because the doors were there. They were patients with frontal lobe damage suffering from field-dependent behavior.

In the most extreme cases, field-dependent behavior takes the form of direct imitation, called "echolalia" (imitation of speech) or "echopraxia" (imitation of action). Instead of answering a question (an act requiring the formation of an internal plan) the patient merely repeats the question or incorporates the question into the answer. When asked "What is your name?" Vladimir would sometimes say: "What is my name Vladimir." Other patients imitate the doctor's actions: if I pick up a pen to write a chart note, the patient will pick up another pen and begin to scribble. Like other symptoms, echo behaviors may take subtle forms in naturalistic environments. On numerous occasions I would catch myself, in the middle of interviewing a patient, doing something entirely unrelated: scratching my nose or adjusting my glasses. The next thing I would notice is the patient engaging in the same unrelated act.

Field-dependent behavior is a complex phenomenon, which may take many forms. Sometimes field-dependent behavior is driven by external stimuli in the outside world, and sometimes it is driven by internal out-of-context associations. As we follow Vladimir's narrative, it takes a turn that finds no ready explanation in the external environment. Following the mention of the tape-recorder and of number 5 "spinning there," Vladimir begins to describe the route of city bus number 5 in downtown Moscow. This is also field-dependent behavior, but now the distractor is found not in the world outside but among the internal associations in Vladimir's own memory. Thus the ability of a frontal lobe patient to stay mentally on course can be disrupted by both external and internal distractors.

Vladimir talks on and on in a monotonous, detached tone of voice. His tale spins by itself, through no apparent mental effort or intentional contribution on his part, one association or external stimulus leading to another. Finally I turn off the tape-recorder and begin to leave. Vladimir continues to ramble for a few more minutes and finally stops.

As noted earlier, Vladimir's ability to act according to an internal plan is severely impaired. But in many cases this deficit takes very subtle forms, not apparent through simple observation and requiring special tests to detect. One such test is known as the Stroop Test, after the name of its inventor.[31] Here the subject is asked to look at a list of color names printed in discordant colors (e.g., word "red" printed in blue or the other way around) and to name the colors, instead of reading the words.

What makes the Stroop Test so interesting? It requires that you contravene your immediate impulse. The impulse is to read the words; this is the natural tendency of every literate person on seeing written material. But the task is to name the colors. To successfully complete the task, you must follow the internal plan, the task, *against your natural, entrenched tendency.*

Most of us can exercise the ability to guide behavior by internal representation so effortlessly that we take it for granted. Bombarded by a myriad of incidental external stimuli and unrelated internal associations, we nonetheless stay on the "mental course" with ease, until the task is brought to successful conclusion. But trivial as it may appear, this ability arises relatively late in evolution.

The capacity to respond to external stimuli is the first attribute of a primitive brain. In an environment rich with events, however, such a primitive brain will be immediately overwhelmed by a plethora of random distractors. In a more complex brain, this will be balanced by a mechanism protecting the organism from the chaos of randomness and allowing it to stay on track in pursuing a particular behavior. Evolution of the brain is characterized by the slow, painstaking transition from a brain simply reacting to a brain capable of sustained, deliberate action.

Saying that life is full of distractions is so obvious it is almost cliché. However, the ability to stay on a course charted by an internal plan, a "memory of the future," arises quite late in evolution, as does the capacity for sustained attention. Their advent parallels the development of the frontal lobes.

Most of us have had encounters with a canine, or simply a dog. Suppose a dog is exploring an object when there is a distracting noise. This causes the dog to turn its head away from the object, toward the source of noise. Unless the object is food, the chances that the dog will go back to exploring the same object after the interruption are slim to nonexistent. This does not mean that the dog failed to form an internal representation of the object, since on subsequent encounters it will exhibit familiarity with the object. It does mean, however, that the mental representation fails to exert an effective control over canine behavior. One of the most prominent students of the frontal lobes, Patricia Goldman-Rakic of Yale University, referred to this "afrontal" behavior as "out of sight, out of mind."[32]

There were always dogs in our household when I was growing up, and I can generally anticipate and "understand" their behavior to the extent that a middle-aged Manhattan intellectual can. But nothing in my canine encounters prepared me for my first truly interactive experience with an ape, albeit a "lesser" ape. As we shall see, an ape's behavior is strikingly different from that of a canine in response to a distractor.

While on vacation in Phuket, an island off the coast of southern Thailand, a number of years ago, I was befriended by a young black male gibbon from Laos, a pet of the owners of a restaurant next to my hotel. For about a week, I spent a few hours with him every day. Every morning the gibbon rushed forth to shake hands. All limbs and a small body, he would then engage in a brief spiderlike dance, which, in my self-flattering way, I interpreted as an expression of joy at seeing me. But then, despite his proclivity for restless play, he would settle next to me and with extreme concentration would study the minute details of my clothes: a watch-band, a button, a shoe, my glasses (which, in one of my unguarded moments, he took off my face and tried for lunch). He stared at the items intently and systematically shifted his gaze from one detail to another. When one day a bandage appeared around my index finger, the young gibbon studiously examined it. Despite his status of a lesser ape (in contrast to the bonobos, chimpanzees, gorillas, and orangutans, which are known as the great apes), the gibbon was capable of sustained attention.

Most remarkably, the gibbon invariably turned back to the object of his curiosity following a sudden distraction, say, a street noise. He would resume his exploration precisely where it had been interrupted, even when the interruption was more than a split second in length. The gibbon's actions were guided by an internal representation, which "bridged" his behavior between before and after the distraction. "Out of sight" was no longer "out of mind." My neuroscientific preconceptions aside, as a past owner of several dogs and as a lifelong dog lover, I can vouch that this behavior was utterly uncanine. Not surprisingly, the canine frontal lobes account for approximately 7% of the total cortex, whereas in the gibbon it is 11.5%.[33]

The interaction with the gibbon was so qualitatively different from, and so strikingly richer than, anything I had ever experienced with dogs, that I briefly entertained the idea of buying the gibbon and bringing him to New York to be my pet and companion. The restaurateurs were game and the price was discussed. But in the end, sanity prevailed and I returned to my fiftieth-floor midtown Manhattan apartment alone.

In humans, the capacity for "staying on track" takes on an even more complex dimension. Not only can we stay on track in attending to external objects, but we can also stay on track with respect to our own thoughts, not allowing random associations to derail our thought processes from their course. The canines, lesser apes, and humans (*Homo sapiens sapiens*) do not represent successive stages on the same branch of the evolutionary tree. Nonetheless, they can be used as examples of different levels of development of the frontal lobes and of the correlation between frontal lobe development and the capacity for guiding behavior by internal representations, "the memories of the future."

When neurological illness affects the frontal lobes, the ability to stay on track becomes lost, and the patient is completely at the mercy of incidental environmental stimuli and tangential internal associations. It does not take much imagination to see how disruptive this disability can be. Easy distractability is a feature of many neurological and psychiatric disorders, and it is usually associated with frontal lobe dysfunction. As we will see later, attention deficit hyperactivity disorder (ADHD), with its extreme distractability, is usually linked to frontal lobe dysfunction.[34]

In psychiatry, susceptibility of thought processes to irrelevant associations has long been termed "tangentiality" and "loose association." These phenomena are among the most dramatic symptoms of schizophrenia. As we will see later, this is more than a coincidence. Schizophrenia is now regarded as a form of frontal lobe disease.

And then there is the everyday distractibility of the proverbial "absent-minded professor." Are we dealing with outright frontal lobe damage or with a variation of normal cognition? In the latter case, do the individual differences related to one's mental focus correspond to the individual differences in the "normal" function of the frontal lobes? Jan de Fockert and his colleagues at the University College in London have shown that by overtaxing the prefrontal cortex, it is possible to increase distractibility even in normal subjects.[35]

Rigidity of Mind

The ability to stay on track is an asset, but being "dead in the track" is not. One may very easily deteriorate into the other if the ability to maintain mental stability is not balanced by mental flexibility. No matter how focused we are on an activity or a thought, there comes a time when the situation calls for doing something else. Being able to change one's mindset is as important as staying mentally on track.

The capacity to switch with ease from one activity or idea to another is so natural and automatic that we take it for granted. In fact, it requires complex neural machinery, which also depends on the frontal lobes. Mental flexibility, the ability to see things in a new light, creativity, and originality all depend on the frontal lobes. When the frontal lobes are damaged, a certain "stiffness of the mind" sets in, and this, too, can be a very early manifestation of dementia.

We all occasionally encounter particularly inflexible people. We call them "rigid," and based on what we have already learned, their rigidity may be a "normal" individual variation of frontal lobe functions. More profound forms of mental rigidity produce obsessive-compulsive disorder (OCD), in which the dysfunction of the caudate nuclei closely linked to the frontal lobes has been implicated.[36] But outright frontal lobe damage produces extreme mental rigidity, which may completely paralyze the patient's cognition. This becomes strikingly clear when one watches Vladimir draw simple designs. In a regularly paced voice I dictate to Vladimir the names of the shapes to be drawn: "a cross, a circle, a square," and he draws them one by one, following my instructions.

Think about what this task entails. First, Vladimir has to decide whether the task requires *drawing* the shapes or *writing* their names. Given our current knowledge of the brain, this task engages the language areas involved in the understanding of verb meaning, found immediately in front of Broca's area. Second, the meaning of the shape name has to be interpreted. This is accomplished in the left temporal lobe. Third, the image of the shape has to be accessed in long-term memory. Such images are probably stored in the temporal and parietal regions of the left hemisphere. Fourth, this image must be translated into a sequence of motor acts. This probably involves the premotor cortex. Fifth, each motor act must be executed. This is accomplished by the motor cortex. Sixth, the outcome of the action must be evaluated against the goal and the decision must be made of whether the goal has been successfully accomplished. Finally, a smooth transition must be made to the next task and the cycle must be repeated. The last two tasks, evaluation and transition, are accomplished by the prefrontal cortex itself.[37] The cortical regions involved in these tasks are outlined in Figure 10.2.

To pursue our orchestra analogy, even the seemingly simple task of drawing to dictation involves the concerted effort of several brain regions (the "players"), directed and supervised by the frontal lobes (the "conductor"). More complex behaviors require the coordinated action of far larger "ensembles"—also under the direction of the frontal lobes.

A closer look at a frontal patient's performance clarifies the relationship between the conductor and the orchestra. Complete transition from one task to another is

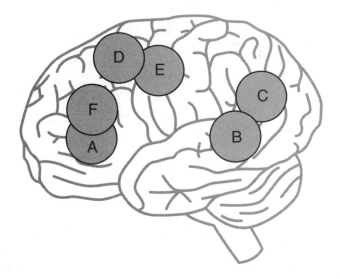

Figure 10.2 Cortical regions involved in drawing to dictation. (*A*) Selection between drawing the shapes and writing their names. This task engages the left prefrontal cortex found in front of Broca's area. (*B*) Interpreting the meaning of shape name. This is accomplished in the left temporal lobe. (*C*) Accessing the appropriate shape representation in the long-term store. It is contained in the left temporal and parietal regions. (*D*) Translating the retrieved long-term representation into a motor sequence. This involves the left premotor cortex. (*E*) Executing each motor component of the sequence. This is accomplished by the motor cortex. (*F*) Evaluating the outcome of the action against the goal and deciding if the goal has been successfully accomplished. Making a smooth transition to the next activity. The latter two tasks are accomplished by the dorsolateral prefrontal cortex.

impossible, and fragments of a previous task attach themselves to the new one, resulting in strange, hybrid designs. This phenomenon is called "perseveration." Different kinds of perseveration are depicted in Figure 10.3.

In Vladimir's brain, only the conductor, the frontal lobes, is damaged. All the players (the motor cortex, premotor cortex, and language areas in the left parietal and temporal lobes) are intact. Yet the performance of each player suffers as the result of frontal lobe damage. This is illustrated by the variety of forms that perseveration may take. Each of them reflects the failure of the frontal lobes to guide the behavior of a particular player. In other words, each type of perseveration in Figure 10.3 is caused by the breakdown of the executive control exerted by the frontal lobes over a distinct, far removed part of the cortex.

When asked to draw a circle (a loop requiring a single movement), a frontal patient keeps repeating the loop (Fig. 10.3A). This perseveration reflects the failure of the frontal lobes to guide the motor cortex.

When asked to draw a cross, a circle, and a square in sequence, the patient draws a cross and then, instead of "letting go" of it, attaches it to the circle and the

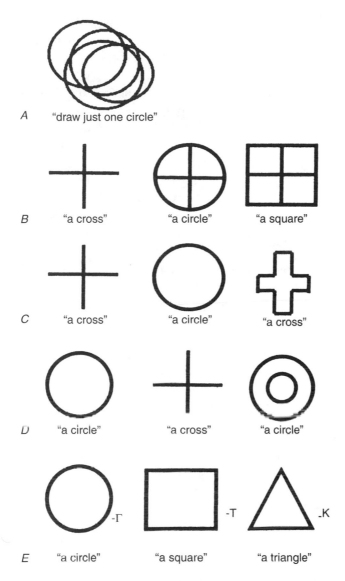

A   "draw just one circle"

B   "a cross"   "a circle"   "a square"

C   "a cross"   "a circle"   "a cross"

D   "a circle"   "a cross"   "a circle"

E   "a circle"   "a square"   "a triangle"

Figure 10.3 Types of perseveration. (A) Hyperkinetic perseveration reflects the failure of the prefrontal cortex to control motor output. (B) Perseveration of elements reflects the failure of the prefrontal cortex to control the output of premotor cortex. (C, D) Perseveration of feature reflects the failure of the prefrontal cortex to control the output of the left temporoparietal cortex. (E) Perseveration of activities reflects the dysfunction of the prefrontal cortex itself. [Adapted from Goldberg and Tucker (1979).[38] Reprinted with permission from Swets and Zeitlinger.]

square (Fig. 10.3B). Here a whole sequence of movements perseverates, rather than being a single movement. This perseveration reflects the failure of the frontal lobes to guide the premotor cortex.

On a different occasion, the task is to draw a shape, a second shape, and then the first shape again. In Figure 10.3C, the first cross and the circle are drawn correctly, but the second cross acquires the property of the intervening circle—an area. In Figure 10.3D, the first circle is drawn correctly, but the second circle acquires the property of the intervening cross, or "two-ness." These strange hybrids reflect the failure of the frontal lobes to select the mental representations of simple geometric forms stored in the temporal and parietal lobes and to complete the switch from one mental representation to the next one according to instructions.

On a different occasion, the task was to draw a circle, a square, and a triangle, all of which the patient did well. He was then asked to write his name and his age. He did that too. Then he was again asked to draw a circle, a square, and a triangle. The result was a sequence of hybrid forms—half-shapes and half-letters (Fig. 10.3E). The juxtaposition of shapes and letters was not random. Attached to each shape was the terminal letter of its Russian name. In this task, the required sequence of activities was drawing–writing–drawing. With the frontal lobes failing to guide the process, this seemingly trivial transition could no longer be smoothly executed and the intervening writing impinged on the subsequent drawing, leading to hybrid performance. These hybrids reflect the failure of the frontal lobes to guide the interpretation of the verbal instruction given to the patient.[38]

The latter examples are particularly instructive. They hint at the role of the prefrontal cortex in selecting task-appropriate specific mental representations and whole classes of mental representations. Damage to the prefrontal cortex interferes with both, as reflected in Figure 10.3C,D (specific representations) and Figure 10.3E (classes of representations). My interest in the minutae of perseveration going above and beyond the needs of clinical diagnosis was directed precisely at trying to understand the role of the prefrontal cortex in the selection and manipulation of mental representations, since the perseveration seemed to provide a unique window into the breakdown of these processes. I was so captivated by this possibility that I made it the subject of my master's thesis at the University of Moscow in the late 1960s. This was obviously before the advent of functional neuroimaging, when lesion studies was the only tool available to neuropsychologists interested in the brain mechanisms of normal cognition (the term *cognitive neuroscience* was still about 20 years away). A more direct demonstration of the role of the dorsolateral prefrontal cortex in the selection of mental representations was provided with event-related fMRI by James Rowe and colleagues at the Wellcome Department of Cognitive Neurology in London.[39] This relationship between the prefrontal cortex and the posterior association cortex, presumed to be the "storehouse" of mental representations, is not unique to humans; it was demonstrated in the macaque monkey by Hyoe Tomia and colleagues at the University of Tokyo.[40]

But back to Vladimir. Throughout the process, he was completely oblivious of his strange performance and unperturbed by its inconsistency. He remembered the task and could draw each of the shapes individually. Yet he was unable to compare the outcome of his labor to its goal.

The extreme inflexibility of mental operations evident in Vladimir's and other patients' performance is among the most devastating consequences of frontal lobe disease. In severe cases it is pervasive and disrupts the work of virtually every other system in the brain. Vladimir's mental rigidity was extreme; in more subtle forms it permeates the mental processes of patients with even "mild" head trauma, early dementia, and other conditions. In those cases, the neurological basis of the symptoms is not always apparent, the subtle change in the patient's mental processes often being attributed to "personality" or "depression," when in fact subtle damage to the frontal lobes is present.

Vladimir's impairment exemplifies the effects of frontal lobe damage very well. He could not initiate activities. Having begun them, he could not terminate them. He could not form a plan; he could not follow a plan. His behavior was at the mercy of incidental distractions, both external and internal. He could not switch from one activity or thought to the next, and his mind became stuck. When, as the result of all these difficulties, his behavior became totally disintegrated, Vladimir lacked any awareness of his impairment.

At the same time, Vladimir's language was grammatically correct, as were his articulation and choice of words. He could read, write, and draw. He could engage in simple computations. His movements were unimpaired. His basic memory was intact. The musicians were spared; the conductor was gone.

Of course, Vladimir exhibited an extreme degree of mental rigidity. Nonetheless, his example captures the mechanism of a disorder which, even in much subtler forms, may deprive mental processes of their dynamism and agility. As stated earlier, loss of mental flexibility is among the very early, and difficult-to-recognize, manifestations of dementia.

A seemingly simple test has turned out to be quite sensitive to subtle impairment of mental flexibility. The test, known as the Wisconsin Card Sorting Test,[41] requires the subject to sort cards with simple geometric forms into three categories according to a simple principle. The classification principle is not revealed in advance and the subject must establish it through trial and error. But when the principle is finally mastered it abruptly changes, unbeknownst to the subject. Once the subject catches up with the new principle, the principle is changed without forewarning again, and again, and again. The task requires planning, guidance by internal representation, mental flexibility, and working memory—in short, all the aspects of frontal lobe function discussed earlier.

Lesion studies have been instrumental in linking mental flexibility to the prefrontal cortex. Now functional neuroimaging methods allow us to attain a greater degree of neuroanatomical precision in characterizing this connection.

Nakahara and colleagues compared the patterns of activation in humans and in macaque monkeys performing a modified version of the Wisconsin Card Sorting Task. In both species posterior aspects of the ventrolateral prefrontal cortex were activated.[42]

Mind Blindspot: Anosognosia

Our success in life depends critically on two abilities: the capacity for insight into our own mental world and into that of other people. These abilities are closely interrelated, and both are under frontal lobe control. Both abilities suffer following frontal lobe damage or poor development, leading to peculiar clinical syndromes. In Chapter 9 we discussed the role of the frontal lobes in the ability to form insight into other people's minds, and how this ability suffers following damage to the frontal lobes. It is time now to consider the role of the frontal lobes in forming the insight into one's own cognitive world.

Again, Vladimir's case is very instructive. The most striking feature of Vladimir's condition was his complete unawareness of his disorder and of his drastically changed life circumstances. Vladimir suffered from *anosognosia*, a devastating condition that strips the patient of the capacity for insight into his or her own illness.[43] A patient with anosognosia may be severely impaired, yet will have no inkling of it and will continue to claim that everything is fine. This is different from being "in denial," when it is assumed that the patient has the capacity to comprehend his or her own deficit but "chooses" to look the other way. Following frontal lobe damage the cognitive capacity for insight into one's own condition is genuinely lost.

Anosognosia may take many forms. For some reason that is not fully understood, anosognosia is more common following damage to the right hemisphere than to the left hemisphere. Some scientists believe that this is because only language-mediated cognition is available for introspection, or because introspection itself is a language-based process. Therefore, according to this belief, any alteration of language-mediated cognitive processes due to brain damage would be available for introspection, and any alteration of nonverbal cognition due to brain damage would not be. This would limit the scope of introspection to left hemisphere–mediated mental processes.

I have always felt, however, that the connection of anosognosia with right but not left hemispheric lesions reflects a broader distinction between the functions of the two hemispheres.[44] The cognitive processes of the right hemisphere are less routinized, less dependent on stable codes, and involve more de novo computations. This is what makes their operational content less available to introspection, more "fuzzy" even in healthy individuals. Since the individual awareness of the right-hemispheric cognitive operations is "fuzzy" to begin with, their changes following brain damage are also less apparent.

Whatever the explanation, one patient, a successful international entrepreneur who suffered a massive right-hemispheric stroke, is unforgettable. His performance on language tasks was perfectly intact, indicating the sparing of the left hemisphere. His performance on visuospatial tasks, requiring drawing or manipulation of visual forms devoid of meaning, was devastated, indicating severe damage to the right hemisphere. He was spatially disoriented to such a degree that he was completely unable to learn the layout of my modestly sized office and kept getting lost between the examination room, the reception area, and the bathroom. Yet he insisted that he had fully recovered, that nothing was the matter with him, and that he had to immediately fly to Cairo to finalize a business deal. There was no chance that he would have gotten anywhere near Cairo. He would have become hopelessly and completely lost the moment he got out of the taxicab at Kennedy International Airport. His wife and daughter understood this very well and, to their credit, arranged for his involuntary hospital admission despite his furious protestations.

But even this degree of anosognosia pales in comparison with the clinical picture common in severe frontal lobe damage. At least the traveling entrepreneur acknowledged that he had been ill. But Vladimir did not have the slightest inkling that his life had been catastrophically and irreversibly changed by the illness. No form of anosognosia is more complete and impermeable than the one caused by severe frontal lobe damage.[45]

The mechanisms of frontal lobe anosognosia are poorly understood. In a broad sense, they probably have to do with the impaired editorial function of the frontal lobes: comparing the outcome of one's operations with one's intentions. Or they may reflect an even deeper aspect of frontal lobe disease: the fundamental loss of intentionality inherent in it. An organism with no desires, no goals, no objectives will by definition experience no sense of failure. Awareness of the deficit is the basic prerequisite of any effort on the patient's behalf to improve his or her condition. A patient with anosognosia experiences no sense of loss or deficiency, and therefore no urge to strive to correct it. Since the patient's cooperation is critical to the success of any therapeutic effort, anosognosia turns the treatment process into an uphill battle, which makes the consequences of frontal lobe disease particularly devastating.

As is the case with virtually every clinical symptom, anosognosia may take a variety of forms and be characterized by degrees of severity. Vladimir's total oblivion of his circumstances represents its most severe extreme. But it may also take much more subtle forms of the failure of monitoring one's performance and of error detection. From the standpoint of rigorous research, uncovering the brain mechanisms of self-monitoring and error detection on specific tasks is a much more tractable enterprise. Based on extensive literature review, Richard Ridderinkhof and his colleagues concluded that posterior medial frontal cortex (including the anterior cingulate cortex) is particularly important in error monitoring and detection of an unfavorable outcome of one's actions.[46] Anterior cingulate cortex appears also to be important in detecting any incongruence in the task context.[47] It somehow sends a signal to the lateral prefrontal cortex, which then adjust behavior accordingly. In the massive frontal injury suffered by Vladimir, both the medial and lateral prefrontal lesions were undoubtedly present. In less severe cases of frontal lobe pathology, subtle dissociations between the capacity for error monitoring and the discrepancy (between the desired and the actual action outcome) signal implementation may be present.

11

Social Maturity, Morality, Law, and the Frontal Lobes

Orbitofrontal "Pseudopsychopathic" Syndrome and the Loss of Self-Control

Among the myriad of anthropomorphic qualities lavished on the frontal lobes, they have been proclaimed the ultimate seat of morality. Does this mean that the underdevelopment of or damage to the frontal lobes will result in immorality? Probably not, but how about amorality?

Enter the orbitofrontal syndrome. This syndrome is in many ways the opposite of the dorsolateral syndrome. Patients with orbitofrontal syndrome are emotionally disinhibited. Their affect is rarely neutral, constantly oscillating between euphoria and rage, with impulse control ranging from poor to nonexistent. Their ability to inhibit the urge for instant gratification is severely impaired. They do what they feel like doing when they feel like doing it, without any concern for social taboos or legal prohibitions. They have no foresight of the consequences of their actions.

A patient afflicted with the orbitofrontal syndrome (due to head injury, cerebrovascular illness, or dementia) will engage in shoplifting, sexually aggressive behavior, reckless driving, or other actions commonly perceived as antisocial. These patients are known to be selfish, boastful, puerile, profane, and sexually explicit. Their humor is off-color and their jocularity, known as *Witzelsucht*, resembles that of a drunken adolescent.[1]

If dorsolateral patients are in a sense devoid of personality, then orbitofrontal patients are conspicuous for their "immature" personality. Not surprisingly, European neurological science around 1900 dubbed the orbitofrontal syndrome the "pseudopsychopathic" syndrome. But in this case the untoward traits are caused by damage to the orbitofrontal regions of the brain and are not under the patient's control. Anyone who has encountered a patient with severe orbitofrontal damage could not escape the impression that the whole motivational structure and value system of cognition, the ability to discern what is important and what is not, what is good and what is bad, was missing. Indeed, extracellular recordings in monkeys have shown that the firing characteristics of the orbitofrontal neurons in response to various stimuli are determined by the reward strengths and reward values associated with the stimuli.[2] We already know that in humans, orbitofrontal activity is associated with "rational" choices, and amygdala activation with "emotional" choices in "framing" experiments modeling economic decision-making.[3]

Whereas the dorsolateral cortex is connected mostly with the neocortical regions supporting the neural representation of the outside world, the orbitofrontal cortex is connected to a large extent with the subcortical structures important for monitoring the organism's internal states. This makes the orbitofrontal cortex a logical candidate for playing a critical role in forming neural representations of the organism's needs.

The unkind term *pseudopsychopathic* is no longer in use. Although some patients with the orbitofrontal syndrome engage in criminally antisocial behaviors, most such patients come across as lacking in inhibitions, "loose" but harmless. Very often their disinhibition borders on the comical. An elderly patient walked into my office many years ago and said with a broad grin by way of greeting, "Doctor, you are a very hairy man!" Aside from this being untrue (I wish), this is obviously no way to greet a stranger who also happens to be your new doctor. My immediate diagnostic hunch was subsequently confirmed. The good man suffered from an early stage of dementia affecting particularly the frontal lobes.

In another case, an elderly wealthy country gentleman was brought by his wife to see me after he had bought 100 horses "on an impulse." He, too, was diagnosed with dementia, a relatively advanced case. When I asked his wife why she had not brought him to the doctor sooner, she conceded that he had been acting "silly" for the last few years, but she thought he was merely "sloshed" on his martinis. Both cases encapsulate the more benign form of "orbitofrontal disinhibition" (and the difficulty that lay people, even family members, have in recognizing it as a clinical disorder).

The jolly, unconcerned quality of the orbitofrontal syndrome (or sometimes the term *ventromedial syndrome* is used, alluding to a somewhat larger area) occasionally produces a paradoxical impression in significant others that the patient has become "a nicer guy" following traumatic brain injury, having "shed" his pre-injury demanding, driven, competitive traits. In a similar vein, it has been shown that combat veterans who suffer ventromedial frontal damage are less susceptible to post-traumatic stress disorder.[4]

Society holds an individual responsible for certain actions but not for others. The scope of our responsibilities is defined by the scope of our volitional control. Vomiting in public by a drunk will be punished, but vomiting following a heat stroke will be excused. A traffic accident caused by speeding will be punished, but an accident caused by a driver's heart attack will be excused. Profanities spouted publicly in anger will be punished, but the same profanities uttered involuntarily by a coprolalic Tourette's patient might be excused. Bodily harm inflicted in assault will be punished, but bodily harm inflicted by a seizure patient who fell on a child will be excused.

Society draws a legal and moral distinction between the consequences of actions presumed to be under the individual's volitional control and those presumed to be outside such control. Drunkenness, speeding, rudeness, and aggression are usually presumed to be under volitional control, thus avoidable and punishable. The effects of seizures, tics, fainting spells, and heart attacks, by contrast, cannot be controlled by the patient at the time of their happening and thus will not be punishable by law.

Volitional control implies more than conscious awareness. It implies the ability to anticipate the consequences of one's action, the ability to decide whether the action should be taken, and the ability to choose between action and inaction. A Tourette's patient and a hapless heatstroke-stricken vacationer may be fully aware of what is happening to them, but they cannot control it.

It appears that, at a cognitive level, the capacity for volitional behavior depends on the functional integrity of the frontal lobes. The capacity for restraint in particular depends on the orbitofrontal cortex.

Social Maturity and the Frontal Lobes

We recognize that the capacity for volitional control over one's actions is not innate, but that it emerges gradually through development. A temper tantrum thrown by an adult will trigger a very different reaction from one following a temper tantrum thrown by a child. The capacity for the volitional control over one's actions is an important, perhaps central, ingredient of social maturity.

Allan Schore, a psychiatrist from southern California, has proposed a provocative hypothesis about this.[5] He believes that early mother–infant interaction is important for the normal development of the orbitofrontal cortex during the first months of life. By contrast, early-life stressful experiences may permanently damage the orbitofrontal cortex, predisposing the individual to later-life psychiatric diseases.

If true, this is a mind-boggling proposition, since it implies that early social interactions help shape the brain. Scientists have known for years that early sensory stimulation promotes the development of visual cortex in the occipital lobes, and early-life sensory deprivation retards its development. Is it possible that social stimulation is to the development of the frontal cortex what visual stimulation is to the development of the occipital cortex? A rigorous answer to this question may be hard to obtain in humans, but it lends itself to a pretty straightforward animal model. Aside from the role of early social interaction, I would like to see another question addressed: is there a relationship between environmental orderliness (as opposed to chaotic environment) and the maturation of the frontal lobes? The role of the frontal lobes in the temporal organization of cognition has been very well established. It has also been established that the lateral prefrontal cortex is critical for extracting and storing information about abstract properties of complex behavioral sequences.[6] An early exposure to temporally ordered environments may prove to be crucial for these abilities to develop.

An even more audacious question may be asked: is it possible that moral development involves the frontal cortex, just as visual development involves occipital cortex and language development involves temporal cortex? A moral code can be thought of as the taxonomy of sanctioned actions and behaviors. The prefrontal cortex is the association cortex of the frontal lobes, the "action lobes." Recall that the posterior association cortex encodes generic information about the outside world. It contains the taxonomy of the various things known to exist and helps recognize a particular exemplar as a member of a known category. Could it be that, by analogy, the prefrontal cortex contains the taxonomy of all the *sanctioned, moral actions and behaviors*? Just as damage or maldevelopment of the posterior association cortex produces *object agnosias*, could it be that damage or maldevelopment of the prefrontal cortex produces, in some sense, *moral agnosia?*

Although these far-reaching possibilities await further exploration, a report by Antonio Damasio lends them some support. Damasio studied two young adults, a man and a woman, who suffered damage to the frontal lobes very early in life. Both engaged in antisocial behaviors: lying, petty thievery, truancy. Damasio claims that not only did these patients fail to act according to the proper, socially sanctioned moral precepts, but they failed to recognize their actions as morally wrong.[7] In a more recent study Damasio and his colleagues demonstrated that moral judgement requiring an emotional component was particularly impaired in patients with damage to the ventromedial prefrontal cortex (VMPF; an area roughly similar to the one I refer to as orbitofrontal).[8] Ventromedial prefrontal cortex has been implicated in moral reasoning by neuroimaging studies in normal subjects as well.[9] In particular, it appears that the VMPF is critical for injecting the emotional component into moral reasoning. Patients with damage to the VMPF approach hypothetical moral dilemmas with the dispassionate utilitarianism of an automaton (e.g., it is OK to throw a human being on the railroad tracks to save the lives of several people).[10] Of course, the important limitation of such experiments presenting "frontal" patients with hypothetical situations requiring a verbal response is that they offer no direct indication as to how such patients would behave in comparable real-life situations. Patients with frontal lobe damage are notorious for the disparity between their rhetorical pronouncements and their actual behaviors.

The orbitofrontal cortex is not the only part of the frontal lobes linked to socially mature behavior. The anterior cingulate cortex occupies a midfrontal position and is closely linked to the prefrontal cortex. Together with the prefrontal neocortex and the basal ganglia, the anterior cingulate cortex is part of what I like to call the "metropolitan frontal lobes." The anterior cingulate cortex has been traditionally linked to emotion. According to Michael Posner, the doyen of North American cognitive psychology, it also plays a role in social development by regulating distress.[11]

The ability to inhibit distress is fundamental to social interactions. The goals and needs of different members of a social group are never in perfect agreement, and the capacity for compromise is a critical mechanism of social harmony and equilibrium. This capacity depends on our ability to harness distress, the negative emotion arising from an inability to find immediate gratification. Negative emotions involve the amygdala, located deep within the temporal lobe. According to Posner, the anterior cingulate cortex reins in the amygdala, and by exerting this control tempers the expression of distress. A society of individuals with the active amygdala unrestrained by the anterior cingulate cortex would constantly be at each other's throats. According to this view, the anterior cingulate cortex makes civilized discourse and conflict resolution possible.

The role of the anterior cingulate cortex in self monitoring is not limited to humans, however; in rudimentary forms it is evident in other primates. This was demonstrated by Shigehiko Ito and colleagues in a saccade-countermanding task in macaque monkeys.[12] In fact, observations of lesion effects in the monkey suggest that damage to the anterior cingulate cortex, more than of the orbitofrontal cortex, is responsible for ensuing breakdown of socially appropriate behaviors.[13] Clearly, this distinction is virtually impossible to make in relatively large natural lesions caused by tumors, stroke, or traumatic brain injury in humans, so the whole notion of "orbitofrontal syndrome" may be a misnomer. Considering how coarse the notion of "social behavior" is, it is most likely that both the orbitofrontal cortex and the anterior cingulate cortex contribute to its different aspects.

Does all this mean that the prefrontal cortex and the anterior cingulate cortex contain certain hard-wired representations of "moral behavior," or that early immersion into an "ethical" environment is necessary for the proper development of the prefrontal cortex, just as early immersion into a visually rich environment is necessary for the proper development of the occipital cortex? I believe that neither of these two claims is correct. Human history contains enough examples of "moral relativism" and it would be far-fetched to think that members of a society operating on moral premises vastly different from our own (e.g., a society of cannibals or racists) have differently wired or underdeveloped frontal lobes. As pointed out earlier, however, I do believe that proper development of the frontal lobes at early stages of ontogenesis benefits from immersion into an environment characterized by predictable and consistently replicable sequences of events, and it suffers from immersion into chaotic, unpredictable environments. Since the prefrontal cortex is critical for making predictions, its development will be fostered by environments where predictions are readily possible and hindered by environments where predictions cannot be readily made. To put it in Bayesian conditional-probabilities terms, environments dominated by high and low conditional probabilities (those close to 1 or 0) are beneficial for the proper development of the frontal lobes. By contrast, environments dominated by middle-range probabilities (those close to .5) are detrimental to the proper development of the frontal lobes. While this hypothesis is strictly a conjecture, it can be easily tested in animal experiments.

At the level of clinical observations, the role of the frontal lobes in grasping temporal and causal relationships and in using this knowledge to guide goal-oriented behavior has been well established for a long time. More recent research has begun to elucidate the neural mechanisms of such processes and their role in predictive cognition. Kenji Masumoto and colleagues from RIKEN Brain Science Institute in Japan have demonstrated the existence in the monkey medial frontal cortex of neurons, whose firing pattern suggested an anticipation of particular rewards following particular cues.[14] So it is only logical to assume that for an ability to engage in predicitive cognition to develop and for the underlying neural substrate to mature, the environment surrounding the growing organism must allow predictions to be made. These neurons should be more prolific in the medial than dorsolateral prefrontal regions, since the former are the neuroanatomical point of convergence of inputs from the internal and external mileus.

What, then, is the relationship between moral behavior and the frontal lobes? I would argue that the appreciation of temporal relations is the prerequisite for the appreciation of causal relationships, and appreciation of the consequences of human actions is the prerequisite for the development of moral reasoning and moral behavior. Indeed, a growing body of literature exists demonstrating the role of the prefrontal cortex in learning complex causal relationships.[15] Of particular interest is the capacity for inferential reasoning captured by the logical "if . . . then . . ." structures. This capacity, which is at the cornerstone of complex human cognition and supports the generative, model-building function of language, is absent in nonhuman primates.[16] One can argue that this capacity is also essential for moral reasoning. It is also very likely that this capacity is mediated by the prefrontal cortex.

So-called counter-factual reasoning is another interesting form of causal reasoning. It involves the ability to consider the consequences of hypothetical alternative actions: "What would have happened had I done Y instead of X?" This ability, which is necessary for moral reasoning as well as for social learning from previous situations, has been shown to be impaired following orbitofrontal damage.[17]

Biological Maturation and Social Maturity: A Historical Puzzle

The implicit definition of social maturity changes throughout the history of society, as so does the time of "coming of age." In various cultures, the time when a boy becomes a man has been codified through rituals, and the change of this time in history is quite revealing.

In the Jewish tradition the age of 13 is celebrated by the *bar mitzvah*. In modern times, it is a joyous ritual full of symbolism. However, when the celebration is over, the boy remains a boy. The ritual of bar mitzvah probably reflects the reality of three millennia ago, when the age of 13 was the age of transition from boyhood to manhood with all its profound connotations.

Initiation rites symbolizing the passage into adulthood are also found in other cultures. On the Indonesian island of Bali, I observed the ceremony of *mepanes* (tooth filing). Mepanes is performed in late adolescence, around the age of 16, and is the prerequisite for entering any adult institution, such as marriage. Surrounded with colorful ritual heightened by the sound of ceremonial gamelans, the young man's or woman's teeth are filed by a *sangging* (a junior Hindu priest). The symbolism of the ritual is revealing.

Ida Bagus Madhe Adnyana, a young Brahmin who had had his own teeth ritually filed a few years earlier, explained the meaning of the ceremony as follows. By acquiring flat and even teeth, the teenager is set apart from animals, whose teeth are sharp and uneven. Flattening the teeth symbolizes joining the world of civilization. Six front upper teeth are filed, corresponding to six vices: *kama* (lust), *krodha* (anger), *lobha* (greed), *moha* (drunkenness), *mada* (arrogance), and *matsuya* (jealousy). Flattening the teeth symbolizes the tempering of these impulses and bringing them under the control of reason. We already know that many of these socially undesirable traits are tempered by the frontal lobes and become unmanageable with orbitofrontal injury.

As society became more complex and increasingly governed by brain rather than brawn and as the life span increased, the age of maturity was pushed up. In modern Western societies the age of 18 (or thereabout) has been codified in the law as the age of social maturity. This is the age when a person can vote and is held responsible for his or her actions as an adult.

The age of 18 is also the age when the maturation of the frontal lobes is relatively complete. Various estimates can be used to measure the course of maturation of various brain structures. Among the most commonly used such measures is pathway myelinization.[18] Long pathways connecting different parts of the brain are covered with white fatty tissue called "myelin."

Myelin insulates the pathway and speeds the neural signal transmission along the pathway. The presence of myelin makes communication between different parts of the brain faster and more reliable. Obviously, long-distance communication is particularly important for the frontal lobes, the CEO of the brain, since their role is to coordinate the activities of its many parts. The frontal lobes cannot fully assume their leadership role until the pathways connecting the frontal lobes with the far-flung structures of the brain are fully myelinated. Evidence exists that myelinization continues until about the age of the mid-30s,[19] or perhaps even as late as the age of 50, and then begins to gradually decline.[20] Synaptic pruning is another index of brain maturation. According to this index, the prefrontal cortex is the last to mature, only by the early 20s.[21]

The agreement between the age of relatively complete maturation of the frontal lobes and the age of social maturity is probably more than coincidental. Without the explicit benefit of neuroscience, but through cumulative everyday common sense, society recognizes that an individual assumes adequate control over his or her impulses, drives, and desires only by a certain age. Until that age, individuals cannot be held fully responsible for their actions in either a legal or a moral sense. This ability appears to depend critically on the maturity and functional integrity of the frontal lobes.

The relationship between the age of social maturity and maturation of the frontal lobes through history raises interesting questions. In ancient and medieval societies social adulthood was achieved at a much earlier age than it is today. Kingdoms were often ruled and armies routinely led into battle by teenagers. Pharaoh Ramses the Great of Egypt, the biblical King David, and Alexander the Great of Macedon all embarked on their major military campaigns while in their early 20s. In fact, Alexander was barely 20 when he crossed the Bosphorus, invaded Persia, and by this act began the fusion of East and West. He was dead at 32, having created one of the greatest empires on earth, from modern-day Libya to India. Peter the Great of Russia set about tearing down and transforming his country while in his late teens. By all available accounts, none of these historical figures was a puppet in somebody else's, more "mature" hands. Each was a decisive, visionary leader of his people at a very young age, and each of them left an indelible trace on civilization. Yet in most developed countries today people their age are prevented from occupying high offices by law, on the assumption of their "immaturity." By law, a president of the United States must be at least 35, which would have disqualified many great historical political figures from occupying the leadership position in our society.

Does this mean that some of the most important decisions in history were made by biologically immature brains? To take it a step further, could it be that much of human history is the neurological equivalent of a juvenile mob scene, and that the most fateful conflicts in ancient and medieval history are best modeled on William Golding's *Lord of the Flies*?[22] The role of elders as arbitrators, moderators, and generally "wise men" was paramount in ancient societies. Is it because the elders were the bearers of neurological, and not just social, maturity?

Or is it possible that the biological rate of frontal lobe maturation is at least partly controlled by environmental (and, in the human case, cultural) factors, such as an early pressure to assume "adult" roles and engage in complex decision making (a hypothesis proposed by my student John Solerno)? The frontal lobe nature–nurture question is interesting for theoretical and practical reasons in this age of rapid social change. Obviously, we do not have brain-imaging data from the times of antiquity. Nor does the idea of imaging the brains of the youthful tribal chiefs in the few remaining primitive societies in the Amazon jungle or Papua New Guinea highlands seem particularly practical. But nonhuman primate experimentation may help answer the question.

Frontal Lobe Damage and Criminal Behavior

We all behave in impulsive and irresponsible ways at times, but most of us have the ability to stay clear of outright criminality. By contrast, behavior devoid of social inhibitions for neurological reasons is much more likely to cross the line. Extreme violations of human norms of behavior intuitively strike us as abnormal; that they are "abnormal" by definition is a truism. It is not by coincidence that we use the word *sick* to describe such behaviors. Instinctively, we refuse to accept them as part of "normal" behavior and try to understand them in "clinical" terms. One reads speculations about Lenin's and Idi Amin's tertiary syphilis, Stalin's paranoia, Hitler's von Economo's encephalitis, and so on. But by inflating the concept of criminal insanity, we devalue fundamental legal and ethical concepts. One must tread very carefully in drawing the line between criminality and mental illness, between morality and biology.

The relationship between frontal lobe damage and criminality is particularly intriguing and complex. We already know that damage to the frontal lobes causes the impairment of insight, impulse control, and foresight, which often leads to socially unacceptable behavior. This is particularly true when the damage affects the orbital surface of the frontal lobes. Patients afflicted with this "pseudopsychopathic" syndrome are notorious for their urge for instant gratification; they are unrestrained by social mores or fear of punishment. It would be logical to suspect that some of these patients are particularly prone to criminal behavior. But is there any evidence for this? More important, is there any evidence that some of the individuals indicted, convicted, or sentenced for criminal behavior are, in fact, unrecognized cases of frontal lobe damage?

Several marginal groups in society exhibit the peculiar trait of relinquishing their executive functions to external institutions, where their options are maximally constrained and the decision-making power over them is exercised by someone else.

Some chronic psychiatric patients feel uncomfortable outside mental institutions and seek readmission; some criminals feel uncomfortable in the outside world and seek ways for being reincarcerated. This could be construed as a peculiar form of self-medication, as an attempt to compensate for an executive deficit rendering them incapable of making their own decisions.

It has been suggested, based on several published studies, that the prevalence of head injury is much higher among criminals than in the general population, and in violent criminals than in nonviolent criminals.[23] For reasons of brain and skull anatomy, closed-head injury is particularly likely to affect the frontal lobes directly, especially the orbitofrontal cortex. Later in the book I will argue that direct damage to the frontal lobes is not necessary to produce significant frontal lobe dysfunction (see Chapter 12). Damage to the upper brain stem is likely to produce a similar effect by interrupting the critical projections into the frontal lobes. Damage to the upper brain stem is extremely common in closed-head injury, even in seemingly "mild" cases, and it is likely to produce frontal lobe dysfunction even in the absence of direct damage to the frontal lobes. Many years ago I described this condition under the name "reticulo-frontal disconnection syndrome."[24]

Contemporary research bears out the designation of certain frontal lobe syndromes as "pseudopsychopathic." Adrian Raine and his colleagues studied the brains of convicted murderers with positron emission tomography (PET) scanning and found abnormalities in the prefrontal cortex.[25] Raine and colleagues also studied the brains of men with antisocial personality disorder and found an 11% reduction in the gray matter of their frontal lobes.[26] The cause of this reduction is uncertain, but Raine believes that this reduction is at least in part congenital, instead of being caused by environmental factors such as abuse or bad parenting.

If this assertion is true, then it appears that people with certain congenital forms of brain dysfunction may be particularly predisposed to antisocial behavior. On the face of it, this assertion is not implausible. We have long recognized the existence of congenital predisposition to brain dysfunction due to aberrant patterns of neural cell migration and other causes. But it is only logical to assume that such "genotypic" predisposition can be quite broad and devoid of neuroanatomical specificity and that its individual "phenotypic" expressions are highly variable and may affect different parts of the brain in different individuals. Just as in certain cases this predisposition may affect the temporal lobe, leading to language-based learning disability, so in other cases it may affect the prefrontal cortex, producing a "social learning disability" of sorts.

The link between frontal lobe dysfunction and asocial behavior raises an important legal issue. Suppose a criminal is found to have structural evidence of frontal lobe damage on a magnetic resonance imaging (MRI) or computerized axial tomography (CAT) scan; or suppose physiological evidence of frontal lobe dysfunction is found on PET, single photon emission computerized tomography (SPECT), or electroencephalography (EEG), all commonly used and widely available diagnostic neuroimaging devices. Or suppose that a criminal is found to perform particularly poorly on the neuropsychological tests sensitive to function of the frontal lobes.

Suppose further that the nature of the crime suggests spur-of-the-moment impulsivity and lack of premeditation. (Obviously, premeditation and intricate planning would argue strongly against severe frontal lobe dysfunction.) In a legal sense, a "frontal" patient may be competent to stand trial, since he or she can understand the court proceedings. Rhetorically, the patient may also know right from wrong, and will correctly answer the questions about which actions are socially acceptable and which are not. In all likelihood, the patient would have had this knowledge in a token form even at the time of the crime. Therefore, the insanity defense will not be conventionally applicable. Yet the frontal damage would interfere with this person's ability to parlay this knowledge into a socially acceptable course of action. Although the difference between right and wrong is known, the knowledge cannot be translated into effective inhibitions.

The discrepancy between rhetorical knowledge and the ability to utilize this knowledge for guiding behavior is conspicuous in frontal lobe patients. This can be demonstrated very dramatically with a simple bedside test introduced by Alexandr Luria.[27] A patient is seated in front of the examiner and asked to do the opposite of what the examiner does: "When I raise my finger, you raise your fist. When I raise my fist, you raise your finger." This task is particularly difficult for frontal lobe patients. Instead of doing "the opposite," they tend to lapse into direct imitation. To help the patient with the task, one may encourage him or her to say aloud what needs to be done. At this point the disparity between rhetorical knowledge and the ability to guide behavior with this knowledge becomes strikingly obvious. The patient will say the right thing but make the wrong move at the same time. With my colleagues and former students Bob Bilder, Judy Jaeger, and Ken Podell, I developed the Executive Control Battery, a collection of tests to elicit precisely such phenomena.[28]

An orbitofrontal patient may know right from wrong, yet be unable to use this knowledge to regulate his or her behavior. Likewise, a mesiofrontal patient with damage to the anterior cingulate cortex will know the rules of civilized behavior but will be unable to *follow them*. The potential legal ramifications of this condition are vast, and the recognition of this possibility represents a legal new frontier.

What is the likelihood of an asocial individual suffering from some form of orbitofrontal or mesiofrontal dysfunction? Under what conditions should this possibility be directly ascertained through neuropsychological and neuroimaging means? What is the legal significance of such evidence? When does it override criminal responsibility? Two legal decisions rest on cognitive evidence: *(1)* is the defendant competent to stand trial, and *(2)* is the defendant sufficiently sane to be held criminally responsible for his or her actions? Based on the standard criteria used in courts in such decisions, a frontal lobe patient may be pronounced both legally competent and legally sane. But whether these legal constructs adequately cover the peculiar potential for asocial behavior related to frontal lobe damage is arguable. The third relevant legal concept is "diminished capacity." This broad concept may be applicable by virtue of its vagueness, but for the same reason it eludes clear-cut criteria to guide legal decision making.

A bizarre criminal case was reported in New York a number of years ago. An obstetrician had carved his initials into a woman's belly after performing a caesarean section. According to the press reports, when challenged, the doctor said nonchalantly that he felt that his surgery had been such a masterpiece that he had to sign it; then he took off on vacation to Paris. As soon as I read about the incident in the *New York Times*, I said to myself that it was too bizarre, too "sick" to be "merely" criminal. And true enough, as a defense, the doctor's attorneys claimed that he suffered from frontal lobe damage due to Pick's disease.

Curiously, the mutilated woman—also a doctor—opposed the obstetrician's criminal prosecution, evidently recognizing that his behavior had been more tragic than criminal. The doctor would have faced up to 25 years in prison had he been convicted of the most serious charge brought up by the prosecution, first-degree assault. Instead, he was sentenced to 5 years' probation and barred from applying for a medical license for 5 years. It is unlikely that he will ever attempt to practice medicine again.

A new legal construct of "inability to guide one's behavior despite the availability of requisite knowledge" may be needed to capture the peculiar relationship between frontal lobe dysfunction and the potential for criminal behavior. Studies of frontal lobe disorders bring into a single focus neuropsychology, ethics, and law. As the legal profession becomes more enlightened about the workings of the brain, the "frontal lobe defense" may emerge as a legal strategy on a par with the "insanity defense."

The exact limits of such a defense have yet to be tested and its legitimate boundaries established. It is almost inevitable that attempts will be made to stretch it beyond its legitimate boundaries. On the other hand, constructive multidisciplinary debate will be fostered. Is it possible that certain types of subtle frontal-lobe dysfunction may render an individual amoral while sparing his or her capacity for planning and temporal organization (admittedly a far-fetched conjecture, but an interesting one)? In that case, is it a likely mechanism of sociopathy ("moral blindness")? Is it possible that sociopathic behavior may be caused by a neurodevelopmental disorder of the frontal lobes, just as dyslexia may be caused by a neurodevelopmental disorder of the temporal lobe? Are we trivializing and debasing the notion of morality by setting on this path, or merely pointing to its "biological basis"? Are we further diluting the notion of personal responsibility? Or are we finally acknowledging that, whereas moral and criminal codes are extracranial, moral and criminal cognition and behaviors are not? They are the products of our cerebral machinery, intact or abnormal, every bit as much as they are the products of our social institutions.

The Hapless Robber

Charlie was a happy-go-lucky guy and everybody's friend, bright and personable, who dropped out of school, got a job, and earned his high school equivalency diploma. His parents, upright people from rural Pennsylvania, encouraged him to join the marines to keep him "on the straight and narrow." Charlie joined, served, was discharged, returned to Pennsylvania, and got a job as a salesman.

Then, at the age of 25, his very ordinary life was shattered in a single instant. One night, when Charlie and a friend were returning from a party, their open vehicle rammed into the metal support of a small bridge. Charlie's friend, the driver, was killed instantly and Charlie was found unconscious in a pool of blood on the side of the road.

Charlie did not regain consciousness until two and a half months later. Then he began several months of cognitive and physical therapy in a rehabilitation hospital. Several CAT scans conducted right after the accident showed signs of damage in the right temporal lobe and in the brain stem, general swelling (edema) of the brain, and blood in the lateral ventricles. There were also multiple skull fractures, including a basal skull fracture. A CAT scan repeated 6 years later showed substantial but incomplete recovery. It was probably damage to the upper brain stem, and the consequent reticulofrontal disconnection syndrome, that was largely responsible for all Charlie's troubles that followed. The presence of basal skull fracture also raised the possibility of direct damage to the orbitofrontal brain regions, even though it was not seen on CAT scans.

Released from the hospital, Charlie returned to his mother's home (his parents had been divorced for some time) and embarked on an idle, vacuous existence. He spent his days watching television, drinking beer, and taking drugs. Eventually, in a state of total exasperation, his mother threw him out. Charlie's father took him in, but not for long. One day Charlie brought home a woman with Tourette's syndrome and the two settled in his grandmother's bed. The woman's noisy tics gave the lovers away, and Charlie was told to leave again.

Charlie married the woman with Tourette's and embarked on a chaotic existence. At times he lived in the woman's house. At other times Charlie hit the road, wandering around the country, drunk and drugged much of the time, occasionally engaging in petty robberies. Charlie had recovered his physical faculties and, to a superficial observer, his mental faculties. He was reasonably articulate and had no obvious stigma of a neurologically impaired patient. Despite his wild ways, he was generally a good-natured fellow. He had a short fuse, however, and got into arguments easily. Charlie occasionally found menial jobs, but he could never hold one for long and ended up on the road again.

Charlie was able to get by until one day he ran out of cash and decided to hold up a convenience store. In this pursuit, Charlie enlisted the help of a companion, also brain damaged, whom he had met earlier at the rehabilitation hospital.

Pointing a Bic lighter through his pants pocket in lieu of a gun, Charlie was able to get some $200 in cash. With the holdup in progress, his partner in crime was patiently waiting in the escape car in front of the store, the license plates fully exposed. Charlie was tracked down and arrested within 2 hours of the robbery, as he was settling down to enjoy the booze and the drugs acquired with the ill-gotten money.

Charlie's misadventure is an excellent example of "frontal lobe crime," precisely because of his utter ineptness. The most remarkable feature of the whole episode is a total lack of precision, foresight, or contingency planning. The crime was so pathetically bungled that it engendered more pity than outrage.

The court was unaware of Charlie's brain damage and he went to jail. Although the prison officers were also unaware of Charlie's neurological condition, he was perceived as "odd" and spent most of the time in the prison infirmary until he was let out on parole. This time his aging mother made the connection between Charlie's behavior and his old brain damage. Charlie was placed in a long-term rehabilitation center run by my former student, Dr. Judith Carman. This is where I met him.

Trim and neatly dressed, Charlie did not show the signs of a neurological patient. He entered Dr. Carman's office with an athletic stride and a friendly smile, nothing in his demeanor betraying the history of either brain damage or crime. Superficially articulate and gregarious, he offered no obvious hint at a cognitive deficit. He seemed to be self-conscious about his appearance, immediately challenging me to guess his age (he was 42 but looked younger), and asked me whether I liked his goatee.

Charlie knew that I was the program director's former professor, was writing a book, and wanted to include Charlie's story in it. He had been expecting our meeting for some time and was determined to put his best foot forward. He was quite excited about being in my book, and he was disappointed to find out that it would take me a while to finish it. He kept prodding me: "C'mon, get on with it, doc!" Charlie proceeded with a jolly delivery of his life's story, dwelling on its more delinquent details with particular relish, and sprinkling his narrative with casual profanities. This left the uncanny impression of a tipsy teenager in the body of a middle-aged man, the famous orbitofrontal *Witzelsucht*:

"Do you like it here in this program?" I asked

"No."

"Why not?"

"'Cause I am horny, doc, and this witch [points at Dr. Carman with a grin suggesting that his choice of the word is a concession to my presence] isn't much help. . . . Do you have any daughters for me, doc?" [slaps me on the knee, winks, and laughs genially]. . . . "You don't mind my free thinking, do you?"

Charlie is known at the center for his roving eye and fancies the idea of marrying one of the center's female residents (he has been divorced from his tourettic wife for some time), because "once you fall off the horse you get right back on it." Charlie's sexual tension took a variety of forms. Once he somehow obtained lollypops in the shape of a penis and went around offering them to the center's female employees. Charlie recounted the episode fondly and with flourish, laughing at the memories of the scandalized women and referring to the lollypops as "dick candy," not in the least inhibited by Dr. Carman's presence.

In the course of the conversation, Charlie casually put his hand on Dr. Carman's behind. When asked to account for his behavior, Charlie's answer was that "it [his hand] just happened to be in motion." While this explanation would have sounded gratuitous coming from a neurologically intact individual, Charlie had unwittingly captured the essence of his condition. In Charlie the *it*, or shall we say the *id*, was no longer under effective neural control by the frontal lobes.

Yet his upright preaccident background came through in incongruous ways. When one of the therapists suggested that he consider doing what men have done since the beginning of time when lacking female companionship, Charlie was first appalled by the idea, since it was contrary to his Christian upbringing. I am told that he has since adopted a more secular view of his options, and his life at the rehabilitation center has been more under control.

During the interview, much as Charlie would have liked to talk about sex, I changed the subject, asking, "Do you feel that you have recovered from your accident?"

"Nobody recovers from an accident 100%, but let us say 99.9%," he said.

But then came a stunningly eloquent revelation, demonstrating more insight into his circumstances than Charlie's bravado would suggest:

"Head injury is like an eternal spring of youth. It stops you from growing up. It happened to me at 25 and I still feel 25. . . . A 42-year-old would have more common sense."

Charlie seems to enjoy his "eternal spring of youth" and the insight proves to be shallow: "The car accident was a blessing."

This surreal conversation coming to an end, Charlie gave me a tour of his room, with photographs of family members and two aquariums with exotic fish. I kept thinking that he was a warm, genial person without a hint of malice or deceit, a teenager in a grown man's body, that despite his crude language there was a certain charm and innocence about him, and I liked him. We shook hands and he slapped me on the back, reminding me to send him a copy of the book.

At the time of this writing, Charlie continues to live at the rehabilitation center and work in the community. Jobs are found for him through a placement program run at the center. Most of the time Charlie is a conscientious worker and does a good job fixing and cleaning things. He tends to get into trouble with his employers, however, because of his short fuse and loose tongue. His uninhibited behavior got him fired from his previous job and he is now a janitor in a department store. Now and then Charlie transgresses, like when he stole the center's car and went for a ride (he does not have a valid driver license).

Most of the time Charlie is an amiable fellow and has no intention of hurting anyone. He is generally funny and gregarious. But true to his orbitofrontal syndrome, Charlie has a volatile temper, which tends to bounce precipitously from one extreme to the other. If someone is in his way, he is likely to turn around and punch that person out, without warning or deliberation. And since Charlie has physically recovered from his injury and now lifts weights for recreation, he is capable of doing real damage. It does not take much provocation to get Charlie going. When another center resident appropriated his ice cream by mistake, Charlie's fists began to flash in a scary fit of rage, and it took four people to subdue him.

Under the circumstances, Charlie's recovery was quite remarkable. He is athletic and articulate, showing no obvious memory impairment. Today, most people would think of Charlie as "odd," "immature," a "loose cannon," "obnoxious," or "vulgar." But very few people would realize that Charlie is brain damaged. I suspect that many psychologists and physicians would miss that as well. The neuropsychological evaluations administered repeatedly several years after the accident suggested average intelligence (Wechsler Adult Intelligence Scale–Revised IQ values within the 90s) and low-average memory (Wechsler Memory Scale–Revised values within the 80s).[29] Charlie's performance on language tests was also within a normal range. All the test results were probably lower than they would have been without the accident, but nothing in them betrayed the extent of Charlie's injuries. Yet Charlie's core was gone, and so was his mooring. Charlie's case captures the essence of the frontal lobe syndrome: specific skills spared, but inner guide gone.

Frontal Lobe Damage and the Public Blindspot

Charlie's story is instructive in more ways than one. For years Charlie moved in and out of menial jobs and lived intermittently with various people, and nobody suspected that Charlie's oddities had a neurological cause, despite the fact that many people around him knew about Charlie's accident.

This raises the broad issue of general-public awareness of cognitive impairment. Although rhetorically the educated public understands today that cognition is a function of the brain, this abstraction often fails to inform specific, real-life situations. As a result, Cartesian dualism prevails when it comes to everyday encounters with brain-damaged people. This naive dualism is evident even at the level of health-care policymaking and health coverage, when physical health is treated seriously whereas "mental" health is given short shrift.

Everyday public attitudes betray a sharp division between "physical" and "nonphysical" symptoms and between "physical" and "nonphysical" bodily organs. Problems with vision or hearing, limp, and weakness on one side of the body will be unfailingly perceived as physical and will engender sympathy and readiness to help. The bodily nature of these symptoms will be immediately grasped, but curiously, most lay people will be very slow to attribute them to the brain.

By contrast, patients with higher-order cognitive impairments are often denied the sympathy accorded people with physical infirmities and are treated instead in moralistic, almost puritanical terms. Forget the hapless criminal Charlie. Consider the common situation of a demented elderly individual whose whole life has been an example of civic responsibility and moral rectitude. Now she is old and very forgetful. Having diagnosed early dementia, I try to explain the implications of my findings to the eager family members. I tell them that their mother suffers from amnesia, that her forgetfulness is caused by brain atrophy, that she cannot help it, that it is likely to get worse, and that they have to be patient with their loved one. The family members listen intently. They nod. They seem to understand—and then comes an irate comment: "But how come I give her breakfast in the morning and she comes back asking for her breakfast again!" When I encounter this lack of understanding, I feel like tipping my hat to my friend Oliver Sacks, who has done more than anyone else to enlighten the general public about the effects of neurological injury on cognition. I urge people to read *The Man Who Mistook His Wife for a Hat.*[30]

But if the neurological nature of impaired memory, perception, or language usually can be grasped by the general public, the executive deficit caused by frontal lobe injury almost never is grasped. Point to the patient's impulsivity, volatility, indifference, and lack of initiative, and the common response will be, "This is not his brain, this is his personality!" Such a response reflects a total retreat three and a half centuries back to Cartesian dualism, as if "personality" were an utterly extracranial phenomenon. The notion of "personality," of course, is something that, on a par with apple pie and spring water, carries moralistic, righteous connotations. If you were born into an honest family and went to a good school, then you must have an upright personality!

Just how oblivious even many highly educated members of the general public are of the biological determinants of personality became strikingly apparent to me during an event described in my book *The Wisdom Paradox.*[31] In the year 2000, I participated in a meeting, organized by my friend Allan Snyder at University of Sydney, right before the Olympic Games being held in Australia that year.[32] The puprose of the meeting was to bring together distinguished individuals, each at the top of her or his field, and to engage them in a discussion of the secrets of great success. The title of the meeting was "What Makes A Champion." Organized into several panels, the participants—Nobel Laureates, famous politicians, past Olympic medalists, leaders of industry and finance—debated the secrets of "championhood" in front of a large group of spectators. As I was listening to the panelists' presentations, they were shot through with a single leitmotiff. Great success rests on two prerequisites. One is a field-specific talent that you have to be born with: a great musical, literary, or athletic gift. Without this gift you are not likely to reach the pinnacle of success, no matter how motivated you are or how hard you try. In this regard, biology is indeed destiny. The other prerequisite is of a more general kind. It is your personality, your drive, your ability to subordinate your life to the pursuit of a single, lofty, often distant goal, and to make a necessary sacrifice. Unlike the subject-specific talent (or lack thereof), all the presentations implied, this general personality type conducive to great success is not ruled by our biological makeup; it it "up to us" to mold it.

When my turn to speak came, I began very gently to argue that our "personalities" are also to a great extent the products of our respective biologies, and that they are specifically related to the frontal lobes. As I was warming up to the theme of the individual differences among our respective brains, and how these differences shape our cognitive profiles, and how our "personalities" vary as a function of the individual differences involving our frontal lobes, I was interrupted by a fellow panelist, a famous international public personality, who said impatiently: "What you are telling us about, Professor Goldberg, is very interesting, but this conference is about the mind, it is not about the brain." Another panelist, a famous scientist, winked in my direction both sympathetically and in amusement, as if to say, "Good luck dealing with this!" I responded to the extent that the social decorum permitted and the discussion moved on, but the experience was an eye-opener for me.

It is my hope that this book will help put "personality" and related expressions of the mind where they belong: inside the brain, so to speak, in the eyes of the general public. By helping accomplish this, I hope the book will help correct the unintended public insensitivity, and sometimes outright cruelty, toward persons with the most devastating of all forms of brain damage, that to the frontal lobes. It will also help us to understand that the complex interplay between "nature and nurture" affects the everyday differences between our personality types, just as it affects so many other aspects of our respective mental makeups.

12

Fateful Disconnections

The Fallen Horseman: A Case Study

When my neurosurgeon friend Jim Hughes called me late one night, I had no idea that the consequences of this call would profoundly affect my career. Jim wanted me to consult on his patient, a man in his late 30s who was recovering from a head injury. It sounded like a pretty routine clinical case and I agreed to see the patient.

Kevin (a fictional name) was a fabulously successful entrepreneur and entertainment executive, a happy husband and father of three. An all-round athlete, he was an accomplished equestrian, but had been riding an unfamiliar horse in New York's Central Park and was thrown on hard basalt rock, hitting his head against a tree in the process. He was rushed to the nearest hospital, where Dr. Hughes performed emergency surgery. Kevin had been comatose for 2 days and was slowly recovering.

I first saw Kevin briefly approximately 2 months after his accident. He was disoriented, confused, and overwhelmed by his surroundings. His general demeanor was panic-stricken, and if there ever was an embodiment of the expression "shell-shocked," Kevin was it. He was severely aphasic and responded to every question addressed to him by saying, "Thank you . . . thank you . . . thank you." That was his only utterance. There was something extremely childlike and pleading in his demeanor and in his "thank you"—he was a man who had lost his core, defenseless like a child. I was struck by the thought that in some metaphoric sense he was in a fetal position, even though physically he was not. He wandered aimlessly on the unit, walking through any open door—just because the door was there. He was very thin, almost emaciated, the hair on his head barely beginning to grow back after neurosurgery. Nothing in this fragile visage was evocative of the supremely confident, buoyant, and physically imposing persona that the old Kevin had been.

Kevin was discharged from the hospital, and 3 months later I was asked to see him again. He was a different person, his wavy hair regrown into a rich mane, his weight regained, with a broad smile on his face and gregarious manners returned. His language was fluent and his mood relaxed. Dressed in one of his expensive suits, his hair blown dry, Kevin appeared the epitome of a palpably successful dweller of New York's Upper East Side. Superficially, his demeanor of a man in control of his environment had returned, and one could imagine the old Kevin—a self-confident, charismatic, and slightly glib, upper-crust New Yorker.

In reality, Kevin was far from recovered. He still had significant memory impairment, which affected both his ability to learn new information (anterograde amnesia) and his ability to recall information learned well before his accident (retrograde amnesia). His language, while generally fluent and even articulate, revealed slight word-finding difficulties that were not likely to be noticed by the uninitiated but were certainly apparent to me.

As I continued to observe Kevin, I was particularly struck by the severity of his "frontal lobe syndrome." Kevin was perseverative—that is, his behavior invariably fell into repetitive stereotypes. Every evening, he would arrange his clothes for the following day and the clothes were always the same. As winter passed and spring began, and well into the summer, Kevin continued to prepare his sheepskin jacket to wear the following day and could be found walking around the Upper East Side of Manhattan clad in his sheepskin on a sweltering July day. It took a lot of persuasion to get him to wear anything else. Despite his superficial flair, any conversation with Kevin rapidly deteriorated into a rather vacuous activity such as simple card games. He had a small repertoire of rehearsed stock topics, and the conversation would predictably and quickly drift toward one of them, for example, discussion of some of his friends. Having run through his repertoire of a half-dozen topics, Kevin would start from the beginning, repeating everything almost verbatim again and again.

Kevin was not only perseverative but also field-dependent. Accompanied by a family member or an aide, Kevin occasionally ventured into a neighborhood restaurant for lunch. In the restaurant he tended to order every item on the menu, 10 or 20 items in all. He did so not because he was that hungry but because the items were there. He spent most of his time, though, languishing in his apartment, occasionally asking people to play simple card games and backgammon with him. His behavior during the games was childlike. He would clap his hands with joy after winning and throw temper tantrums after losing. He was not above cheating.

Kevin's affect was constantly oscillating between euphoria and superficial rage. These mood swings were abrupt, extreme, and could be precipitated by the most trivial events, such as a waitress in a restaurant asking him if he wanted more coffee.

His personality took on childlike characteristics in virtually every respect. He related to his wife like a 12-year-old and competed with his children for her attention. In many ways he interacted with his children as an equal. Like a little child, he demanded instant gratification, although his needs were not those of a child. On several occasions he approached his female acquaintances with rather explicit propositions, an odd combination of the old charming Kevin and the socially inappropriate frontal patient.

Kevin had no insight into his condition. When questioned about the effects of the accident, he would mention his physical injuries but maintained that his mind was sound. He was convinced that he was ready to go back to work. When asked why he had not done so, he would say that he did not feel like it, or that he had been busy doing other things. Eventually Kevin was encouraged to spend a few hours a day in his old office, engaged in various cognitive exercises designed to help his recovery. He enjoyed going to the office and chatting with his old colleagues. His sense was that he was "back to work"—despite the fact that the way he spent his time in the office bore little similarity to his activities before the accident.

Kevin's mind was astoundingly concrete. When I once said that it was time to repeat the CAT (computerized axial tomography) scan, this was met with genuine puzzlement. Why the CAT scan, Kevin marveled, if he had been hurt by a horse, not a cat? On another occasion, somebody used the metaphor "increasingly interconnected isles of communications" to refer to the growing role of communications in North America. This threw Kevin into a fit of rage, since the United States "has never consisted of a bunch of islands."

The more time I spent with Kevin, the more convinced I became that his cognition was a textbook case of the frontal lobe syndrome. The puzzling thing was that not a single one of the several CAT scans administered to Kevin could detect a frontal lobe lesion. This is not to say that Kevin's brain was normal—far from it; Kevin suffered severe and multiple brain damage.

The damage affected the temporoparietal regions in both hemispheres. The ventricles (spaces within the brain containing cerebrospinal fluid) were enlarged. There was also a shunt surgically placed in his brain to help the drainage of cerebrospinal fluid. But the frontal lobes were clear—an amazing finding in a patient with such strong clinical evidence of frontal lobe dysfunction.

The discrepancy between the clinical picture of Kevin's behavior and his CAT scans presented an intellectual challenge, and Kevin became another important patient on my career path who influenced and even shaped its direction. With the help of my research assistants Bob Bilder and Carl Sirio (now a prominent neuropsychologist and a prominent physician, respectively), I embarked on a detective mission of sorts, trying to unravel the mystery of Kevin's condition. Since no such condition had ever been described before, we were on our own.

If the frontal lobes themselves were structurally intact, I reasoned, is it possible that the problem lay with the pathways connecting them to some other structures? Could it be a frontal disconnection syndrome? The concept of a "disconnection syndrome" was introduced by Norman Geschwind,[1] one of the preeminent American behavioral neurologists, whose numerous students continue to shape the field. The idea was that a severe cognitive deficit could be caused not by the damage to a brain structure per se, but by the damage to long connecting nerve fibers between two brain structures, interrupting the information flow between them. But the classic disconnection syndromes were "horizontal," affecting the connections between two or more cortical regions. I had the inkling that in Kevin's case we encountered a "vertical" disconnection syndrome. Could it be that Kevin's condition was caused by damage to the massive pathways projecting from the brain stem into the frontal lobes?

The brain stem contains the nuclei thought to be responsible for the arousal and activation of the rest of the brain. Collectively some of these nuclei are called the "reticular formation," a bit of a misnomer and a conceptual anachronism, since the term implies a diffuse undifferentiated action. Today we know that the brain stem machinery of arousal and activation consists of distinct nuclei and pathways, each with its own biochemical properties. The whole design of the arousal and activation machinery provides a treasure trove of an argument in support of Steven Jay Gould's notion of "dumb" evolution and against the creationist notion of "intelligent design."[2] The design of the arousal and activation machinery is anything but "intelligent" and would not have passed the graduate project requirements in any self-respecting school of engineering, because it is woefully devoid of redundancy. The critical nuclei in charge of general arousal are tightly packed in the ventral pons, thus the damage to this area produces deep coma. Some degree of redundancy is present at a higher level, as the arousal and activation system bifurcates into two components: the ventral tegmental area of the mesencephalon, and the midline thalamic reticular nuclei. Either of these two components appears to be capable of supporting arousal for much of the brain, which is why the stimulation of either the ventral brain stem or the midline thalamic nuclei has been shown to help arouse patients from vegetative states.[3]

The complex relationship that exists between the frontal lobes and the brain stem nuclei responsible for arousal and activation is best described as a loop. On the one hand, the arousal of the frontal lobes depends on the ascending pathways from the brain stem. These pathways are complex, but one component—the mesocortical dopamine system—is thought to be particularly important for the proper function of the frontal lobes. It originates in the ventral tegmental area (VTA) of the brain stem and projects into the frontal lobes. If the frontal lobes are the decision-making center of the brain, then the ventral tegmental area is its energy source, the battery, and the ascending mesocortical dopamine pathway is the connecting cable.

On the other hand, there are pathways projecting from the frontal lobes to the nuclei of the ventral brain stem. Through these pathways the frontal lobes exert their control over the diverse brain structures by modulating their arousal level. If the frontal lobes are the decision-making device, then the reticular formation and other arousal nuclei of the ventral brain stem are amplifiers helping to communicate these decisions to the rest of the brain in a loud and clear voice. The descending pathways are the cables through which the instructions flow from the frontal lobes to the critical ventral brain stem nuclei. Elsewhere in the book (Chapter 14) I comment on the fashionable notion of dopamine transmission as the "reward" system. It is important to distinguish between the originator of the signal and it amplifier. I believe that the ventral tegmental area is critical for broadcasting via its dopaminergic projections the "reward" signal actually computed in the prefrontal cortex and related structures.

In Kevin's case, I suspected that as a result of the accident a small lesion had occurred in his brain somewhere along these pathways, probably in the ventral upper brain stem, where the critical pathways originate. Even a small lesion in that area could produce a devastating effect, and it could easily remain undetected by the relatively crude, first-generation CAT scans available to us at the time. On the strength of this hunch, we ordered a new CAT scan and asked the radiologists to examine the brain stem with the highest resolution possible. And there it was, a lesion sitting exactly in the ventral tegmental area and effectively destroying it (Fig. 12.1). I called this condition the "reticulo-frontal disconnection syndrome."[4]

Today the close functional link between the prefrontal cortex and the ventral tegmental area is among the most high-profile themes in the studies of executive functions,[5] but in the late 1970s, when we first examined Kevin, this link was barely appreciated. Writing this book now 30 years after my encounter with Kevin, I think that on balance he did more for us, his doctors, than we were able to do for him. Our treatments worked to a point, and a slight but quantitatively demonstrable improvement did take place. But the old Kevin was gone and we could not bring him back. We tried very hard to help restore Kevin's shattered executive functions, but our success was modest at best. Yet by giving us the opportunity to observe and describe the reticulofrontal disconnection syndrome, Kevin helped us, through his personal catastrophe, to better understand the workings of the frontal lobes and its connections. This understanding, in turn, sheds light on many disorders affecting the frontal lobes.

The pathways connecting the frontal lobes and the ventral brain stem are particularly subject to shearing and tearing even in "mild" traumatic brain injury. As discussed later in this chapter, there are good reasons to expect that these pathways may be aberrant also in certain subtypes of schizophrenia and of ADD and ADHD.

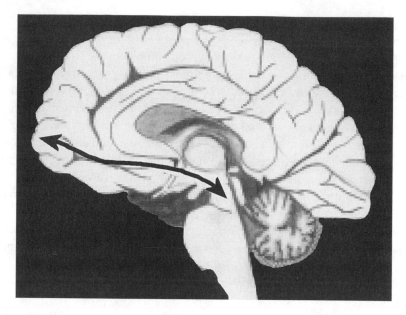

Figure 12.1 Schematic representation of the reticulofrontal pathway (arrow) connecting the ventral tegmental area with the prefrontal cortex. This pathway was damaged in Kevin's case.

Furthermore, since the frontal lobes succumb to the effects of normal aging more rapidly than does the rest of the brain (see Chapter 13), and since the myelin coating of long pathways is also highly susceptible to the effects of aging (a process known as "demyelinization"), the fate of these pathways in aging is of particular interest and should be closely studied and correlated with cognitive and neuropsychologal findings.

Kevin's condition was unusual and highly informative in yet another respect. His was the first well-documented case of remote memory impairment without a comparably severe deficit of new learning (retrograde amnesia without anterograde amnesia). This allowed us to propose the existence of an "isolated retrograde amnesia" syndrome. The scope of Kevin's retrograde amnesia was also unusual, much broader than was thought possible at the time. It concerned not only his episodic memory, but also significant aspects of his semantic memory. With my former student Bill Barr we were later able to demonstrate that retrograde amnseia commonly affected significant aspects of semantic memory. This in turn led to the conclusion that the true scope of retrograde amnesia is best described by the distinction between singular and generic knowledge, and not by the difference between episodic and semantic knowledge, as was thought at the time. Perhaps most importantly, Kevin's case enriched our understanding of the brain mechanisms of normal and abnormal memory by pointing to the role of the ventral tegmental area in memory. In addition to the well-known limbic and diencephalic amnesias, we were able to introduce the concept of mesencephalic amnesia. But this is a separate story, told in my book *The Wisdom Paradox*[6] and elsewhere.[7]

Schizophrenia: A Connection That Was Never Made

Schizophrenia is a devastating disorder of the mind that affects approximately 1% of the population. It is at least in part a hereditary disorder, although environmental factors play an important role in its clinical expression and course. Schizophrenia seems to be more prevalent and has an earlier onset in males than in females. The first overt manifestations of schizophrenia usually take place in the late teens to early 20s. Hallucinations (mostly auditory, "hearing voices") and delusions set in. They are usually paranoid, threatening in nature. The psychotic episodes are intermittent, interspersed with periods of relative mental health.[8]

In addition to the psychosis, schizophrenia is characterized by a cognitive deficit, which is permanent, present even between the psychotic episodes, and is often even more debilitating than psychosis. Two early students of schizophrenia, Emil Kraepelin and Eugen Bleuler, were well aware of this, as is reflected in the original term for schizophrenia, *dementia praecox*, or "early loss of mind." The functions of the frontal lobes are particularly disrupted in schizophrenia. In his classic book *Dementia Praecox and Paraphrenia*, Kraepelin wrote:

> On various grounds it is easy to believe that the frontal cortex, which is especially well developed in man, stands in close relation to his higher intellectual abilities, and these are the faculties which in our patients suffer profound loss in contrast to memory and acquired capabilities. The manifold volitional and motor disorder . . . makes us think of finer disorders in the neighborhood of the precentral convolution. On the other hand, the peculiar speech disorders resembling sensory aphasia and the auditory hallucinations . . . probably point to the temporal lobe being involved. We must imagine that the speech disorder is more complicated and less circumscribed than is sensory aphasia. The auditory hallucinations, which exhibit predominantly speech content, we must probably interpret as irritative phenomena in the temporal lobe.[9]

Contemporary neuropsychological and neuroimaging methods highlight the severity of frontal lobe dysfunction in schizophrenia. Of all the neuropsychological tests, schizophrenic performance is particularly impaired on the Wisconsin Card Sorting Test (WCST).[10] Since patients with frontal lobe damage find the WCST particularly vexing,[11] this is taken as evidence of frontal lobe dysfunction in schizophrenia.

Even more direct evidence of frontal lobe dysfunction in schizophrenia has been provided by the methods of functional neuroimaging. In healthy people the frontal lobes are usually more physiologically active than the rest of the cortex.[12] Neuroscientists refer to this pattern as "hyperfrontality." Hyperfrontality in normal individuals is a robust, highly replicable phenomenon, which does not depend on the method of neuroimaging used. It can be demonstrated with electroencephalography (EEG), positron emission tomography (PET), and single photon emission computerized tomography (SPECT).

In certain disorders, however, the pattern of hyperfrontality disappears. It is replaced with "hypofrontality," which means that the frontal lobe activity deteriorates relative to other parts of the cortex. Hypofrontality is a sure sign of severe frontal lobe dysfunction. Daniel Weinberger and his colleagues at the National Institute of Mental Health used PET to study brain activation patterns in schizophrenia. And true enough, severe hypofrontality was revealed.[13]

Popular conceptions of schizophrenia emphasize hallucinations and delusions, the so-called positive symptoms. But mental health professionals increasingly realize that the "negative" symptoms are far more debilitating. The negative symptoms of schizophrenia are the telltale symptoms of frontal lobe dysfunction. They include lack of initiative and drive and affective flatness. Schizophrenic patients tend to perseverate, which we know by now to be a frontal symptom. They are notorious for "loose" and "tangential associations," which are remarkably akin to the field-dependent behavior common in frontal lobe damage. Just think of Vladimir's monologues.

The first overt psychotic manifestation of schizophrenia usually takes place at about the age of 17 or 18, which is also the age of the functional maturation of the frontal lobes. Is this coincidental? Probably not. It is possible that the organism is able to compensate for a faulty development of the frontal lobes to a point. But once the disparity between the required adaptive frontal lobe function and its actual limited contribution hampered by disease is too great, the whole system decompensates and clinical disorder becomes evident.

Why are the frontal lobes particularly affected in schizophrenia? This question leads to a broader question: what is the cause of schizophrenic disorder? The puzzle is far from solved, but some of the pieces are already in place. Beginning at the turn of the twentieth century, various treatments have been tried to cure schizophrenia, without much success. Some of these treatments were, in retrospect, pretty horrific: shaking therapy, fever-inducing animal blood and syphilis-infected blood transfusion, and insulin coma among them.[14] Finally, in the 1960s a class of medications was introduced that appeared to have a genuine therapeutic effect. These "neuroleptics" acted on the neurotransmitter dopamine (DA). Neuroleptics were quite successful in reducing the so-called positive symptoms of schizophrenia, hallucinations and delusions.

The discovery of neuroleptics marked a turning point in not only the treatment of schizophrenia but also the understanding of its mechanisms. The reasoning followed a simple syllogism. Neuroleptics relieve psychotic symptoms in schizophrenia. Neuroleptics act on the dopamine system. Therefore, schizophrenia is a disorder of the dopamine system. The logic behind this argument is patently flawed. According to this logic, an accident victim in a wheelchair had lost a pair of wheels, not a pair of legs. Drug efficacy does not always mean that the drug acts directly on a disordered ingredient.

Yet, despite the logical flaw behind its rise to prominence, the dopamine theory of schizophrenia has taken hold and received support from other experimental sources. Today it is widely accepted that the dopamine system is somehow impaired in schizophrenia, either by itself or as a consequence of a mismatch in the way dopamine interacts with other neurotransmitters, such as gamma-aminobutyric acid (GABA) and glutamate.[15] But which dopamine system is impaired? Several are known to exist in the brain. Of particular interest to us are the nigrostriatal and mesolimbic–mesocortical dopamine systems.

Both systems originate in the brain stem, the nigrostriatal dopamine system in the nucleus, or *substantia nigra*, and the mesolimbic–mesocortical dopamine system in the *ventral tegmental area*.[16] The nigrostriatal dopamine pathway projects into the basal ganglia, a group of nuclei found below the frontal lobes, which are important for the regulation of movements. This pathway is not affected by schizophrenia itself, but it may be affected by the drugs used to treat schizophrenia.

The current thinking about schizophrenia focuses on the mesolimbic–mesocortical dopamine system. As mentioned earlier, the disorder is presumed to either originate within this system or be expressed through it as the remote effect of a disorder affecting glutamate, GABA, or other neurotransmitters.[17] The system diverges into two components: mesolimbic and mesocortical. The mesolimbic dopamine pathway projects into the deep (mesial) aspect of the temporal lobe. The mesocortical dopamine pathway is already familiar to us—it is the pathway that is disrupted in the reticulofrontal disconnection syndrome and which was presumably damaged in the fallen horseman. Dysfunction within this pathway probably also accounts for much of frontal lobe dysfunction in schizophrenia.[18]

Of course, the analogy between a schizophrenic patient and the fallen horseman is limited. In Kevin, the mesolimbic–mesocortical dopamine system had functioned properly up to the age of 36, when it was destroyed as a result of head injury. Kevin's cognitive development had completed its normal course before the injury. By contrast, in a schizophrenic patient the deficit is presumed to be neurodevelopmental. The mesocortical dopamine pathway fails to develop properly from the outset, due to some combination of genetic and environmental factors. This means that in schizophrenics the whole cognitive development is likely to be subtly different from that of healthy people. The cognitive development is abnormal from the beginning, long before the first overt clinical symptoms of schizophrenia are recognized. In Kevin the lesion was structural, caused by mechanical impact to the head. In schizophrenia the deficit is biochemical.

Despite the obvious differences between the two conditions, the neuroanatomy of the deficit is somewhat similar, in both cases affecting the projections from the ventral tegmental brain stem into the frontal lobes. Frontal disconnection appears to be central to both disorders, neurodevelopmental in one case, acquired in the other.

Abnormal dopamine biochemistry is probably not the only factor behind the frontal lobe dysfunction in schizophrenia. Fine quantitative CAT and magnetic resonance imaging (MRI) studies of schizophrenic brain have revealed numerous structural abnormalities as well, including the decrement of the gray matter cortical volume.[19] This decrement is quite widespread and does not appear to be limited to any particular part of the brain. Still, some studies suggest that it is particularly pronounced in the frontal lobes.[20]

To conclude, both biochemical and structural factors may play a role in frontal lobe dysfunction in schizophrenia. Whatever the exact mechanisms of this dysfunction are, Kraepelin's prescient conclusion has been confirmed by modern neuroscience. Schizophrenia is to a large extent a frontal lobe disease.

Kraepelin was prescient in yet another respect, by implicating the temporal lobe, in particular the left temporal lobe. Subtle difficulties of perceptual organization have been well documented in certain forms of schizophrenia. To use the vernacular of cognitive science, these difficulties seem to reflect a breakdown of "top-down" control over perception, or "filtering": previously formed, generalized perceptual representations fail to exert their organizing influence on the incoming sensory information. We encountered this condition in Chapter 5, under the name "associative agnosia." This is caused by damage to the left hemisphere, a finding that can be easily explained and even predicted by the novelty-routinization principle of hemispheric specialization. A typical case of associative agnosia results from a neurological event, such as stroke or a penetrating gunshot wound to the head, acquired in adulthood. But in an article published in *Brain and Behavioral Sciences*,[21] I argued that certain aspects of the perceptual disorganization in schizophrenia can be best understood as neurodevelopmental associative agnosia caused by the neurodevelopmental dysfunction of the left hemipshere. The understanding of the interaction between the frontal-lobe and the lateralized aspects of schizophrenic disorder has been advanced by the work of several leading neuroscientists, notably Timothy Crow and his associates at Oxford University.[22]

Head Trauma: A Broken Connection

Traumatic brain injury (TBI) is a particularly poignant condition, since it is largely a disease of young people. In the beginning and middle of the twentieth century, TBI involved mostly penetrating gunshot wounds. But in the Western world today, TBI is usually caused by car accidents and job-related accidents. In the popular lore, TBI lacks the drama of Alzheimer's disease, acquired immune deficiency syndrome (AIDS), or schizophrenia, but it is an epidemic of similar proportions. Since more than 2,000,000 people sustain TBI annually in the United States alone, it is sometimes referred to as the "silent epidemic."[23]

In the majority of cases, the so-called mild head injury, a seemingly complete recovery occurs within a few weeks of the injury. There is no lasting loss of movement, language, or perception. Deficit of memory and attention may persist longer, but eventually they also disappear. These patients are pronounced "fully recovered" and sent off to enjoy life.

Yet, in subtle ways, these young people are no longer their own selves. Drive, initiative, and competitive edge are often gone. They become passive and indifferent. Frequently they become inappropriately jocular, emotionally volatile, irritable, fractious, and impulsive. To an ordinary observer, these changes usually do not signal neurological impairment. In the tradition of naive dualism, they are often dismissed as "personality changes," as if "personality" were an extracranial trait. But in fact these changes reflect subtle impairment of the executive functions, subtle dysfunction of the frontal lobes.

The CAT and MRI scans are usually normal in these patients. For years, this contributed to the belief that the patients did not suffer lasting brain damage. Indeed, in most of these patients there is no structural lesion *within* the frontal lobes. But with the advent of functional neuroimaging, it became possible to study the physiology of the frontal lobes, in addition to its structure. Joseph Masdeu and his colleagues used SPECT to study brain blood flow patterns in patients with mild head trauma.[24] Invariably, blood flow was abnormal, and often it was reduced in the frontal lobes. This pattern of "hypofrontality" was present even when the MRI scan was normal.

Like schizophrenia, closed head injury often presents a puzzling picture of frontal lobe dysfunction without a frontal lobe lesion. And again, the mechanism is likely to be damage to the bidirectional projections between the brain stem and the frontal lobes—the reticulofrontal disconnection syndrome. Many neurologists have always felt that such damage is likely to occur in head injury. Today it is finally possible to understand both its causes and its consequences.

Kevin's case was relatively unique in that the lesion disrupting these connections was large enough to be seen on the CT scan. In most cases, however, the "shearing and tearing" damage to the pathways is too microscopic to be captured on CT or even on conventional MRI scans. But today new neuroimaging tools are increasingly available, capable of ascertaining the condition of long pathways directly. Diffusion tensor imaging MRI (DTI) is one of them. It allows one to trace the diffusion vectors of water molecules in biological tissues, and by so doing to infer the direction and integrity of long pathways. DTI is being used increasingly to characterize various neurocognitive disorders,[25] and I believe that damage to the long projections interfacing ventral brain stem and the frontal lobes will be found in many, perhaps even most, cases of "mild" traumatic brain injury.

The news emanating from this understanding is both good and bad. The bad news is that the prevalence of lasting impairment following even "mild" head trauma is higher than had been thought. Almost invariably, the impairment affects frontal lobe functions. The good news is that identifying the cause is the first step toward developing effective therapies. The effects of reticulofrontal disconnection are presynaptic. Since there is no lesion *within* the frontal lobes, the receptors for the critical neurotransmitters (the chemicals in charge of signal passage between neurons) are largely intact.

This opens the door for truly "cognotropic" pharmacology in closed head injury.[26] By *cognotropic* I mean the kind of pharmacology that is directed specifically at the cognitive deficit. There is nothing new about giving medications to patients recovering from head injury. However, the traditional rationale behind these treatments was directed at the control of seizures, depression, or other common consequences of head injury, but not at the cognitive deficit itself. It was not until the mid-1990s that the first attempts were made to use pharmacology directly to improve cognition of patients recovering from traumatic brain injury. Not surprisingly, in light of the previous discussion, this pharmacology targets mostly the dopamine system.[27]

Attention Deficit/Hyperactivity Disorder: A Fragile Connection

If one were to run a "disease of the decade" contest, attention deficit disorder (ADD) and attention deficit hyperactivity disorder (ADHD) would be among the plausible contenders.[28] At the close of the twentieth century and the beginning of the twenty-first, the diagnosis has been made generously and casually, often with little understanding of the underlying mechanisms, and sometimes with none at all. Parents actively seek the ADD diagnosis for their children to explain their school failures, and adults seek it for themselves to explain their life failures. It is not uncommon for a patient to ask the doctor "to diagnose my ADD." The proposition, of course, is utterly oxymoronic, about as sensible as asking, "What is the color of my green sweater?" But many doctors oblige, and those who do not often run the risk of losing their patients to those who do (it happened to me). It is not unheard of for a patient to shop for a doctor until the magic diagnosis is obtained.

When a diagnosis is not merely suffered but sought, clearly we have more than a clinical disorder; we have a social phenomenon. The reasons for ADD becoming a social phenomenon may well be worth a separate sociological and cultural anthropological treatise. I believe that it has to do with a complex combination of several cultural factors.

First, it has to do with the guilt, parental or personal, for one's child's or one's own failures. A clinical diagnosis removes the guilt and even the sense of responsibility. In an age when diagnostic labels proliferate, this offers a convenient way of unburdening the responsibility for life's failure. Second, it has to do with the ever-expanding scope of perceived individual rights and antidiscrimination. A clinical diagnosis earns all kinds of concessions and exemptions in wide-ranging situations. Third, the ADD phenomenon is true to the indefatigable American belief that anything can be fixed with the right pill (in this case, Ritalin). This may explain why another heavily inflated diagnosis of our time, learning disability (LD), is nonetheless nowhere nearly as commonly made or sought after: there is no ready promise of a magic pill.

Finally, the general-public appeal of the ADD diagnosis has much to do with the illusory transparency of the very notion of "attention." Just as with "memory," everyone has an immediate, albeit often misguided, sense of the word's meaning. This, in turn, leads to an equally misguided sense of confidence in one's self-diagnosis. Nobody has introspection into one's pancreas, but everybody has introspection into one's own mind. As a result, very few lay individuals would presume to make the self-diagnosis of pancreatitis, but most people would have no compunction in self-diagnosing their ADD.

Together with verbal and nonverbal learning disabilities of various stripes, and probably even more so, ADHD is among the more elastic diagnoses even when made by qualified professionals. This is inevitable, given that ADHD is a syndrome not linked to any single, well-defined pathogen. Disorders caused by distinct pathogens can be thought of in inherently discrete terms. Any notion of "continuity" between hepatitis B and hepatitis C would strike an infectious disease expert as nonsensical. But syndromes defined as constellations of cognitive symptoms are inherently idiosyncratic, particularly when the syndromes in question may be caused by a number of different pathologies. These syndromes' definition is further complicated when all these pathologies have broad and overlapping ranges of neuroanatomical expressions. Since the pattern of cognitive deficit depends more on the neuroanatomy of the disorder than on its biological cause (a circumstance that many physicians and psychologists fail to fully grasp), the relationship among cognition, neuroanatomy, and the biological cause of the disease becomes particularly complicated. As a result, cognitively and behaviorally constructed syndromes should be thought of not as intrinsically discrete entities but as regions on continuous multidimensional symptom distributions with inherently arbitrary boundaries.

The additional complication, both conceptual and practical diagnostic, is that the pathological processes that produce the neurodevelopmental disorders in question are almost never focal, since mother nature is under no obligation to adhere to our discrete taxonomic manuals. This leads to the so-called comorbidity of different learning disabilities and ADHD, which is really not comorbidity at all, since the different symptoms in question seen in combination in a single individual are usually all caused by a single, albeit neuroanatomically distributed, pathological process rather than separate pathological processes.

With such a cluttered background, it is important to restore some measure of precision to the terms *attention* and *attention deficit*. Attention deficit hyperactivity disorder is a genuine and highly prevalent condition, which can be precisely diagnosed and treated. A substantial body of rigorous research into this disorder exists, much of it summarized in an excellent book by Torkel Klingberg, *The Overflowing Brain*.[29] A genuine deficit of attention can indeed have quite devastating effects on cognition. This has been highlighted by the relatively recent findings challenging the notion that highly overlearned mental operations are completely "automatic" and do not require attention at all; it turns out that even such highly overlearned processes remain under attentional control at least to some degree.[30] Attention has often been compared to a flashlight illuminating a certain aspect of our mental or physical world against the background of competing distractors. Is there any biological reality behind the flashlight metaphor? There just may be. As we explore the analogy, we will see that attention involves complex neural machinery consisting of the prefrontal cortex and its connections. For this reason, I prefer "a set of stagelights" to "a flashlight" as a metaphor, since a mulitude of pathways is at play, rather than a single pathway.

Once we link ADHD to frontal lobe dysfunction, its very high prevalence (even when the diagnosis is made rigorously and conservatively) should come as no surprise. As we already know, frontal lobes are particularly vulnerable in a very broad range of disorders, hence the very high rate of frontal lobe dysfunction. The diagnosis of ADD or ADHD commonly refers to any condition characterized by mild dysfunction of the frontal lobes and related pathways in the absence of any other, comparably severe dysfunction. Given the high rate of frontal lobe dysfunction due to a variety of causes, the prevalence of genuine ADHD should be expected to be very high. But saying merely that ADHD is a mild form of the frontal lobe disorder oversimplifies the matter.

To pursue the stagelights analogy further, let us remind ourselves that a set of stagelights is an instrument. Someone (or something) must be responsible for choosing which stagelight to turn on and for how long. In neural terms, this means that the goal of action must be identified and it must effectively guide behavior for a period of time. We already know that goal setting and goal maintenance are provided by the *prefrontal cortex*. This is the actor, the lighting operator whose hand controls the stage set keyboard.

The stagelights analogy also implies the stage in need of illumination. The stage is found in the brain, mostly in the *posterior aspects of the cortical hemispheres.* These are the structures most directly involved in processing the incoming information. Depending on the goal at hand, distinct, particular parts of the posterior cortex must be brought into the state of optimal activation (illuminated by an appropriate stagelight, so to speak). The selection of these areas is accomplished by the prefrontal cortex, which selects the appropriate stagelight accordingly.

The stagelights themselves are found in the nuclei of the *ventral brain stem,* which can selectively activate vast cortical regions through their ascending projections. The prefrontal cortex guides the "stagelights" through its own descending pathways into the ventral brain stem. Finally, the prefrontal cortex *modifies* its control over the stagelights, based on the *feedback* it receives from the posterior cortex.

In sum, attention can best be described as a looplike process involving complex interactions among the prefrontal cortex, ventral brain stem, and posterior cortex (Fig. 12.2). Breakdown anywhere along this loop may interfere with attention, thus producing a form of attention deficit disorder.

The first consequence of this analysis is that the deficit of attention is among the most common consequences of brain damage. The second consequence of this analysis is that a number of distinct variants of attention deficit disorder exist, some with and others without hyperactivity. Yet a third consequence is that this understanding of attentional mechanisms allows one to develop a unified understanding of two sets of disorders that traditionally have been regarded separately: attention deficit disorder and hemiinattention. Attention deficit disorder has been regarded mostly as a neurodevelopmental disorder, the purview of child and adolescent psychiatrists and neurologists. By conrast, hemiinattention and hemineglect, a peculiar condition in which a patient underattends to or even completely ignores one half of the stimulus space, which may affect half of the visual space or even half of the patient's own body, has been the purview of neurologists treating the effects of stroke or other focal lesions. I tend to think of these two conditions as being closely related, affecting different sides of the triangle depicted in Figure 12.2. Damage (structural or biochemical) to the connections between the prefrontal cortex and the brain stem machinery of arousal and activation produces the condition we call ADD or ADHD, whereas damage to the connections between the posterior association cortex and the brain stem and/or thalamic nuclei in charge

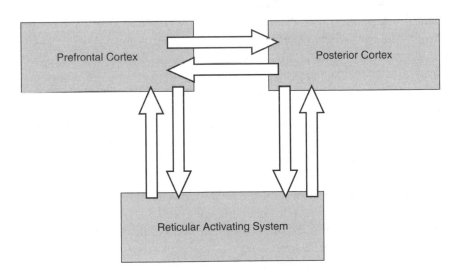

Figure 12.2 Fronto-reticular-posterior cortical attention loop (see text for explanation).

of arousal and activation produces the condition known as hemineglect or hemi-inattention. Both sets of pathways project into both hemispheres. However, the frontoreticular pathways are characterized by a relatively midline trajectory, the left- and right-hemispheric projections traveling in close proximity to each other. By contrast, the pathways connecting the brain stem and thalamic nuclei with the posterior portions of the left and right hemispheres follow distinctly separate trajectories and thus can be affected separately by a stroke or other focal lesion, resulting in distinctly lateralized, "hemi" manifestation.[31]

The aspects of attention mediated by the frontoreticular pathways and the brain stem and thalamic pathways projecting to the posterior protions of the hemispheres are functionally distinct, however. The former set of pathways is most likely involved in the "top-down" forms of voluntary attention internally driven by the cognitive context at hand. By contrast, the latter set of pathways is most likely involved in the "bottom-up" involuntary forms of attention driven by external stimuli. This division of labor is consistent with extracellular-recording findings in the monkey, reported by Timothy Buschman and Earl Miller.[32]

The prefrontal cortex and its connections to the ventral brain stem (the hand controlling the stagelights) play a particularly important role in the mechanisms of attention. Precisely because the ventral brain stem contains a number of nuclei involved in arousal and activation, a stage set may provide a more accurate analogy than a single flashlight. When we talk about attention deficit disorder we usually implicate these systems. The exact causes of damage to these systems vary. They may be inherited or acquired early in life. They may be biochemical or structural. In the latter case it may be possible to detect damage with diffusion tensor imaging MRI, and I believe that the DTI methodology will prove very powerful in elucidating the mechanisms of attentional disorders. More recently, an even more advanced methodology was developed at New York University School of Medicine, diffusion kurtosis imaging (DKI), which, unlike DTI, is not constrained by the assumption of normal distribution and is more powerful in separating different pathways' contribution to a composite bundle.[33]

It should come as no surprise that the features of ADD are usually combined with some aspects of executive deficit. When the executive deficit is severe, the diagnosis of ADD becomes superfluous. But when it is mild, when the attentional impairment stands out and the executive deficit is minimal, then the diagnosis of ADD is properly made. In most such cases biochemical disorder affecting the frontal lobe connections is present, but there is no actual structural damage to the frontal lobes. In some cases the attentional deficit is highly encapsulated and may coexist with supreme capacity for planning and foresight. Winston Churchill may have been a case in point. Numerous descriptions of his behavior are strongly evocative of ADHD. Yet he was the man who foresaw the danger of Lenin, then Stalin, then Hitler, then Stalin again, ahead of most other political leaders of the free world. Thus he can hardly be faulted for a lack of foresight.

Of course, we know that the term *executive functions* is quite broad, subsuming a wide range of more specific cognitive functions. Some of these functions, like working memory, intrinsically imply real-time processing. Other functions subsumed under the broad ruberic of *executive control* are less closely linked to real time. Strategic military planning or strategic corporate planning usually do not require unflagging, split-second alertness and thus may be successfully executed even when attention is somewhat compromised, hence the Winston Churchill phenomenon. From a neuroanatomical standpoint, the pathways we have discussed here are complex. They comprise both ascending and descending pathways. Within the medial forebrain bundle interconneting the frontal lobes and the ventral brain stem, the descending components are more closely linked to the "guiding hand" and the ascending components to the "stage lights." To the extent that these pathways are biochemically distinct (e.g., the ascending components are mostly catecholaminergic, norepinephrine, and dopamine dependent, and the descending components are glutamate/GABA dependent), it is conceivable that certain neurodevelopmental disorders may selectively affect some biochemical systems while sparing others, thus having a different impact on different aspects of attention and executive functions. By contrast, acquired brain dysfunction due to a macroscopic lesion, as in traumatic brain injury, is likely to have a less differentiated impact, affecting the ascending and descending pathways to an equal degree, thus producing more global impairment impacting both attention and executive functions.

Attention deficit in ADD is often selective. It is present only in the "uninteresting" activities but is absent in "interesting" activities. If the patient enjoys the task (a computer game or sporting event) and derives pleasure from it, his or her attention is on the mark. But attention drifts on any task devoid of instant reward, such as listening to a lecture or reading a textbook. This observation clearly links ADD to frontal lobe dysfunction, given the role of the prefrontal cortex in goal setting, volition, and delayed gratification.

The attention deficit disorder comes in a variety of forms. Functionally the prefrontal cortex is diverse (left–right, dorsolateral–orbitofrontal); thus different anatomical patterns of frontal lobe dysfunction will disrupt attention in different ways. The pathways connecting the prefrontal cortex with the ventral brain stem nuclei are biochemically complex. Damage to different biochemical components within these pathways will also disrupt attention in different ways.

The *H* between the *D*'s is a case in point. It is common to distinguish between attention deficit disorder (ADD) and attention deficit hyperactivity disorder (ADHD). It may very well be that the *hyperactive* form is most commonly associated with subtle dysfunction of orbitofrontal cortex and its pathways. This is why ADHD is often associated with the volatility of affect commonly seen in orbitofrontal damage. By contrast, the *nonhyperactive* form is more likely to be associated with subtle dysfunction of dorsolateral cortex and its pathways.

The distinction between ADD and ADHD is only the beginning. Numerous forms of attention deficit probably exist, requiring different remedies. As we learn more about the frontal lobes and their connections, we will be able to identify these forms and their remedies with growing precision.

ADHD Conquered: How Toby from Down Under Reclaimed Himself

Toby used to say that he is an anomaly by definition, since he consists of three halves: half black, half Jewish, and half gay. Toby used the word *black* generically, referring to all people of color, and the "half" in question is not African but Polynesian. Nonetheless, all three "halves" represent minorities persecuted in many societies, with Toby at the intercept.

Toby was adopted at the age of 6 days, so his exact background is unknown. Based on the information from his adoptive parents and his own research, his bio-logical father was a French Jew and his biological mother was a Maori from New Zealand. They were college students in Sydney, and Toby was the obviously unwanted product of a date rape. His adoptive parents were a middle-class Welsh couple who immigrated to Australia from Great Britain. They wanted a daughter but adopted Toby because their older child (also adopted) was a boy and they did not have a separate room for a girl. This background of "unwantedness" haunted Toby all his life, and he talked about it movingly in a documentary made about him many years later. The documentary, entitled *Alias*, was shown to critical acclaim at several film festivals in Australia, including the Bondi Film Festival and Sydney Short Film Festival (both in 1998).

Toby was a precocious child. He studied voice, the flute, and dance. Singled out for his exceptional talent, he performed solo at various gala events. But Toby was also a difficult, willful child. On many occasions, when his parents clashed with Toby, they practiced "tough love." They would pack a little bag with Toby's posses-sions and tell him to get out of the house and return only when he "repented."

Predictably, Toby would walk around the block and return knocking at the door, "repentant," until the next time. But once, at the age of nine, Toby did not return. Instead, he walked several miles in the middle of the night, clutching his little bag, from the suburb where he grew up to downtown Sydney. There he joined other homeless children and began his life as a street urchin.

For several years Toby was making a living as a hustler, a male street prostitute. Many years later he took me on a tour of "his" Sydney and brought me to the "Wailing Wall," a yellow sandstone structure, the exterior of Sydney's first jail off Oxford Street next to St. Vincent's Hospice, where the child hustlers used to congregate waiting for "johns." At first, I found my Jewish sensibilities offended by this sacrile-gious reference, but then I acceded to its bitter accuracy. On the Wall, Toby showed me a faded graffiti "Toby, 1976," made during his life on the streets.

For all the other cases in this book I use fictitious names to protect my patients' confidentiality. "Toby," however, is in a sense a real name. It is one of several "noms de guerre" that Toby used in his profession as a child sex worker on the streets of Sydney. All these years Toby has visited his graffiti periodically, spending some silent time with it and making sure it had not faded or been erased. He invited me to join him on this pilgrimage to his Wall, and I chose not to pry into the complex emotions that must have surrounded the ritual, and just stood silently by.

In the course of his street life, Toby became addicted to numerous drugs— heroin, cocaine, speed, barbiturates, and anything else that he could find. Feeling increasingly desperate and trapped, Toby wrote this poem, "My Love for My Lady Sin," at the age of 16, likening his drug addiction to "Lady Sin":

A tale of sadness was born
In my love for my Lady Sin.
A story of trouble and woe,
And loneliness found within.

My lady stepped into my life
One night when I was alone,
And in the void she found in my heart
She quietly made her home.

The first year was fantasy, fiction.
The second a gay carousel.
By the third, the signs started showing,
By the fourth, my friends all could tell.

But still I worshipped my lady,
And one day I made her my wife.
And in my woe, with words "I do,"
I quietly gave up my life.

So my body and soul are now twisted,
That which did not waste away.
And I cry as I quietly remember,
It's the price we all have to pay.

This devotion doth turn to obsession,
My body as torn as my heart.
But still to my ear she whispers,
"Till death do us part."[34]

At the age of 19, Toby sought out his adoptive parents, made peace with them, and embarked on an effort to rejoin the mainstream. Over the next few years he learned several trades. At various points he worked as a horticulture and hydroponics specialist, a nurse practitioner, a hairdresser, a makeup designer, a counselor for homeless children. By all accounts, he became quite accomplished in each of these trades. The only graduate with perfect test scores in the history of his agricultural college, Toby was invited to teach at the college immediately upon graduation, an unprecedented appointment. Faced with students often much older than himself and looking even younger than he was, Toby grew a beard to look "professorial." Toby also became increasingly interested in creative writing and photography, and his work was beginning to meet with modest success. He had an amazing knowledge of animals and plants, and he used to maintain a menagerie consisting of several dogs, lizards, birds, and mice, as well as fish and frogs in the pond of the little Japanese garden he created in front of his house in a suburb of Sydney.

Despite his obvious and numerous talents, however, Toby was unable to hold a job. Sooner or later (usually sooner) Toby would get into violent arguments with his co-workers and end up fired or he would quit in a huff. He was restless and could not stick with any one activity. His adoptive parents hoped that Toby would take advantage of his obvious talent and become a veterinarian. But just as he was unable to settle in a job, Toby was unable to settle on a profession. The restlessness was pervasive and it played itself out in numerous ways. Toby attributed this restlessness to being multitalented, but it was clearly maladaptive.

Toby's personal relationships were also volatile and tumultuous, and his social persona was full of contradictions. He was known to be warm, loyal, and generous, someone who would never turn away a friend in need. At the same time he was explosive, quarrelsome, and belligerent even with his closest friends. He had a daughter out of wedlock and acted the part of a caring, devoted, and involved father, yet he was unable to settle into a marriage or any other sort of long-term relationship. When he finally did, the relationship was punctuated with volatility and outright violence, yet it was characterized by strong mutual commitment. He continued to fight his drug addiction, joined a methadone clinic, and finally, after several setbacks, was able to kick the habit.

I first met Toby during one of my frequent visits to Sydney, and then again when he visited New York. He was now in his 30s and full of contradictions. Immediately, Toby struck me as uncommonly intelligent and articulate, yet also uncommonly immature. Without actually having measured his IQ, I would guess it to be somewhere around 140–150, within a "very superior" range. Yet he was constantly caught unprepared for the consequences of his own and other people's actions, apparently unable to anticipate them. Things tended to constantly "happen" to Toby "all of a sudden," suggesting a glaring lack of foresight. Toby possessed an amazing amount of knowledge on an amazingly broad range of subjects, yet it was haphazard and unsystematic. At the same time, Toby was capable of an uncanny insight into people and situations at hand, and he was an exceptionally keen judge of human character. It appeared that his weakness of judgment was limited to the temporal domain, when some projection into the future was required. Toby was the most striking example in my personal experience of how noninterchangeable "insight" and "foresight" are, and how sharply divided these two abilities could be in the same individual. Toby was a man with superb capacity for *insight* and virtually zero *foresight*.

Restlessness was the dominant feature of Toby's personality, and it was evident in every interaction. The pressure to act, to move on, was palpable. He had a dozen competing plans and thoughts at any given time, all tripping over one another. In a group social setting, he had to talk with everyone simultaneously and then rush out in the middle of the dinner to do something else. A telephone conversation was invariably and suddenly interrupted in half-sentence with "I have to run." He had a volatile temper, with precipitous oscillations between gregarious charm one moment and brooding hostility the next. As I observed Toby's interactions with other people, I found his outbursts disturbing—extreme, unprovoked, almost frightening. Yet he was so obviously intelligent and gifted. He knew Sydney like the palm of his hand and was an insightful and witty guide.

Increasingly, I got the impression that Toby's outrageous behaviors had a life of their own, that Toby was engaged in them *in spite of himself*, and that he was in pain. As a result, my sympathy for Toby overrode my irritation at his antics. It was this combination of intelligence and pain that I connected with, and it made Toby attractive despite his very unattractive traits. Toby seemed to engender this reaction in other people as well. He was, on balance, well liked and had many friends of all ages and from every walk of life who let him get away with behaviors not usually forgiven.

The clinician in me became more and more intrigued by what I saw. Toby was clearly hyperactive and also possibly suffered from a bipolar disorder. His affect fluctuated constantly and wildly. On a few occasions Toby made allusions to "highs" and "lows," confirming my observations. That Toby's life consisted of extreme states with very little in between was reflected in the diary he kept, true to his literary bent. The diary notes were entered from both ends of a big book: the "day section" and the "night section," referring to Toby's high and low points. In this context, Toby's past drug history looked like a desperate attempt at self-medication, a phenomenon not uncommon in people with subtle, undiagnosed conditions. I felt that I should talk to Toby and urge him to seek professional help, but an occasion did not present itself and I left Sydney without having this conversation.

I returned to Australia half a year later and Toby joined me for dinner at the Russian Accent restaurant in Sydney's Darlinghurst section. He seemed different. As if reading my mind, Toby started the conversation by recounting the events of the past few months. On his own, Toby had reached the conclusion that something was clinically wrong with him and that he was in need of professional help. He found a psychiatrist who put him on Dexedrine, a stimulant in the amphetamine family often prescribed to treat ADHD.

Dexedrine worked. Toby remained on it throughout my 6-week stint as a visiting professor at the University of Sydney, and I was able to observe its effects on several social occasions (which included a visit to the Wailing Wall). Toby was calmer, more thoughtful, less argumentative, and no longer visibly hyperactive. There were no racing, competing, or conflicting ideas and no impulsive changes of mind every 5 minutes. There was no rush from one activity to another. Toby was able to sit and relax through a dinner, something he had not been able to do before; now it was usually I who finished our telephone conversations with "I have to go." His affect no longer bounced from one extreme to another and was most of the time where it should be, at a pleasant, neutral level. For the first time since I had known Toby, he was predictable in a normal kind of way. Toby's capacity for organized, goal-oriented behavior had clearly improved as well. He no longer projected the image of immaturity and was talking and acting in a way that was, well, mature.

As I found out later, 3 months into treatment Toby developed depression, a known side effect of Dexedrine. He was switched to lithium but felt "lifeless," his "thought processes slowed down." With his doctor's consent, Toby decided to go completely off medications. He joined a support group and sought supportive psychotherapy. He feels that finally understanding his condition gives him power over it, and he is, on the whole, a much happier man. As of this writing, Toby continues to do reasonably well. He seems to have conquered his demons and successfully reclaimed himself.

For the first time in his life, Toby has been able to pursue things in a relatively systematic and methodical way. He bought a farm and is in the process of turning it into a thriving horticultural business. For the first time in his life he is making a considerable, steady income. At the end of my last visit to Australia, Toby showed up with a half-dozen bottles of my favorite Australian reds, mostly Shiraz blends, as a parting gift. The wines were young and had to mature for 4 or 5 years, and Toby made a point of bringing this to my attention. "Could *you* delay gratification for so long?" I asked. "Now I could," came the answer.

As a friend, I was delighted to witness Toby's success. As a professional, I found it instructive that hyperactivity and attention deficit were so closely interwoven in this exceptionally bright individual with the textbook features of orbitofrontal dysfunction: poor planning and foresight, combined with diminished impulse control and exaggerated affective volatility. I could also place Toby's past drug addiction in a different perspective. It is not uncommon for people with various biochemical imbalances to self-medicate, usually with self-defeating results (although, admittedly, there were many factors in Toby's life on the street that may have contributed to his multiple addictions). With successful treatment, these symptoms disappeared, or at least receded, in concert. Although we do not fully understand how Dexedrine (or, for that matter, Ritalin, Adderall, or other stimulants used to treat ADHD) works, it somehow helped strengthen the fragile frontal lobe connections to other parts of the brain.

Toby's life continued to be a struggle, stretches of success being interspersed with painful reversals. The problem has not disappeared, but he has learned how to manage it, at least to a degree. The knowledge that his problem is biochemical helped Toby cope with it and removed the guilt and the shame. He no longer perceived it as a personal failure of character, but merely as a medical condition. Toby has learned to cope and to prevail.

Jerky Tics and Ticky Jokes

Frontal lobes are particularly closely linked with subcortical nuclei called the basal ganglia, especially with the caudate nuclei. This functional relationship is so close that the term "greater frontal lobes" may be warranted, by analogy with "greater New York," which includes Westchester, parts of Long Island, parts of Connecticut, and so on. Dysfunction within the frontal-striatal system results in one of the most fascinating neurological conditions, Tourette's syndrome.[35] Tourette's is a disorder associated with, among other symptoms, involuntary motor tics and involuntary verbalizations, often highly inappropriate and offensive. It is precisely this provocative productive quality that makes it so intriguing.

Our culture traditionally approaches a neurological disorder as a deficit, a loss. This is reflected in our terminology: aphasia—loss of language; amnesia—loss of memory. Hypermnesia and hyperverbality, when they occur, are viewed by society as a mnemonic or literary gift, not as pathology. But if the norm is defined as the population average, then talent is, by definition, a deviation from the norm. The relationship between talent and psychopathology has intrigued and beguiled both clinicians and those afflicted (or blessed). Edgar Allan Poe, himself suffering from episodes of confusion, paranoia, and possibly seizures, wrote poignantly about genius and madness intertwined.[36]

It is common to distinguish in neurological and neuropsychological conditions between "negative" and "positive" symptoms. Negative symptoms reflect the loss of something that should normally be present, such as the ability to walk, talk, and see things. Positive symptoms reflect the presence of something that is not part of normal cognition, such as hallucinations or tics. Negative symptoms are more readily comprehensible, easier to conceptualize, measure, quantify, and subject to rigorous scientific examination. Positive symptoms are usually more elusive, more mysterious but also more intriguing and challenging. They hint at an inner world that is different and not merely impoverished—at the presence of a neurological condition that not only robs but also endows.

The link between creativity and mental illness is strikingly apparent in the lives and genius of van Gogh, Nijinsky, and Rimbaud. This is true also for some leaders with a particularly visionary brand of leadership, who shaped the history of our civilization in a way that suggests an exceptionally powerful "executive talent." Alexander the Great of Macedon, Julius Caesar, Peter the Great of Russia, and possibly Akhenaton (the Egyptian pharaoh who founded the first known monotheistic religion in the history of human civilization) suffered from epileptic seizures. Peaks of creativity and productivity were interspersed with nadirs of despair and mental paralysis in the lives and work of Byron, Tennyson, and Schumann, all of whom suffered from the bipolar manic-depressive disorder. On a more ordinary plane, I have often felt that the more gifted people in my personal surroundings paid a price for their talent in other areas of their mental life, and that the balance between gift and deficit is ruled by some unforgiving zero-sum equation.

If talent tends to come at a price, then certain neurological and psychiatric conditions may sometimes bring their own rewards. These conditions remain the source of fascination and intellectual challenge. Among such conditions, Tourette's syndrome is particularly intriguing and remains a source of fascination for scientists and the general public alike.

What makes Tourette's so intriguing is the richness and variety of positive symptoms associated with it. Originally described by George Gilles de la Tourette in 1885, this condition is characterized by uncontrollable facial and bodily tics, compulsive grunting vocalizations, profane verbalizations, and incessant exploration of the environment. These symptoms appear in various combinations, which often change over time. They may be subtle and masked or highly conspicuous. In the latter case they are often perceived as offensive and asocial.

Clinical observers of Tourette's patients also note a particular quickness of wit reminiscent of a fencing match and a peculiar cognitive style. Over the years of observing people with Tourette's, I came to recognize a unique and unmistakable mental quirkiness, quickness, and jerkiness of their thought processes. There are also peculiarly wicked, singularly irreverent and risqué, jousting flashes of humor. At the height of the Bill Clinton–Monica Lewinsky scandal a tourettic acquaintance of mine appeared, accompanied by his girlfriend, at a party in the house of a mutual friend and announced with a flourish: "Neither I nor my girlfriend had sex with the president." As a visual metaphor of tourettic cognition, Balinese dance comes to mind. This quick quirkiness of the mind goes hand in hand with the quick quirkiness of the movements. This is not all curse: some Tourette's patients are known to be gifted in sports like karate and basketball despite their condition.

The symptoms of Tourette's usually appear in childhood, sometimes triggered by a traumatic event, and often disappear with age. However, in many cases the symptoms persist through the life span. Tourette's tends to afflict males more often than females.[37] Because of the diversity of manifestations, it is increasingly common to talk about the "Tourette's spectrum" rather than a single Tourette's.[38]

Tourette's syndrome affects the neuromodulator dopamine, which is one of the major biochemical systems in the brain, and neuroanatomical structures called the caudate nuclei and the putamen, critical for the initiation of movements and more complex behaviors. In many cases Tourette's seems to have a hereditary basis. Anecdotally, Tourette's syndrome and Parkinson's disease (both disorders of the nigrostriatal dopamine system) sometimes run in the same families.

Some scientists believe that in Tourette's syndrome the caudate nuclei or/and putamen (major basal ganglia) somehow escape from the control normally exerted over them by the prefrontal cortex. Together with the thalamus, the basal ganglia can be thought of as the evolutionary antecedents of the neocortex. In the course of evolution their original role was superseded by the frontal cortex, which in developed mammals exerts an influence over the caudate nuclei and the putamen. It appears that in humans the caudate nuclei and the putamen trigger certain behaviors and that the frontal cortex puts these behaviors through a complex system of cognitive filters, "permitting" some of them and curtailing others.

I also believe that in Tourette's syndrome the moderating influence of the frontal cortex on the caudate nuclei and the putamen is weakened. As a result of this disinhibition, peculiar behaviors arise, bearing a distinct similarity to frontal lobe syndromes. These behaviors are often so socially provocative that the patients are met with derision, ostracism, and sometimes even physical assault.

The most provocative among them is coprolalia, from the Greek words "copra" for "feces" and "lalia" for "utterance." The patient makes profane exclamations in socially inappropriate situations. Many years ago I salvaged from a likely arrest a decently dressed young man who was walking up and down a line of passengers (myself among them) waiting to board an Amtrak train at the 30th Street Station in Philadelphia and cursing us out in the foulest conceivable language. He was also exhibiting characteristic motor tics, which I immediately recognized as tourettic. As the cops were about to converge on him, I approached one of them and quickly explained what was going on. The officer listened and I was thankful to see him merely tell the man to get lost.

But coprolalia is not the only form of the characteristic tourettic "verbal incontinence." To understand the nature of this incontinence, we must again consider a loss of inhibition, which we discussed in connection with the orbitofrontal syndrome. At times we all have thoughts that social norms prevent us from voicing in public. Walking down the street I may note to myself in passing that someone is "fat," someone else is "ugly," and someone else again looks "dumb." I am able to contain these thoughts and they do not leave the sanctum of my cranium, so to speak. Not so with a Tourette's patient. What is on his mind may immediately be also on his lips. It may be unflattering epithets, slurs of various kinds, obnoxious editorial comments—anything forbidden. "Forbidden" seems to be the key to understanding the particular inability of some tourettic patients to contain the unprintable lexicon.

This brings up an interesting psycholinguistic question. Why would a language contain words that are culturally forbidden from being uttered? This sounds like an oxymoronic feature of the language. Yet as far as I know, most, and most likely all, languages contain such "forbidden" lexicon. It could be that they serve the function of emotional release, and it is precisely the act of discarding the barrier of prohibition that accomplishes the release. Forbidden fruit is sweeter! It seems that in Tourette's the urge to release internal tension may be ever present and unquenchable.

As we learn more about Tourette's, different subtypes of this disorder begin to emerge, which may reflect different patterns of the aberrant interaction between the basal ganglia and the frontal lobes. Oliver Sacks talks about the duality of Tourette's symptoms: "stereotypic" and "phantasmagoric."[39] These symptoms clearly parallel the two most conspicuous features of "afrontal" cognition, discussed earlier in the book: perseveration and field-dependency. In most cases of Tourette's, stereotypic and phantasmagoric symptoms do not appear in isolation but are combined in tourettic behavior in various proportions.

I believe that the relative severity of these symptoms reflects the relative involvement of the left or right caudate nuclei and the putamen in any individual case. In many patients both symptoms are present, reflecting the bilateral nature of the disorder. However, relatively pure cases also exist, suggesting the existence of relatively lateralized caudate/putamen dysfunction. On the whole, the stereotypic symptoms seem to predominate, probably due to a particularly close relationship between dopamine and the left hemisphere.

Tourette's syndrome is often associated with obsessive-compulsive disorder (OCD) and attention deficit disorder (ADD). In OCD, repetitive thoughts (obsessions) and behaviors (compulsions) dominate the patient's life, frequently in an extremely disruptive way. Manifestations of OCD resemble perseveration; in fact, they are perseveration. Interestingly, cognitive inflexibility reminiscent of OCD-like behaviors can be caused by the depletion of serotonin in the prefrontal cortex,[40] and can be reversed by the administration of serotonin-reuptake inhibitors.[41] By contrast, ADD is characterized by extreme distractibility, often with equally devastating consequences for cognition. This distractibility is a mild form of field-dependent behavior. I suspect that Tourette's is accompanied by the symptoms of obsessive-compulsive disorder when the left striatum is particularly involved. And it is accompanied by the symptoms of attention deficit disorder when the right striatum is particularly involved. In this sense, the notion of Tourette's—ADD comorbidity may be a misnomer, since "comorbidity" implies co-occuring but separate mechanisms, whereas the "ADD" in Tourette's is likely to be caused by the same mechanism as the tics, both implicating the basal ganglia but in varying left–right gradients. The tics of Tourette's and obsessive-compulsive manifestations of OCD are similar in that both are forms of peseveration, but they differ in the size of the behavior subject to perseveration: smaller in Tourette's and larger in OCD. Careful mapping of the functional neuroanatomy of these two disorders may provide an interesting insight into the hierarchic nature of cognitive control exerted by the striatum.

The stereotypic aspects of Tourette's take the form of forced repetitive behaviors, such as motor tics and grunting vocalizations. These behaviors can be extremely conspicuous, branding the patient as "weird," a social pariah. The tics are often perceived as intentional grimacing and taunting. A friend of mine who developed symptoms of Tourette's at the age of five recalls being chased away from the playground by other children's mothers because they thought he was deliberately teasing them with his "grimaces."

The phantasmagoric symptoms are often expressed as an excessive (and often grotesquely so) urge to explore every incidental object in the environment. These symptoms are less common than the stereotypic ones, but they can be equally conspicuous. I was particularly struck by them many years ago as I was walking on Manhattan's Upper West Side with Oliver Sacks, who has always been interested in Tourette's syndrome, and a tourettic friend of Oliver's by the name of S.F., an extremely intelligent and articulate man, then in his early 30s. The young man's exploratory behavior was extreme and he was drawn to everything in his path: a tree, an iron gridwork, a trash can. As we were walking down the street, he bounced from object to object, checking them out with all his senses. He looked, listened, touched, smelled, and licked them with his tongue. The whole spectacle was so bizarre that I turned to Oliver at some point and said, "I hope you have a picture ID on you, in case we all get arrested!" When we walked into a neighborhood restaurant, the young man immediately felt up the owner, an upright-looking middle-aged woman from Germany, under the scandalized stares of other guests. This was done with casual innocence, in passing. Since I was a regular, the German lady laughed it off and let it go, instead of throwing us out of her establishment or calling the police.

But it is not always easy to categorize a tourettic behavior as clearly stereotypic or clearly phantasmagoric. Often it appears as both. My friend L.H. is an acclaimed photographer, filmmaker, and author, with an award-winning film, *Twitch and Shout*, and a book of the same title to his credit.[42] He has a relatively mild form of Tourette's. No matter whom he is talking to, several times in the course of the conversation L.H. will make a jerky fencing movement touching the other person with his hand and immediately withdrawing it. His friends are so used to this touching behavior that they ignore it completely. But it raises eyebrows and creates tensions with strangers. Is L.H.'s urge to touch an exploratory behavior? Is it a perseveration? Or is it both?

I asked L.H. and S.F. to give an insider's view of their unusual urges and behaviors. This is what they said.

EG: You often have an urge to touch an object or a human being. What goes through your head at the moment and right before?

LH: It is heightened sensory curiosity and lack of inhibition. I become focused on a body part or an object. Once I focus on it, the urge becomes uncontrollable. It is an urge that I cannot resist.

SF: It is tactile curiosity, an urge to explore. I am attracted to a leather chair, plastic surface, or some other object that I must touch. It may take extreme forms. I once gagged on a toothbrush because I wanted to swallow it to find out what it feels like in my mouth. When I eat I sometimes have an urge to put my face in the food to feel the texture. Sometimes I have an urge to probe the roof of my mouth with utensils like a knife and a fork until it bleeds. This is why I like to eat sandwiches, to stay away from the utensils, because even though it does not happen every time, sooner or later it will happen. I often eat with my hands; I don't care what people think. I can do it elegantly.

EG: Suppose the object of your interest is out of your reach. Would you climb over things to get it?

LH: I will be able to inhibit the urge, but SF may not be.

SF: Sometimes when I see an object which I cannot touch at the moment I come back hours later to touch it. A few times I had an urge to touch things as I was moving heavy furniture. So I would balance the furniture with one hand and touch with the other.

EG: How extreme is this urge? Would you touch an object or a human even knowing full well that it may lead to destructive consequences? Or will you be able to inhibit the urge?

LH: I will probably be able to inhibit the urge.

SF: I constantly touch light bulbs and burn my fingers.

EG: Why the light bulbs?

SF: Because they are particularly shiny.

EG: How about people? Will you touch a cop on the street if you have the urge?

LH: I might touch his nightstick (laughs).

SF: I try to avoid places where I am surrounded with people, like the subway. Sometimes I would imitate a person instead of touching him.

EG: Is this urge to explore limited to the tactile sensations? Or does it involve other senses?

LH: It involves all of the senses. But for me it inevitably ends up being tactile.

sf: Also taste and smell. I sometimes used to put my face into the toilet bowl to taste the water. I do not do it anymore.

eg: What do you experience before and at the time of a tic?

lh: Sometimes there is a precursor to a tic, sometimes a quasi-sensation, like an "itch for a twitch." There is often a tension going through my body.

eg: As I am talking to SF, I hear these barking sounds at almost regular intervals. Tell me more about this urge to vocalize (part of the interview was conducted over the phone).

sf: I am drawn to mimicking sounds. Sometimes I mimic animals, or some odd sounds idiosyncratic to particular people. I imitate them for hours, can't get rid of them. Sometimes I imitate fragments of a word. And sometimes the word doesn't suit me, but even when it is not "native" to me, I will still repeat it. If I listen to you long enough, I will incorporate your way of speaking into my own . . . probably not your accent but your verbal mannerisms.

eg: I can see that you are hypersensitive to sound. You keep interrupting me and asking me about every background street noise that reaches you over the phone.

sf: This hypersensitivity is true not just for noises but also for speech. I often adopt other people's stereotypic phrases and postures. . . . I once read Constantine Stanislavski about imitation leading to a metamorphosis in an actor . . . when somebody else's mannerisms become yours . . . something like that. When I used to spend a lot of time with Oliver Sacks I adopted some of his mannerisms.

eg: Did he notice that?

sf: I don't think so.

eg: So your extreme sensory curiosity is tactile and gustatory and auditory in nature. How about visual? And how synthetic, or synesthetic, does it all get?

sf: All the senses play a role together. When I walk down the hall I want to feel everything, like a cold wall. I will pick the mood of it. I want to see left side and right side simultaneously. I want to wear the environment like clothes. I experience the disappearance of a person behind me like physical weight removed. When I move from a big room to a small room, I feel physical change like pulsating light.

LH: It is very visual with me also. I am incredibly visually oriented by what I do because I am a photographer. I am influenced by visual things and I am tempted by them.

EG: How about coprolalia? Why do some people with Tourette's have the urge to use profanities?

LH: Fuck you . . . That was a joke . . . Because it is forbidden. Tourette's is a lack of inhibition.

SF: I have this urge only to a very limited degree. I understand that only 12%–14% of people with Tourette's develop strange phrases. With me it is not coprolalia, but saying things without feeling inhibited.

EG: If it is the lack of ability to inhibit forbidden thoughts, then how about other inappropriate utterances? If you see a fat person on the street will you say "fat," or if you see an ugly person will you say "ugly"?

LH: I won't but some people with Tourette's may. I knew a woman with coprolalia. We went to a very upscale Manhattan restaurant together, and as we were talking she would shout something derogatory about every person who walked in. Two gay guys were sitting next to us and she said "faggots," a black guy was sitting nearby and she said "nigger"; two guys with pony tales walked in and she said "hippies." This was not directed only at others; she was making derogatory comments about herself and me, too. She said "My family are . . . spicks," and "you, LH are a . . . kike." Then we finished lunch and walked down Eighth Avenue and somebody bald walked by and she shouted out "baldie." She was trying to inhibit these slurs but they were very audible.

SF: No, I won't make slurs, but I may do a pantomime, like I may have a barely perceptible movement in my belly to imitate an extended belly when I see a fat person on the street.

EG: Does your Tourette's affect your mental processes also? Is there such a thing as a "tourettic cognitive style" or "tourettic personality"?

LH: Tourette's produces a higher-order lack of inhibition. This makes it difficult to concentrate, makes me very distractible. There is a low frustration threshold in Tourette's. I used to slam things into walls, break and smash things. I also think that my irreverent sense of humor is part of my Tourette's. I was once at a party and someone said that he was gay. To which I said that I was trisexual: males, females, and animals.

SF: Increased risk taking is part of Tourette's. I once stopped when I saw a man mugging a little girl and intervened.

EG: Some doctors working with Tourette's believe that Tourette's is associated with hypersexuality. What to do say to that?

LH: I consider myself hypersexual and think it is part of my Tourette's. But to me hypersexuality is just a special case of being generally hypersensitized to any experience. In sex you deal with a sensory enhancer and Tourette's enhances attraction to everything.

SF: In this culture everything is sexualized, but I do have huge energy and wide tastes, certainly for a 40-year-old.

EG: Does Tourette's make your life difficult?

LH: Yes, because of the stigma. Ignorant people misconstrue the symptoms and try to explain them within their own limited frame of reference. Once somebody asked me if I was dancing. On another occasion somebody told me to shut up.

SF: Tourette's does make my life difficult, less because of the tics and other symptoms themselves and more because of social issues. The social issues easily eclipse Tourette's itself. I had violence directed at me at college, at the karate school. In addition to assaults I have been arrested many times, once while visiting my father in the hospital, while they were looking for someone else. I was suspected of rape for no good reason. I have been harassed by cops for doing nothing, just for ticking. . . . A man once tried to push me off the subway platform. I did not call the police, because I did not think police would believe me because of my tics. And some time later the same man pushed a girl under a train. . . . And I felt bad about not reporting him earlier. . . . But not all cops are like that. There are some very enlightened cops.

EG: Does Tourette's add anything positive to your life?

LH: Definitely, but it takes a certain talent to turn it into an asset. The compulsions and obsessions of Tourette's give me an edge in getting work done, in bringing things to a closure. There is a compulsion to complete work, to go an extra step. Tourette's makes me hypersensitive, it gives me sensory curiosity, really a multisensory curiosity. This is important in writing and photography. It gives me an extrasensory component, it sensitizes me, clues me into things. My inner world is richer because of this.

SF: Now I know that it does. A higher degree of athletic ability is common in Tourette's. The sense of smell is very acute. I once smelled freshly cut grass far from the place where it was being cut, way before anyone else could smell it. People with Tourette's are much more inquisitive than other people. . . . Tourette's gives you a great sense of humor. . . . Tourette's gives you energy, but it is merciless.

EG: How does Tourette's affect your relationships with other people?

LH: It sort of scans out certain people who would not be interested in me anyway. So I am left with the people to whom my Tourette's does not matter. And these are the people I want to be with.

SF: I lost a few friends, but I was able to help other people. When I worked in a summer camp, I once saw a boy, 17–18 years of age, who could not stop washing his hands. He had an extreme case of obsessive-compulsive disorder. He was washing his hands for literally an hour and could not stop. I was the only one who understood what was going on. I turned off the faucet, gently dried his hands with a towel, and escorted him out of the bathroom.

EG: How does Tourette's affect your identity?

LH: My identity is definitely one of a touretter. There is a Tourette's culture of being on the outside and I have a sense of brotherhood with other outsiders. I feel closer to other frowned-upon groups of people with differences of all kinds. I feel that they have a better insight into my condition.

SF: Tourette's is one of my identities, but not the only one. . . . By the way, I dislike the word "touretter." It demeans the condition, makes it sound like a vocation.

EG: There is a certain popular mystique about Tourette's syndrome. How do you explain it?

LH: There is that mystique and I have become a poster boy for Tourette's. Tourette's has a mystique and a cult both glamorized and tainted with infamy. Tourette's is a disability and is off and odd, yet it resonates with our culture of overabundance. Unlike other disorders, Tourette's is not something shortchanged with life, but something overloaded with life. In these times of extreme political correctness and prudishness people tip their hat to us, because we are full of life, intoxicated with it.

SF: One should differentiate between mystique and mystery. What people usually see is a panoply of odd things that have been exploited in movies to dramatize things, often in a way which has nothing to do with the substance of the character or the reality of Tourette's.

EG: Is your Tourette's the defining fact of your life?

LH: It definitely is for me.

SF: Socially, yes to a major extent. Privately less so. My life is not just unidimensional.

EG: How do you cope with your Tourette's?

LH: I try to ration myself a certain amount of quiet time alone in my apartment. An occasional drink helps . . . and a lot of vitamins.

The Cortex and the Striatum

This richness of symptoms has made Tourette's syndrome a favorite of movie-makers and popular media outlets, but it also informs us about the relations between the frontal lobes and the basal ganglia. Over the last few years, this relationship has become one of the hottest topics in cognitive neuroscience and decision-making theory. From an evolutionary standpoint, the basal ganglia are to the frontal lobes approximately what the thalamus is to the posterior cortex: their functional, if not neuroanatomical, precursor. In this capacity, the basal ganglia used to be in charge of initiation and temporal organization of behavior in the miriad precortical species, and for millions of years the buck stopped at the basal ganglia as far as executive control was concerned, or whatever passed for it at those early stages of the evolution of the brain. Then the arrivista neocortex burst onto the evolutionary scene and relegated the basal ganglia to a supporting-actor status. Johan Lauereyns and colleagues at the National Eye Institute have discovered neurons in the monkey's caudate nuclei, which exhibit the anticipatory behavior predicting the rewarded trial on a guided eye-movement task.[43] Therein lies an interesting evolutionary riddle. In humans, neural representation of the future is commonly associated with the prefrontal cortex, and it would be very interesting to see if similarly behaving neurons are found in the monkey frontal cortex as well. Likewise, a functional neuroimaging study with a similarly designed activation task may help determine whether the caudate nuclei are still involved, or whether they have been preempted by the prefrontal cortex in the mediation of such predictive cognition.

A "supporting" role does not mean irrelevant, however. To understand the division of labor between the prefrontal cortex and the basal ganglia in a developed mammalian brain, we must consider a hierarchy of contexts and of context sizes.

In deciding whether to act and how to act, we take a relatively narrow or a relatively broad set of factors into account. This is what I mean by the context size. It appears that the increase of the context size as the basis for decision making has been among the most important developments in the evolution of the brain, and this is precisely what distinguishes the frontal lobes from the basal ganglia. The basal ganglia make their "executive decisions" (to act or not to act and how to act) on the basis of a very narrow context. By contrast, the prefrontal cortex makes its executive decisions on the basis of a much broader, richer context.

Context size as the basis for decision making helps explain the symptoms of field-dependent behavior often seen, in different variations, both in people with Tourette's syndrome and in patients with prefrontal lesions. Most objects in our environment—certainly all the tools and other function objects—have distinct behaviors associated with them: we hold and manipulate a knife in a certain way and a cup in a different but equally standard way. We leaf through a book but we tap a computer keyboard. Does this mean that we grab a knife, lift a cup, leaf through a book, or tap a keyboard every time we encounter one in our environment? Not at all—we do it only when a larger context warrants it: when we need to cut a steak, when we are thirsty and the cup is filled and clean, when we want to extract some information from a book, or send an e-mail to a friend. In fact, most of the time we encounter any of these objects we simply ignore them. A mere encounter with an object does not automaticlally trigger the object-associated behavior. But in patients with severe Tourette's syndrome or with prefrontal damage it often does, the famous "utilization behavior" described by François Lhermitte.[44]

Why do we see "utilization behavior" in both Tourette's syndrome and focal prefrontal lesions? Because in both conditions the basal ganglia escape from the frontal lobe control and begin to operate on their own, the way they had been operating before the frontal lobes arrived on the evolutonary scene. In Tourette's syndrome the basal ganglia are physiologically overactive and in focal lesions the frontal lobes are rendered functionally disabled. As a result, in both conditions the frontal lobes no longer exert their moderating influence over the basal ganglia and the latter revert to their original modus operandi. And this modus opernadi is driven by a very narrow context: an object-appropriate behavior is immediatley triggered by the object's mere presence in the environment even if the behavior is inappropriate to a larger context (e.g., grabbing and drinking from someone else's cup or putting on someone else's jacket just because the cup or the jacket is there).

The parallel between "basal ganglia" action and "thalamic" perception is inescapable. It has been said that the thalamus operates on the basis of isolated features rather than well-organized percepts. Now and again I am reminded of this by my bullmastiff Brit. Impressively intelligent for a canine, he is still a canine, and while canines undoubtedly have the neocortex, their perception remains to a large extent thalamic—driven by isolated features. Brit responds to a life-size window mannequin or to a life-size stuffed animal as if they were alive: he will bark and attempt to engage them in play. Likewise, he will respond to a piece of paper flailing in the wind as if it were alive and will attempt to engage it in play. A certain form by itself or motion by itself, rather than the obligatory conjunction thereof, will be perceived as "alive." As a puppy Brit tried to develop a somewhat intimate relationship with the suede sofa in our living room. Again, his behavior was guided by an isolated feature, the texture, without taking anything else into account. In order to form perceptual conjunctions, more neocortex is required than my Brit possesses. Just as his perception seems to be guided by the thalamus more than by the posterior neocortex, so, too, his action appears to be guided by the stiatum more than by the frontal lobes. Over time I noticed that he engages in very specific behaviors in very specific places. Once we visited an electronic gadget store together, and he will try to enter the door every time we pass by even if the original visit did not entail a reward. After an episode when we had to stop in a totally incidental location on Broadway, he continued to stop there whenever we traverse this route. Having experienced a bout of exuberance on Columbus Circle as a puppy, he invariably gets into an exuberant routine in the same exact spot years later. A very specific action seems to be triggered by a vey simple trigger in a very constant way.

So it appears that the concept of "context size" applies equally to perception and to action, and that the advent of neocortex has ushered in, among other things, the ability to operate on the basis of a larger context, perceptual context owing to the posterior association cortices, and action context owing to the prefrontal cortex. As is usually the case in neurobiology, we should not think about the relation between the basal ganglia and the frontal lobes, or that between the thalamus and posterior association cortex in strictly binary terms: absence of cortical control vs. presence of cortical control. It is more productive to think in continuous terms of relative contributions and the balance between them. My Brit does possess some neocortex and even a certain amount of the frontal cortex, but not as much as a human does.

Does this mean that a brain with no or little cortex was capable only of highly stereotypic behaviors with certain stimuli triggering certain responses in a highly invariable, automatic and predictable fashion? This assumption would fly in the face of evidence that basically acortical nervous systems, like the ones seen in birds, reptiles, and cephalopods, are capable of learning and of exploratory behaviors. Remarkable feats of such abilites have been observed in parrots, squids, and other basically acortical creatures. What do we know about such acortical exploratory behavior? Again, the notion of context size offers a useful heuristic.

We constantly encounter novel stimuli in our environment—new faces, new sounds, new objects. And more often than not we ignore them despite their novelty. Whether we choose to actually examine them depends on a broader cognitive context, and the mere presence in the environment of a novel stimulus is not enough to elicit exploratory behavior. Not so in a patient with frontal lobe damage or in certain patients with Tourette's syndrome. In them any new object in the environment will predictably elicit intense and irresistable exploratory behavior. According to the descriptions of my acquaintances with Tourette's, the uncontrollable urge for exploratory behaviors is as powerful as the urge to discharge tics. It is strikingly reminiscent of the "utilization behavior" described by Francois Lhermitte in patients with prefrontal lesions.[45] To continue our line of reasoning, this is also because the basal ganglia have escaped the frontal-lobe control.

So it appears that behavior driven by the basal ganglia is capable both of discharging overlearned cognitive routines and of exploratory behaviors. Both, however, are driven by a very narrow context. The difference between the basal ganglia–driven behavior and the frontal lobe–driven behavior is in the scope and scale of the cognitive context on which it is predicated. Likewise, the difference between thalamic perception and neocortically driven perception is in the scope of perceptual integration afforded by these two systems.

It has been proposed that the division of labor between the frontal lobes and the basal ganglia is along the lines of "exploration" (dealing with novelty) vs. "exploitation" (discharging overlearned behaviors).[46] This is probably true in the broad evolutionary sense that hard-wired behaviors are likely to be controlled by subcortical structures. It is also true in that many forms of cognition are relegated from cortical to subcortical control as they become automatic. The relationship between the frontal lobes and the basal ganglia in the control over action have much in common with the relationship between posterior neocortex and the thalamus in the control over perception. But this does not seem to capture the whole story. In fact, a study by Anitha Pasupathy and Earl Miller would seem to suggest an oppositie relationship: the basal ganglia learn more rapidly than the prefrontal cortex.[47] But keep in mind the analogy between basal ganglia action and thalamic perception. Thalamic perception is also faster than neocortical perception—this is the basis for the rapid "fear response" studied by Joseph LeDoux.[48] The consideration of context size may be critical for understanding both. There is a trade-off between the speed of learning and the complexity of the situation to be learned. It is very likely that a more complex task would have yielded a relationship between prefrontal and striatal learning rates that is opposite to the one described by Pasupathy and Miller. Kazuyuki Samejima and colleagues from Japan have shown that the striatum is important for learning the reward value of various simple actions in a probabilistic environment,[49] clearly an exploratory activity. But I wouldn't be surprised if a similar experiment involving a more complex probabilistic environment (e.g., Markovian as opposed to simple stochastic) would critically involve the frontal cortex more than the striatum. In fact, the relationship between the prefrontal cortex and the striatum in guiding behavior in probabilistic environments of different complexity levels was examined by Ming Hsu and colleagues from the California Institute of Technology and University of Iowa, who found that when critical information about the probabilistic environment is missing, normal subjects rely more on the orbitofrontal cortex and less on the striatum. Patients with orbitofrontal damage become insensitive to ambiguity and make their decisions without taking it into account.[50]

Admittedly, the view of the striatum as being associated with simple decision making is challenged by the findings of caudate activation in people desiring to inflict "altruistic punishment" on their transgressing peers.[51] Altruistic punishment is a punishment you choose to inflict on the other that has no direct benefit and is perhaps even at direct cost to yourself, as in rejecting a deal that would reward the other party excessively but would also modestly reward yourself. This is clearly a social, emotionally colored behavior, and by no means simple. Perhaps its association with the striatum points to altruistic punishment's early, pre-human evolutionary roots.

Earlier in the book we considered the neural means by which an organism is able to reconcile the needs for cognitive plasticity and cognitive stability, to engage in novel explorations and at the same maintain certain well-established routines. We put forth the idea that at a cortical level a division of labor exists between the two hemispheres, one playing the leading role in dealing with novelty (the right hemisphere), the other with cognitive routines (the left hemisphere). I believe that the prototype of such a division of labor arose early in evolution and was mediated already by the basal ganglia through their functional lateralization. So a hierarchic relationship exists between the basal ganglia and the prefrontal cortex, whereby the balance between "exploration" and "exploitation" exists at each level, both at the level of the prefrontal cortex and at the level of basal ganglia, but driven by contexts of different scales. Presence of "exploratory" and "exploitative" mechanisms at both the frontal-cortical and the striatal level is reflected in the parallel sympomatology seen following damage to the frontal lobes and in Tourette's syndrome. Damage to the prefrontal cortex is capable of producing both perseverative behavior (excessive exploitation) and field-dependent behavior (excessive exploration). Likewise, Tourette's is characterized by tics (excessive exploitation) and by excessive exploratory behaviors of the sort described earlier in this chapter. I believe that the relative prevalence of these two types of symptoms in Tourette's reflects different neuroanatomical patterns and depends on the relative lateralization of striatal involvement in the disease process.

A study by Hisham Atallah and colleagues from the University of Colorado at Boulder supports my point generally but challenges it specifically. Whereas damage to the rat's dorsal striatum interferes with the performance of a learned skill ("exploitation"), damage to the ventral striatum interferes with skill acquisition ("exploration"), even though the authors refer to the two processes as "actor" vs. "director."[52] So it indeed appears that the "exploration—exploitation" synergy exists already within the phylogenetically old striatum. But the neuroanatomical substrate of this distinction reported by Atallah and colleagues is different from the one proposed in this book: it is ventral vs. dorsal, not right vs. left.[53] Considering the close link of the ventral striatum with the orbitofrontal cortex, which is in turn closely linked to the organism's ability to integrate the information about internal states with that about the outside world, it comes as no surprise that the acquisition of skills directly driven by reinforcement should involve these systems. By contrast, dorsal striatum is linked to the dorsolateral prefrontal cortex closely implicated in the execution of behavioral sequences. But I would still not give up on the right–left distinction. In Atallah and colleagues' study, both ventral and dorsal striatum were impacted bilaterally, which would have obscured any possible lateralized effects. If they read this book carefully, they may consider a 2×2, ventral–dorsal vs. left–right design and see what happens.

Both "exploration" and "exploitation" mechanisms are present in the basal ganglia of rodents, according to the study by Terra Barnes and colleagues.[54] In a cogent review of the basal ganglia functions, Henry Yin and Barbara Knowlton[55] conclude that the striatum contains the mechanisms for both goal-directed learning and habits. Goal-directed behavior is mediated mostly by the caudate nucleus, which receives projections from the prefrontal cortex and the posterior heteromodal association cortex. Habit formation is mediated mostly by the putamen, which receives projections from the sensorimotor cortices. So a very close parallel exists between the functional organization of the neocortex and that of the basal ganglia. We already know that the process of familiarization with and routinization of a cognitive task is linked to the gradual transition of cognitive control from the prefrontal cortex to the more posterior (including the premotor) cortices. In a very similar vein, Yin and Knowlton propose that the process of habit formation is linked to the transition of neural control from the caudate nucleus (or its rodent equivalent, the dorsomedial striatum) to the putamen (or its rodent equivalent, the dorsolateral striatum).[56]

We know from the previous chapters of this book that the cortical mechanisms of the novelty–routinization transition are at a minimum two-dimensional: both front-to-back and right-to-left. We also know from the earlier discussion that the heteromodal association cortices (including the prefrontal cortex) are somewhat more extensively in the right hemisphere, and the modality-specific and premotor cotices are more extensively represented in the left hemisphere. I wouldn't be surprised, and would venture to predict, that similar structural and functional asymmetries exist in the basal ganglia. This would entail somewhat larger right than left caudate nucleus (or dorsomedial striatum) and somewhat larger left than right putamen (or dorsolateral striatum). I would further predict that the process of habit formation on the basal-ganglia level is also two-dimensional. It is characterized by a gradual transition of neural control from the right dorsomedial striatum (or the right caudate nucleus) to the left dorsolateral striatum (or the left putamen).

An understandably skeptical reader may ask the following question: how is it that the extensive studies of the basal ganglia in habit formation in various mammalian species have failed to turn up anything even remotely consistent with Goldberg's armchair speculations? I have an (equally speculative) answer to this as well. First, one usually needs to look in order to see; this is as true in science as it is in life. As long as hemispheric differences were construed strictly in terms of the verbal–nonverbal dichotomy, there was no reason to look for such differences outside of our own loquacious species, and certainly not in the basal ganglia. Much of this book has been devoted to the overturning of this premise and to the promotion of novelty–routinization as the defining basis for functional hemispheric asymmetries. The novelty–routinization distinction is central to any process of learning, including habit formation, in any species capable of it. And it can be meaningfully applied to both the cortex and the basal ganglia. So please start looking!

Second, one must take gender into account. As we already know from earlier chapters, functional differences between the left and right frontal lobes are much better articulated in males than in females. Given the the degree of functional unity between the frontal cortex and the striatum, this is probaly true for the striatum also. So in any gender-mixed sample of animals hemispheric differences may be somewhat obscured.

Third, one probably also needs to take handedness into account. In the human literature, most statements pertaining to hemispheric specialization are made to apply predominantly to right-handers. Since the overwhelming majority of humans are right-handed, this caveat is often ommitted as self-evident. Not so in other mammalian species: handedness is also present in any given specimen, but the breakdown across the specimens for the species as a whole is much closer to 50/50. So any predictions pertaining to functional hemispheric asymmetries outside our own species shoud probably be restricted to the right-pawed specimens, be it a monkey or a rat. Is the inverse pattern of functional lateralization to be expected in left-pawed members of the species? Is there a continuum of functional lateralization corresponding to the continuum of the degrees of powedness? These are interesting possibilities. But to assess this experimentally, one needs to assess the animals' paw preference and take it into account in data analysis. This is usually not done. Furthermore, if my armchair speculations are right, then any real functional hemispheric differences—both cortical and striatal—would be washed out in a sample of animals containing both righ- and left-pawed specimens. Unfortunately, pawedness is not only ignored in data analysis, it is usually not assessed in the first place, but it should be.

13

"What Can You Do for Me?"

"Cognotropic" Drugs

For many neuropsychologists, like myself, science is a labor of love, but seeing patients is bread and butter. Traditionally, the clinical contribution of neuropsychology has been mostly diagnostic, with precious little to offer patients by way of treatment. Neuropsychology is not the only clinical discipline for years consigned to helpless voyeurism. Every discipline concerned with cognition shares this humbling predicament. A psychiatrist treating a schizophrenic patient or a depressed patient finds him- or herself in a similar position. There are ample pharmacological tools to treat the patient's psychosis or mood, but very few to treat the patient's cognition. Even though psychiatrists increasingly recognize that cognitive impairment is often more debilitating in their patients than psychosis or mood disorder, traditionally, very little direct effort has been aimed at improving cognition.

A neurologist treating a patient recovering from the effects of head injury does not fare much better. There are adequate means to control the patient's seizures but not his or her cognitive changes, despite the fact that cognitive impairment is usually far more debilitating than an occasional seizure. Society has been so preoccupied with saving lives, treating hallucinations, controlling seizures, and lifting depression that cognition (memory, attention, planning, problem solving) has been largely ignored. Granted, various neuroleptics, anticonvulsants, antidepressants, sedatives, and stimulants do have an effect on cognition, but it is an ancillary effect of a drug designed to treat something else.

Alzheimer's disease and other dementias have been society's wake-up call. Here, in the most affluent country in the most affluent of times, human minds were succumbing to decay before human bodies, a sharp challenge to the tacit popular belief that the "body is frail but soul is forever." This provided an impetus for the development of an entirely new class of drugs, which can be termed familially as "cognotropic." Their primary and explicit purpose is to improve cognition.

Since medical and public preoccupation with dementia focuses on memory, most of the pharmacological efforts have been directed at improving memory. At the time of this writing, a handful of drugs known as "Alzheimer's drugs" or "memory enhancers" have been approved by the U.S. Food and Drug Administration (FDA). In reality, both designations are somewhat misleading. The drugs in question are anticholinesterases. They are designed to inhibit an enzyme necessary for the breakdown of the neurotransmitter acetylcholine in the synapse, and thus to prolong its action after its release into the synapse. Acetylcholine is a neurotransmitter that plays an important role in memory as well as in other cognitive functions. Biochemical processes involving acetylcholine ("cholinergic transmission") are impaired in Alzheimer's dementia, but they are also impaired in many other disorders.

My first encounter with this class of drugs took place in the late 1970s and involved physostigmine (Antilirium), a first-generation anticholinesterase, now out of use as a cognitive enhancer. We gave it to a patient recovering from severe head injury.[1] The problem with physostigmine was that its length of action (half-life) was so miserably short that no sustained therapeutic effect could be reasonably expected. At best, a very fleeting, short-term improvement could be hoped for. To capture this improvement, my colleagues and I designed a brief battery of neuropsychological tests, which my research assistants Bob Bilder and Carl Sirio rushed to administer with clockwork timing during carefully calculated, and very narrow, windows of opportunity. Fleeting though it was (and at times overshadowed by vicious diarrhea), subtle memory improvement was reproducibly present. This was a cause for hope that with some improvements this class of medications could someday have real clinical value.

A number of years later, tacrine (Cognex) appeared on the market, followed by donepezil (Aricept). These drugs are also anticholinesterases, but with a much longer action and a more meaningful therapeutic effect. They should not be thought of as exclusively "Alzheimer's drugs" since their utility is not limited to Alzheimer's disease. I have observed a significant, albeit transient, therapeutic effect of these drugs on cognition in patients with Parkinson's disease and brain damage due to hypoxia.

Although their effect is still transient and inconsistent, the advent of these second- and third-generation anticholinesterase drugs opened a new chapter in pharmacology, ushering in cognotropic medications.

More recently, a new drug, Namenda (memantine), was approved by the FDA. It targets several receptors in the brain: glutaminergic, serotonergic, and cholinergic. Its most pronounced effect is presumed to be one of a glutamate antagonist. Targeting glutamate, a ubiquitous neurotransmitter mediating mostly excitatory processes in the neocortex and elsewhere in the brain, has opened a "second front" in the pharmacological assault on dementia. Interestingly, stimulating GABA, a mostly inhibitory neurotransmitter working in tandem with glutamate, was shown to slow the progression of a dementia-like condition in the monkey.[2]

In the next few years we will undoubtedly witness a boom in the cognotropic pharmacology acting on various biochemical systems. Much further research is needed for it to become established and some controversy is inevitable, but the concept of cognotropic drugs is provocative and timely.

Interesting work on cognotropic pharmacology is being done in Europe as well. An audacious program to investigate neuroanatomically precise effects of various drugs has been under way in Russia for some time. Scientists at the Bourdenko Institute of Neurosurgery in Moscow, where I trained in Luria's lab 40 years ago, have reported an array of specific drug effects. According to them, levodopa (L-dopa), a precursor of the neurotransmitter dopamine, improves the functions we typically associate with the posterior aspect of left frontal lobe: motor sequencing, speech initiation, and expressive language. To put it in technical terms, the Russians claim that L-dopa reduces the symptoms of dynamic aphasia, transcortical motor aphasia, and Broca's aphasia. By the same token, L-dopa seems to retard the functions commonly associated with the parietal lobes (spatial orientation and spatial construction). According to the Russians, L-glutamic acid, an analogue of the neurotransmitter glutamate, improves other functions associated with the frontal lobes. It improves insight into one's condition (reduces symptoms of anosognosia) and improves the sense of humor, time estimation, and time sequencing. L-Glutamic acid also improves the functions commonly associated with the parietal lobes. L-Tryptophan, a precursor of the neurotransmitter serotonin, improves the functions of the parietal lobe but retards the functions of the frontal lobes. At the same time, L-tryptophan interferes with the functions of the frontal lobes, particularly the left frontal lobe. Ameridin, an anticholinesterase not commonly known in the United States, seems to improve the functions of the parietal lobes, particularly the left parietal lobe. It improves comprehension of grammar and reduces the symptoms of "semantic aphasia."[3] These claims made by the Russian scientists associating various neuroactive drugs with particular cortical functions are more specific and in a way more ambitious than most Western claims to this effect. They require careful review and replication, but they are extremely provocative.

But where do the prefrontal cortex and the executive functions fit in? Executive deficit is easily as common and debilitating as memory impairment, and so there should be as much societal pressure for the development of cognotropic frontal-lobe pharmacology. Here, too, developments are at an embryonic stage, but some forward movement is evident. We have discussed the role of dopamine in frontal lobe function, so it should come as no surprise that dopamine-enhancing pharmacology has shown some promise.

The dopamine system is complex, with a number of different receptors. To be truly effective, dopamine pharmacology must be receptor-specific. As we learn more about the variety of dopamine receptors, we are learning about the receptor-specific action of dopamine-enhancing drugs. Bromocriptine (Ergoset or Parlodel), a dopamine D2 receptor agonist, has been shown to improve working memory, a function closely linked to the frontal lobes, in normal adults.[4] The efficacy of two more recently developed D2 receptor agonists, ropinirole (Requip) and pramipexole (Mirapex), has yet to be established.[5]

Currently, a great deal of interest exists in identifying specific dopamine receptors and developing receptor-specific pharmacology. But the thrust of this research is driven by the treatment of schizophrenia, which requires dopamine receptor–specific antagonists. To boost the function of the frontal lobes, dopamine agonists may be required with an affinity to various dopamine receptors, including D1 and D4. This poses a new challenge to pharmaceutical industry and research.

Cognotropic pharmacology of the frontal lobes holds out particular promise in those disorders where frontal lobe dysfunction is present without massive structural damage to the frontal lobes. In such conditions neurotransmitter receptor sites are largely intact, which makes pharmacological intervention more promising. Mild traumatic brain injury (TBI) is such a condition. This is a particularly poignant disease, since it afflicts young people, often in good physical shape and with undiminished life expectancy. Following traumatic brain injury, problems with working memory, decision making, attention, motivation, and impulse control are common. Bromocriptine tends to improve these functions in patients with head injury.[6] So does amantadine (Symmetrel), a drug presumed to facilitate dopamine release and delay dopamine reuptake following its release into the synapse.[7] Mirtazapine (Remeron), typically used to treat depression, has been shown to enhance dopaminergic transmission in the frontal lobes.

The advent of these drugs signals the beginning of frontal-lobe cognotropic pharmacology. Here, too, a second front was recently opened. A new "schizophrenia" drug is in clinical trials at the time of this writing. Developed at Lilly by pharmacologist Darryle Schoepp, this as of yet unnamed agent is supposed to impact in particular the frontal lobes, but by acting on the glutamate system instead of the dopaminergic one. As is the case with the anticholinesterases, even though the motivation behind the development of the drug was triggered by a particular disorder, its biochemical target may have an impact on a wide range of other disorders; these patients may also benefit from the drug.[8]

I hope there is much more to follow. But the true excitement will come when the cutting-edge pharmacology is combined with cutting-edge neuropsychology, when fine cognitive measures are used to guide cognotropic pharmacology in precise, individualized ways. The actor-centered cognitive tasks shown to be so exquisitely sensitive to distinct variants of frontal lobe dysfunction may prove to be particularly useful in guiding custom-tailored cognotropic pharmacology of the frontal lobes.

With the advent of such dramatic cognotropic pharmacological agents, is our society on the verge of embracing it as performance enhancers for the healthy? Are we ready to push the envelope and cross the boundary between treating neurological and psychiatric disorders and boosting normal cognition? Outlandish as this proposition might have sounded even a few decades ago, it is no longer off the table and is a subject of legitimate debate in authoritative scientific literature. In 2004 a position paper titled "Neurocognitive Enhancement: What Can We Do and What Should We Do?" was published by a group of leading neuroscientists headed by Martha Farah.[9] One of the authors, Nobel laureate Eric Kandel, whose work will be discussed later in the book, is somewhat of a role model for me, because of the caliber of his work and because of a shared background: we both escaped from "evil empires," he from Austria after Hitler's Anschluss, and I from the Soviet Union. Kandel helped found the company Memory Pharmaceuticals, aimed at developing innovative memory-enhancing agents.[10]

More recently, the pro's and con's of pushing the envelope of cognitive-enhancing pharmacology were discussed by Barbara Saharian and Sharon Morein-Zamir in a commentary published in *Nature*, one of the most august scientific journals in the world, under the provocative title "Professor's Little Helper."[11] The verdict? More pro's than con's. The authors conclude that under the right set of circumstances the boundary between using pharmacology for treating diseases and using pharmacolody to further enhance normal cognitive performance is acceptable and may even be desirable.

But pharmacology is by far not the only tool available in combatting various forms of cognitive impairment, including the cognitive decline of aging. A range of promising approaches is prompted by the new findings of neuroplasticity. This will be the subjects of the subsequent sections.

Aging Brain and Neuroplasticity

As we age, so do our brains. The sulci become wider and the ventricles, larger.[12] Both are unmistakable signs of atrophy, partial denuding of dendritic branching (connections between neurons), or the loss of myelin sheath covering long axons. There are reasons to believe that all three processes take place as we age. But the decay does not affect all parts of the brain equally. The rates of decay are highly variable; we will discuss some of the sources of this variablity later. Two general rules are apparent. First, the prefrontal cortex is particularly susceptible to normal age-related decay (unlike in Alzheimer's disease, in which the hippocampi are likely to be affected first).[13] Second, the right hemisphere succumbs to the effects of aging more rapidly than the left hemisphere[14] (and the findings of early development complement this picture of later-life decay, with the right hemisphere developing earlier than the left hemisphere).

Susceptibility of the frontal lobes to the effects of aging is a universally accepted fact. Because of the importance of the frontal lobes in handling novel situations, this vulnerability reflects the common observation that the elderly are often stymied by changes in their habitual routines and circumstances, and such changes often unmask an early sign of a dementing process that had remained subclinical and hidden up to that point.[15]

The assertion of uneven rates of hemispheric changes with age is less universally shared, but a growing body of findings, coming from various corners of the world, supports it. I reviewed some of the evidence in *The Wisdom Paradox*[16] and will briefly mention it here.

An uneven rate of sulcar shallowing with age is one such finding. As the cortical tissue "shrinks" with age, sulci, the indentations on the brain's walnut-like surface, become more shallow. The extent of this shallowing tells us about the extent of cortical atrophy. A group of scientists from Johns Hopkins Univrsity and The National Institute of Aging have shown that the sulci in the right occipital and parietal regions exhibit a much greater degree of shallowing with age than do the sulci of the left hemisphere.[17]

A similar asymmetry is apparent with the insula, an enigmatic part of the cortex hidden beneath the meeting point of the temporal, parietal, and frontal lobes and particularly important for multisensory integration. The extent of age-related atrophy is more pronounced in the right than in the left insula, according to findings reported by a group of Australian scientists.[18]

On a related note, interesting age-related changes occur in processing positive and negative emotions. It appears that the amount of activation in the insula and the amygdala associated with the anticipation of monetary gains remains intact with age, but the amount of insular and amygdaloid activation associated with the anticipation of monetary losses is reduced. This may suggest a relatively greater age-related deterioration of these structures in the right than in the left hemisphere.[19]

Yet another study, conducted in Japan, used "voxel morphometry" (a *voxel* is a three-dimensional pixel, the smallest unit of measurement in MRI; one can estimate the size of various neural structures by literally counting the number of voxels contained in them). According to this study, age-related decline in size is present in a number of brain regions and becomes evident in the right hemisphere well before becoming evident in the left hemisphere. In the right hemisphere, decline in the gray-matter volume is apparent already during the fourth decade of life and becomes more pronounced during the fifth decade. By contrast, the decline in the size of the left hemisphere becomes first apparent only durig the fifth decade of life.[20]

Asymmetric rates of atrophy are not limited to the neocortex. In the elderly afflicted with depression, the frontal lobes and the right hippocampus, but not the left hippocampus, exhibit size reduction, according to an MRI study.[21]

Do these two aspects of age-related vulnerability, one affecting the frontal lobes and the other affecting the right hemisphere, have a shared mechanism? If so, what is this mechanism and why does it operate in a way that, at least in relative terms, spares the posterior aspect of the left hemisphere? Remember that both the frontal lobes and the right hemisphere are important in dealing with novel information, and that their relative roles recede once the individual's world of novelty shrinks and the world of well-honed cognitive routines expands, which is what happens when we age. Also, the left hemisphere, particularly its posterior aspect, is the storehouse of well-entrenched cognitive routines; consequently, its relative role in cognition expands with age. Could it be that the relatively rapid decline of the prefrontal cortex and of the right hemipshere, and the relative preservation of the left hemisphere are all somehow related to the shifting balance between novelty and familiarity with age, and consequently to the shifting "balance of use" of different neural structures?

This possibility would have sounded utterly far-fetched even two decades ago and would have remained so, had it not been for our better appreciation for the power and effects of neuroplasticity. For years, the prevailing assumption among scientists was that the brain loses its plasticity and capacity for change as we move from childhood to adulthood. This notion, first introduced at the turn of the twentieth century by the great neuroanatomist Ramon y Cajal[22] acquired an axiomatic status in neuroscience and remained unchallenged for almost a century. Today, however, new evidence is increasingly available that the brain retains plasticity well into adulthood and possibly throughout the life span. The earlier assumption was that in an adult organism, dying neural cells could not be replaced. Although there has long been evidence that new cells could develop in birds (from the work of the Rockefeller University scientist Fernando Nottebohm)[23] and rats (from the work of Joseph Altman at the University of Indiana),[24] it was dismissed as an exception rather than the rule.

But subsequent evidence demonstrated ongoing neuroplasticity across a wide range of mammalian species that increasingly got closer to our own. The work by Elizabeth Gould of Princeton University and Bruce McEwen of Rockefeller University has shown that neurons continue to divide in the adult marmoset monkey.[25] Neural cell division was demonstrated in the hippocampus, the brain structure particularly involved in memory. In another study Elizabeth Gould and her colleagues found an ongoing proliferation of new neurons in the cortex of the adult macaque monkey.[26] The new neurons are added to the heteromodal association cortex of the prefrontal, inferior temporal, and posterior parietal regions, the brain areas involved in most complex aspects of information processing.

Despite the mounting evidence of lifelong neurogenesis across mammalian species, the possibility that it also exists in our own species continued to meet with resistance for a long time. One commonly made argument was that the human species is qualitatively different from other mamalian species, even from other primates, in that we have the ability of accumulating and preserving a huge amount of knowledge, which remains available to us through the life span. It was argued that the preservation of such knowledge requires the conservation of neural circuitry that stores it. But the argument does not withstand even modestly rigorous scrutiny. As we already know, the brain is not a static entity—it changes with age, the ventricles and sulci become larger in a way that is impossible to miss by anyone who compares the MRI scans of a 20-year-old and of a 60-year-old. All this makes the notion of structurally inviolate brain an exercise in neuro-wishful thinking. Knowledge itself is not static either, as psychologists have understood since the days of Bartlett. We constantly reconfigure and re-associate our knowledge, and this undoubtedly is mediated in the changes in neural circuitry. Exactly how knowledge is preserved in the brain despite the constant changes is a fascinating and profound question, one that neuroscience has not even begun to tackle directly. But whatever the mechanism of this ability turns out to be, it is clearly not due to some kind of literal preservation of fixed neural circuitry.

The whole debate on whether the human brain is capable of lifelong neurogenesis or whether it represents an evolutionary exception was finally put to rest by the work of the Swedish neuroscientist Peter Eriksson, who has demonstrated that the human hippocampus (or the dentate gyrus, to be more precise) continues to acquire new neurons well into adulthood.[27] Subsequent research has suggested that adult hippocampal neurogenesis can be influenced pharmacologically and may in fact be one of the mechanisms by which antidepressants exert their therapeutic effect.[28] It has also been shown that adult neurogenesis occurs in the so-called subventricular zone of the adult brain, from which the new neurons migrate to the olfactory bulb.[29]

The extent of human adult neurogenesis outside the dentate gyrus and the olfactory bulb is still being debated. The additional brain regions where it may be present include the neocortex, striatum, amygdala, hypothalamus, and various structures of the brain stem, including the substantia nigra, but the findings are still inconclusive with both positive and negative, sometimes contradictory evidence.[30] Particularly intriguing are the findings that adult neurogenesis is stimulated by brain damage, thus serving as powerful compensatory mechanism of the brain restoring itself.[31]

Subsequent work has suggested that adult neuroplasticity extends into advanced age and may continue even in the presence of Alzheimer's disease, counteracting the detrimental effects of the disease to a degree and for some time. This helps explain the seemingly incongruous observations that sound cognition may inhabit the brain affected with hallmarks of Alzheimer's disease. To my knowledge, the first such finding was reported by Robert Katzman and his colleagues at Albert Einstein College of Medicine in New York and the University of California at San Diego. They studied a sample of people who were periodically evaluated with neuropsychological tests until their death, at which point their brains became available for neuropathological studies. Within this sample, a subset of subjects remained cognitively sound until the very end of their lives, but their brains were marked by distinct neuropathological evidence of Alzheimer's disease. The brains of these people were characterized by unusually great weight and a high number of unusually large neurons.[32] Similar observations of intact cognition in "Alzheimer's brains" in a large number of individuals have been reported by Yakov Stern and his colleagues at Columbia University.[33] The findings of sound minds in Alzheimer's-affected brains also appeared in the nuns from the School Sisters of Notre Dame, who will be discussed later in this chapter. While other possible explanations cannot be discounted, vigorous late-age neuroplasticity is a plausible candidate among the factors that helped offset the effects of Alzheimer's disease in these people.

Assuming that new neurons continue to be born in adult brains, the exact means by which they are incorporated into the pre-existing circuitry remains unclear. It has been argued that adult neurogenesis would be detrimental to information processing, since the insertion of "naïve" neurons into well-integrated circuits would disrupt rather than facilitate them. It is likely that ultimately, the functional ramifications of adult neuroplasticity will be best understood through neural-net modeling more rapidly than through direct experimentation.

Neuroplasticity in Action

What are the factors influencing neuroplasticity? The question is compelling both as a scientific challenge and because of the therapeutic promise of neuroplasticity once we know how to control and harness it. Among such factors, the environmental factors influencing neuroplasticity are particularly intriguing. It turns out that a strong relationship exists between what people do with their brains throughout their lifespan and how their brains age.

Both anecdotal observations and formal research suggest that education confers a protective effect against dementia. Highly educated people are less likely to succumb to its effects. Robert Katzman was the first to note that the prevalence of dementia, including Alzheimer's disease, is lower in people with advanced education.[34] The MacArthur Foundation Research Network on Successful Aging sponsored a study of the predictors of cognitive change in older persons. Education emerged as by far the most powerful predictor of cognitive vigor in old age.[35]

The basis for this relationship is not fully understood. Does the lifestyle associated with education protect against dementia, or is it that some people are born with a particularly robust neurobiology that makes them better candidates for advanced education and protects them against dementia? It is reasonable to assume that it is the nature of activities associated with advanced education that protects against dementia, rather than education itself. Highly educated people are more likely to engage in lifelong vigorous mental activities than less educated people because of the sheer nature of their occupations.

Assuming that neurological dementia-causing illness strikes both groups with equal frequency, then equally severe neurological illness will have a less disruptive effect on the well-conditioned brain than on the poorly conditioned brain, because of the extra reserve that the well-conditioned brain has by way of additional neural connections and blood vessels. Equal amounts of structural damage will produce less functional disruption. Again, the analogy between cognitive conditioning and physical conditioning comes to mind. The case of Sister Mary makes the point with dramatic and remarkable clarity. She performed well on cognitive tests until her death at the age of 101, despite the fact that the postmortem study of her brain revealed multiple neurofibrillary tangles and plaques, the hallmarks of Alzheimer's disease. It would appear that Sister Mary had an intact mind inside an Alzheimer's brain.

Sister Mary was one of the School Sisters of Notre Dame, the much-studied and reported nuns from Mankato, Minnesota. Remarkable for their longevity, they were also known for the absence of debilitating dementia among them. The phenomenon was unanimously attributed to the lifelong habit of being cognitively active. The nuns constantly challenged their minds with puzzles, card games, debates of current policy issues, and other mental activities. Furthermore, the nuns with college degrees, who taught and engaged in other mind-challenging activities on a systematic basis, on average lived longer than their less well-educated counterparts.[36] So compelling were the observations of the nuns' cognitive well-being that a postmortem brain study was designed to examine the relationship between cognitive stimulation and dendritic sprouting.

In the nuns, the protective effect of cognitive exercise on the brain appeared to be cumulative, extending over the whole life span. Old convent records were found, containing the nuns' autobiographies written when they were in their 20s. When the relationship between the nuns' early life writings and the prevalence of dementia in later years was examined, a striking picture emerged. Those nuns who tended to write more grammatically complex and conceptually rich essays in their youth retained their mental vigor until much later in life than those who wrote simple, factual prose as young women.[37]

These findings prompted speculation in the popular press that dementia is a lifelong process that begins to subclinically affect some people early in life, causing them to write simpler prose. But it is just as likely that the aspects of brain organization that make some people "smarter" than others also confer a protective effect against later-life dementia. Then again, it is also possible that the nuns who developed the habit of taxing their minds early in life, and presumably kept doing this, acquired the protective effect on the brain that proved to be of critical importance in their advanced years.

Data are rapidly accumulating that suggest that the effect of experience may actually change brain morphology even at a macroscopic level discernable on MRI. The first such evidence involved London cabdrivers, who turned out to have larger hippocampi than their non-cabdriving contemporaries. British neuroscientists reported a finding that, even a few years earlier, would have been dismissed as a neurological impossibility. They scanned the brains of 16 London taxi drivers and compared them with the brains of 50 control subjects.[38] The taxi drivers, who in the course of their work develop an intricate mental map of their huge metropolis, had larger posterior hippocampi. Furthermore, the greater the number of years spent on the job, the larger the hippocampi were in individual drivers. The hippocampi, of course, are presumed to be critical for learning and memory, including spatial memory,[39] and anyone in a position to memorize multiple routes in the huge metropolis that London is must be straining his or her hippocampi to the utmost. A lifelong denizen of large cities, I am nonetheless stymied by the sheer size and irregularity of the British capital. Whether this finding could be replicated in New York is very much in doubt. In London, a cabdriver cannot receive his licence until he can pass a test identifying nearly every street in the city. This is certainly not the case in New York, where even a basic command of the English language doesn't seem to be a prerequisite. The London cabdriver findings may very well have been the first direct demonstration of a relationship between the size of a macroscopic brain structure and the environmental factors contributing to its use.

As in any correlational observation, the direction of causation between hippocampal size and cabdriving as a vocation is ambiguous. Unlike their New York counterparts, the London cabdrivers are supposed to undergo a very rigorous test and are true professionals. One might say that only those with the oversized hippocampi make the cut. But this argument is undermined by another correlation— between the hippocampal size and the number of years on the job. In other words, the longer a person was employed as a cabdriver, the larger the hippocampi were. This seems to clarify the direction of causation: the hippocampi appear to increase in size as a function of time spent driving a cab on the streets of London. This finding is particularly striking if one considers the fact that more years on the job usually implies a more advanced age, which in turn would predict a certain decrease in size as a result of age-related brain shrinkage. But it appears that the effect of hippocampal stimulation by job demands overrides the effects of aging.

Additional findings of a similar kind were not long in coming. One of them concerns the angular gyrus, a cortical region on the juncture of the parietal, temporal, and occipital lobes. In right-handed people the left angular gyrus is among the most important substrates of language, particularly of the ability to process complex relations. Scientists from the Wellcome Department of Imaging Neuroscience at the Institute of Neurology in London have shown that in bilingual individuals the left angual gyrus contains more gray matter than in people in command of only one language, and the underlying white matter is denser.[40] This means that there are more neurons and/or more connections in the language area of the people who mastered more than one language. This was true both in early bilinguals (people who acquired the second language early in life) and in late bilinguals (people who acquired the second language later in life). Again, one might argue that the direction of causation is in question, but bilingualism is usually a function of personal circumstances (such as resettlement from one country to another) or an accident of birth (being born in a multilingual environment), rather than a function of aptitude-based selection. To the extent that the angular gyrus findings are indeed a reflection of experience-driven plasticity, it appears that these affects are not limited to very young people but are present also at later stages of life.

Yet another study involves Heschl's gyrus (also known as the traverse gyrus), a region of the temporal lobe important for processing acoustic stimuli. It turns out that Heschl's gyrus is larger in professional musicians than in musically untrained people—in fact, twice as large.[41] As with the London cabdrivers, there is a positive relationship between the size of Heschl's gyrus and the amount of time spent practicing an instrument. This latter correlation argues strongly in favor of practice being the cause and Heschl's gyrus size the consequence.

So it appears that cognitive activity promotes neural tissue growth, and that such neuroplastic effects can be quite targeted and specific: certain kinds of mental activity are related to morphological changes in those parts of the brain most directly responsible for supporting them. In the three examples just discussed, London cabdrivers, bilinguals, and professional musicians, the morphometric findings reflected the effects of very long-term cognitive activities of particular kinds, measured in years and perhaps even in decades. But the effects of neuroplasticity can manifest themselves within a much more compressed time frame, as the juggler study has shown. A group of volunteers without any prior juggling experience were trained in a three-ball juggling routine for 3 months, until they reached a certain level of proficiency. MRI scans taken before and after the training period were compared, and a considerable increase in the amount of gray matter was found in the temporal lobes in both hemispheres and in the left parietal lobe. Then the training was discontinued for 3 months and a third MRI scan was performed. It revealed reduction of the amount of gray matter in all the regions that had benefited from training earlier.

This truly spectacular finding shows that even relatively brief but sustained cognitive activity is capable of affecting brain morphology and is detectable in neuroanatomically specific ways. As the findings of this kind continue to accumulate, the existence of lifelong neuroplasticity and its dependence on cognitive activity will be no longer in doubt.

Jogging the Brain

If you embrace the notion of lifelong neuroplasticity as reality and the fact that it can be influenced by the extent and type of your cognitive activities, then the notion of structured, guided cognitive exercise is the logical next step. In August 1994, I picked up a copy of *Life* magazine with a picture of the human brain on the cover.[42] The article suggested that mental exercise may help forestall the onset of mental decline associated with aging. *Life* magazine is not where new ground in neuroscience is usually broken, and the idea sounded a bit sensational. But some of the world's top neuroscientists were interviewed for the feature and stood behind it. Among them were Arnold Scheibel, director of the prestigious Brain Research Institute of the University of California, Los Angeles; Antonio Damasio, then director of the Neurology Department at the University of Iowa School of Medicine, the author of the best-selling *Descartes' Error* and *The Feeling of What Happens*;[43] Zaven Khachaturian, a leading scientist at the National Institute of Aging in Bethesda, Maryland; and Marilyn Albert, then of Boston's renowned Massachusetts General Hospital. A few years earlier the notion of cognitive exercise as a method of prevention of mental decline would have scandalized serious neuroscientists as snake oil. But now the tide was clearly changing.

I was thrilled with the *Life* magazine article because it resonated with my own intuition. As a clinical neuropsychologist, I have spent a significant part of my career studying the patterns of recovery from the effects of brain damage and designing cognitive rehabilitation methods. My mentor, Alexandr Romanovich Luria, was a pioneer of cognitive exercise as a way of spurring the recovery from the mental effects of brain damage, first developing this approach during World War II to help soldiers with head wounds. The neurologist and author Oliver Sacks, my friend and colleague, has written eloquently and poignantly about the therapeutic effects of mental stimulation on dementia in the elderly. My own experience has led me to conclude that cognitive stimulation can serve as a powerful catalyst for the natural recovery from the effects of traumatic brain damage.

Treatment and prevention often call for similar approaches. Vaccines developed to protect against infection with viral diseases such as hepatitis B have been shown to reduce clinical symptoms in those already infected. In the efforts to fight AIDS, some scientists, like Jonas Salk, believed that future vaccines would serve a dual function: they would protect healthy populations and slow down the disease progression in those already infected with human immunodeficiency virus (HIV).

The idea of systematic cognitive exercise as a way of improving mental functions is not new. For decades, people who suffered head injury or stroke have been treated with cognitive therapy as a way of restoring mental functions lost to brain damage. Today we are on the threshold of a conceptual leap from treatment to prevention. A growing number of scientists, physicians, and psychologists believe that vigorous and diversified mental exercise may help in the battle against the decline of mental functions, which ultimately may take the form of dementia. From treatment to prevention—this is the dominant theme of modern medicine, and it is becoming an important theme in the battle against cognitive decline.

The theme has gained currency as the general public is made increasingly aware of the ravages of dementia. Earlier, mental deterioration was assumed to be a normal and inescapable product of aging. "Becoming sclerotic," "getting senile," "losing one's marbles" were the standard popular terms for referring to such "inevitability." But recent scientific research has shown that a large portion of the elderly population never loses mental acuity through gradual, inexorable decline. Instead, scientific research suggests a "bimodal" picture, a distinct difference between those who lose their cognitive powers with age and those who do not. In their influential book *Successful Aging*, John Rowe and Robert Kahn make the point with impressive clarity.[44] From this it follows that cognitive deterioration is not an obligatory part of *normal aging*; it is a *disease* of aging that affects some, perhaps many, but not all. The disease is called "dementia" and several types of dementia exist, each representing a different type of illness afflicting the brain. Therefore, we usually talk about "dementias" rather than "dementia."

A preordained, inexorable progression toward "senility" is a myth. This is the good news. The bad news is that while not inevitable, dementias are very common. Alzheimer's-type dementia is the most common among them, accounting for more than 50% of all dementias. By the age of 65, more than 10% of the population is afflicted with one form of dementia or another. According to the American Medical Association, by the age of 85, some 35% to 45% of people have it to at least some degree. It is estimated that dementias are likely the fourth or fifth most common cause of death in the United States.[45]

The high rate of dementia means that something must be done to treat it, and preferably to prevent it. Unfortunately, mental illness (and dementia is a form of mental illness) has been traditionally associated with stigma. People are more open about their "physical" ailments than they are about their "mental" ailments. Stigma means silence and the illusion of absence. Therefore, the taboo imposed by tradition on the discussion of mental illness has hindered society's ability to grasp its full scope and dimension and thus to assign the battle against it the priority it merits.

Fortunately, attitudes are rapidly changing. With the development of science and public awareness, the distinction between "physical" and "mental" ailments is becoming increasingly obsolete. Until recently, the general public was under the blissful assumption that while the body is frail and subject to decay, the mind is forever invulnerable. Today most people understand that the "mind" is a function of the brain, which is very much part of the "body."

Courageous statements by high-profile figures like the late Ronald Reagan and other public personalities have lent the cause of treating and preventing dementia a sense of urgency and dignity. The growing popular awareness of dementias and an open discussion about this disease are welcome developments, aligning the public sense of priorities neatly with reality.

How can dementias be fought? Again, the thrust must be two-pronged: treatment and prevention. A concerted effort has been launched by scientists and the pharmaceutical industry to develop dementia-treating drugs. Little of immediate clinical utility has been accomplished, but the battle has been joined and the resources mobilized, and there is good reason for optimism in the long run. As discussed in the previous section, several Alzheimer's-fighting medications have been approved, targeting cholinergic and glutaminergic neurotransmitter systems in the brain, and others are on their way.

By contrast, the concept of prevention of cognitive decline is only beginning to take shape in the minds of the scientific community and to enter public consciousness. Over the last few decades, the concept of physical exercise as a way of extending one's physical well-being with age has taken a firm hold in American culture. Today, the notion of cognitive exercise as a way of extending one's cognitive well-being with age is becoming increasingly accepted by scientists and is beginning to connect with the general public. In the last few years we have witnessed a sea change in public attitude toward the notion of cognitive fitness. No longer perceived as a fringe activity for the weird, it is well on its way to becoming a media darling, the next big hype.

While the concern about cognitive decline and how to prevent it naturally increases with age, it need not be limited to the elderly. A certain decline of cognitive powers is already evident at the age that we usually associate with the zenith of our lives and the pinnacle of our careers: the 40s, 50s, and 60s. A green youth is usually more adept at learning a foreign language, computer language, or a complex game like chess than is a corporate or political leader at the height of his or her power and societal influence. We begin to notice subtle memory slippage long before our confidence in ourselves becomes eroded in a global sense. Is this inevitable? Are our lives governed by a cruel Faustian deal, so that as we approach the pinnacle of our lives we lose something of ourselves?

Today a prominent professional or a powerful corporate leader refuses to accept as an inevitable fact of life the tradeoff between the success that comes with age and the loss of physical youthfulness. Physical exercise is viewed as a way of slowing down physical erosion of the flesh. Taking care of one's body enhances the way one is perceived, both professionally and socially. The opposite also occurs: chain smoking and gluttony stigmatize one as a slob out of touch with modernity.

But ours is an "information age." The relative competitive importance of brain versus brawn has been reversed over the centuries, so that today success hinges more on brain than brawn. Corporate duels, political contests, and scientific rivalries are not fought hand to hand or toe to toe. They are fought brain to brain and mind to mind. In modern warfare, too, the sharpness of the minds is decisive, not the sharpness of the steel. The outcome of military conflicts is increasingly decided by technological and scientific sophistication.

Increasingly, the advent of new computational technologies, virtual reality, and the Internet will bring together the human nervous system and manmade computational devices in a fundamentally new interface. We will need our brain more than ever in the brainy new age. How can we protect it from disease and decline?

The body of information essential to the workings of society is increasing exponentially, and never in the course of human civilization has there been an informational explosion as rapid as today's. The history of human civilization can be described in terms of a ratio of the amount of knowledge added to the total knowledge bank by a given generation to the amount of knowledge inherited from the previous generation. In antiquity, this ratio was close to zero, the rate of knowledge accumulation was slow, and the curve was almost flat.

The rate of knowledge accumulation has shot up particularly in the last century, and it continues to increase. It is already true today that much of the knowledge we acquire in school becomes obsolete by the time we reach our career peak. In the past, a university graduate could spend the bulk of a career complacently reaping the fruits of his or her early accomplishments. Today, large amounts of knowledge must be acquired throughout life in order to stay professionally afloat.

The slope of the information curve reflects the degree to which different cultures place a premium on the tradition embodied in the experience of the old compared to the innovation embodied in the daring of the young. The informationally static cultures of antiquity were built on a reverence for the old. Vestiges of this attitude are seen in the contemporary, but traditional, cultures of Asia and part of Europe. By contrast, American society, which among the major contemporary societies is the youngest and least rooted in tradition, is based on a reverence for youth. This is undoubtedly a reflection of its informational dynamism. The message contained in this analysis is clear: retaining mental vigor throughout life has never been as essential to success as today. It will get even more so.

The body of essential information is growing exponentially, but the human brain has remained biologically unchanged, or changed very little. It is commonly said that the computational capacity of the brain is virtually unlimited and can accommodate the body of knowledge of virtually infinite size. This common biological assumption is challenged by history. Whatever the theoretical computational capacity of the brain, in a practical sense it proves to be limited. It was possible for an educated person of antiquity to be in command of virtually all the essential knowledge of the time. This is no longer possible. Around the High Middle Ages or Renaissance the body of essential knowledge in human culture exceeded the mental capacity of a single individual. Knowledge became increasingly distributed and specialized. Paradoxically, the admired Renaissance man was the first human *not* capable of holding all the essential knowledge of the time. The ability to integrate diverse knowledge in an informationally fragmented world is clearly a decisive competitive advantage for those who can do it. This, too, calls for particular mental sharpness.

Middle-aged people engage in physical exercise to improve their odds against having a heart attack, whereas young people exercise to improve their social attractiveness. The criteria of social attractiveness reflect the attributes critical for competitive success, which in turn change through the history of human civilization.

The criteria of physical attractiveness reflect the markers of physical fitness, which has been, and will remain, an important ingredient of success. For centuries the definition of attractiveness has revolved mostly around physical attributes.

This attitude is changing. We are entering an unprecedented era in the development of human society ruled overwhelmingly by information processing. Bill Gates refers to this as the advent of the knowledge-based society. As we move into the twenty-first century and beyond, the attributes of social attractiveness will reflect the prerequisites of success in an increasingly information-driven society. Sharp will be beautiful. Being perceived as "dumb" will be more socially damning than being perceived as "ugly." In this social context, any credible approach to the preservation of cognitive well-being will be met with a public sense of approval and urgency.

History of Cognitive Rehabilitation

What can we learn from the experience of using cognitive exercise as treatment in order to apply cognitive exercise as prevention? The history of cognitive rehabilitation as a way of helping recovery from stroke and head injury is long, and the results are mixed. Several decades ago, Alexandr Luria introduced the concept of a "functional system." Any complex behavior controlled by the brain as a whole, he reasoned, was a result of the interaction between a number of specific brain functions, each controlled by a particular part of the brain. He called such an interactive constellation of specific functions responsible for a complex mental product a "functional system." The same cognitive task can be accomplished by different routes, each based on a slightly different functional system. The simple analogy with skilled movements helps illustrate the point. Most people lock the door with their right hand under most circumstances. However, if your right hand is occupied or injured, you should be able to do it with your left hand. If you need to lock the door while carrying two shopping bags, each in one hand, you can hold one bag with your teeth while quickly pulling the key and locking the door with the free hand.

What will happen to a functional system in brain damage? When World War II was raging, Luria's mandate was to develop ways to help soldiers with head wounds recover their mental abilities. The brain damage is likely to affect only a few, but not all, the components of a functional system. The challenge, then, is to rearrange it so as to replace the impaired components with different, intact ones. The specific composition of the functional system will change, but its overall product will not. A new functional system is introduced through retraining the patient in order to form a new cognitive strategy for the same mental product.

Although this plan sounds good in theory, the method did not always work in practice. The transfer of training was the stumbling block. Imagine the patient who had lost his memory as a result of head injury. A common way to restore functions was to teach the patient various strategies to memorize word lists of increasing length. In the end, the patient became spectacularly successful at memorizing word lists, but what difference would this make in real life? The real-life outcomes of such training were mixed. There was little generalization from one specific use of memory to others. To me, the enterprise had the ring of politically driven Soviet "scholarship," and I noted to myself that in private Luria talked about cognitive rehabilitation somewhat dismissively. By way of a curious historical digression, politicized Soviet science was led by Trofim Denisovich Lysenko, a Stalin-era agronomist and barely literate neo-Lamarckian, who claimed that he had a method for making acquired traits hereditary. This was a typical, if extreme, exercise in "Marxist science" designed to exalt the miracle of Soviet agriculture. By contrast, genetics was declared "bourgeois pseudoscience" and banished. Of course there was no scientific basis behind Lysenko's claims. Meanwhile, genetics was retarded in Russia for many years, despite Russia's early lead in the field.

The relative lack of success of generalization in cognitive retraining was disappointing but not entirely surprising. Research has shown that the capacity for generalization in problem solving is limited even in neurologically healthy people. It is not that they showed no generalization at all, but this generalization tends to be "local" rather than "global." People tend to learn by acquiring situation-specific mental templates.[46] It is thus only logical to assume that the capacity for generalization is even more limited following brain damage.

These considerations led to the rise of a more modest, concrete approach. Instead of attempting to help recover a mental function in a general, open-ended way, very specific, practical situations were identified in which the patient had difficulties. Training was then directed at these situations specifically, and narrowly. This approach worked, but by its very essence it was of inherently limited value. And it held little romantic appeal to the clinicians.

Brain Plasticity and Cognitive Exercise

These early efforts, with their mixed results, were based on the premise, or at least hope, that cognitive training helps change cognitive functions. The field changed radically with the new evidence that cognitive exercise helps change *the brain itself*. It seems almost self-evident that this should be the case. When you engage in an athletic activity, not only do your athletic skills improve, but actual muscle growth takes place. By contrast, lack of exercise leads to not only the loss of athletic skills but also actual muscle tissue reduction. Of more immediate relevance, sensory deprivation of an infant monkey will produce an actual atrophy of the corresponding brain tissue. Furthermore, the evidence of experientially driven neuroplasticity of the sort reviewed on the preceeding pages makes a very compelling case for controlled, structured cognitive exercise designed with the knowledge of neuropsychology and cognitive science.

The critical evidence directly supporting the utility of cognitive exercise began to accumulate gradually, starting with animal models. It has been known that immersion into an enriched environment facilitates recovery from the effects of brain damage in rats.[47] Now the mechanisms behind this recovery are finally becoming clear. The recovery of animals with traumatic brain injury was compared under two conditions: in an ordinary environment and in an environment enriched with an unusual amount of diverse sensory stimulation. When the brains of the two groups of animals were compared, striking differences were revealed. The regrowth of connections between the nerve cells ("dendritic sprouting") was much more vigorous in the stimulated group than in the ordinary group. There is also some evidence that with vigorous mental exercise, blood supply to the brain improves through enhanced growth of small blood vessels ("vascularization").[48] Scientists like Arnold Scheibel believe that similar processes take place in the human brain. Systematic cognitive activation may promote dendritic sprouting in the victims of stroke or head injury; this in turn facilitates the recovery of function.

These findings invite another question: Does cognitive activation slow down the progression of degenerative brain disorders, such as Alzheimer's disease, Pick's disease, and cortical Lewy body disease? These disorders are characterized by progressive brain atrophy and loss of synaptic connectivity, which in turn is associated with the accumulation of pathological microscopic entities, such as amyloid plaques and neurofibrillary tangles in Alzheimer's disease.

Unlike head trauma or stroke, dementias are slow, insidiously progressive disorders. This means that the efficacy of treatment should be judged not just by whether it reverses the course of the disease (this, for the time being at least, would be an unrealistic expectation) but also by whether the treatment slows the disease progression. Evidence exists, however, that for limited periods of time, cognitive exercise can actually improve brain physiology, even in an absolute sense. Scientists at the Max Planck Institute in Germany used positron emission tomography (PET) to study the effects of cognitive exercise and neurostimulant medications on brain glucose metabolism in people at an early stage of cognitive decline. Administered together, the two treatments enhanced brain glucose metabolism.[49] The German study examined the changes of resting brain physiology, its background state, and the changes in the pattern of brain activation when stimulated by a cognitive task. The advent of sophisticated brain-imaging technology gives us a window into the brain basis of mental processes, which would have been deemed unthinkable in the past. It is now possible to observe directly what happens in the brain as the person is engaged in a mental activity.

The new evidence, arising from animal studies and research with humans, opens an entirely new way of thinking about the effects of cognitive exercise. *Rather than attempting to shape or reshape specific mental processes, try to reshape the brain itself.*

While most of us agree that brain processes are mental processes, the logic behind the various approaches to cognitive retraining is different. Early efforts emphasized particular functions in the hope that the brain structures corresponding to that function would somehow be modified as a result. The new approach emphasizes generalized, open-ended effects of cognitive exercise on the brain. A tennis player or a golfer engaged in daily practice may aim at improving a particular stroke. This is akin to a specific task-oriented cognitive training. Or, players may hope that by practicing a few particular strokes, they will improve their other strokes and thus their game as a whole. This is akin to functional system-based cognitive training. Or, finally, they may embark on an exercise regimen with the goal of improving not so much the game in and of itself but the body that plays it—to increase strength, coordination, and stamina in a very general way. This is akin to trying to improve brain function. The third goal is far more ambitious than the first two, but new evidence suggests that it is attainable, at least in principle.

Animal studies show that improvement of "brain power" through cognitive activation is more than a fantasy. Scientists at the famed Salk Institute for Biological Studies in southern California examined the effects of enriched environment in adult mice.[50] They found that mice placed in cages filled with wheels, tunnels, and various toys developed up to 15% more neural cells than the mice left in standard cages. The "stimulated" mice also did better than their "unstimulated" counterparts on various tests of "mouse intelligence." They were able to learn mazes better and faster.

These findings are critical in two respects. First, they further debunk the old notion that new neurons cannot develop in an adult brain—they can. Second, these findings demonstrate with dramatic clarity that structured cognitive enhancement may actually change brain structure and improve its information-processing capacity. The new cell growth was particularly evident in the dentate gyrus of the hippocampus, a structure on the mesial surface of the temporal lobe considered to be particularly important in memory.[51]

The emergence of new nerve cells (*neuronal proliferation*) in the adult brain appears to be linked in the *neuroblasts*, the precursors of neurons, which in turn develop out of generic cell "prefabricates" called *stem cells*. The stem cells and neuroblasts continue to proliferate throughout adulthood, but usually they do not survive to become neurons. The Salk Institute study suggests that cognitive stimulation increases the neuroblasts' chance of survival to become full-fledged neurons.[52]

Among all the applications of cognitive exercise, its preventive role in helping people to enjoy their cognitive health for the longest time possible is particularly exciting. Is the protective effect of prior cognitive stimulation on mental decline universal, present across mammalian species? It appears to be, since the effect can be demonstrated in other species as well, as found by Dellu and colleagues in male Sprague-Dawley rats.[53] Animals with previous experience of learning various tasks were less susceptible to age-related memory deficits than the rats without the history of "mental exercise." Similarly, behavioral enrichment helped preserve the capacity for new learning in older dogs, as a study by Milgram and colleagues has shown.[54]

"Use it or lose it" is an old adage that seems to apply to the mind directly and literally. Among the very first to study the effects of structured cognitive enhancement in the aged, two scientists at the Pennsylvania State University, Warner Schaie and Sherry Willis, published an article with the provocative title, "Can Decline in Adult Intellectual Functioning Be Reversed?"[55] The authors studied a group of individuals, aged 64 to 95 years, who had suffered cognitive decline in a variety of mental functions over a 14-year period. Could a relatively brief cognitive training regimen restore their mental performance to its original level, to compensate for the 14 years of decline in spatial orientation and inductive reasoning? In many instances, the answer turned out to be "yes." Furthermore, cognitive recovery was generalized; it could be demonstrated on several independent tests of the cognitive functions of interest, and not just on the procedures used for training. The effect was lasting; in many participants it could be demonstrated 7 years after the completion of the training regimen. The authors concluded that the training regimen reactivated the cognitive skills, which had become "rusty" from lack of use. Since this early work, a number of similar studies have led to guardedly optimistic conclusions and were published in leading journals, such as *The Journal of American Medical Association*,[56] and *Proceedings of the National Academy of Science*.[57]

If it is logical to expect the therapeutic effects of cognitive exercise, why did earlier attempts at cognitive rehabilitation of the effects of brain damage meet with such mixed success? There are several reasons. The first reason lies in the large difference between the cognitive retraining of a damaged brain and cognitive conditioning of an intact or almost intact brain, between treatment and prevention. Medical knowledge dictates that it is easier to prevent an illness than to treat it. A severely damaged brain is predictably less likely to respond to any kind of remedy than is a basically healthy brain responding to prevention.

The second reason relates to how cognitive exercise has been traditionally designed under the "old" philosophy. In an attempt to target a specific, very narrow, cognitive function, targeted cognitive exercises were used. It is logical that the more broad-based a cognitive workout regimen, the more general the effects. To use a physical fitness analogy, an individual who spends all the exercise time on one machine cannot be expected to improve his or her cardiovascular system. For that, one needs a diverse circuit.

The third reason has to do with the ways in which the effects of treatment are measured. By measuring the effects of one cognitive exercise with the ability to perform on a different cognitive task, we are making an assumption about the specific nature of therapeutic effects being measured. Failure to find an effect may indeed result from the true lack of effect. But it may just as easily reflect our failure to find an appropriate measure to detect it. Since we are trying to enhance the underlying biological processes, it would be better to measure such processes directly. Indeed, when the effects of cognitive exercise were evaluated with PET, improved glucose metabolism (an important marker of brain function) was found.[58]

The fourth reason relates to what constitutes reasonable expectations of the effects of a cognitive workout. If general brain functions are enhanced through such conditioning, then the expected effect may be broad but subtle.

In any event, the recent findings of ongoing neural cell proliferation throughout the life span have breathed new life into the enterprise of cognitive exercise and endowed it with a new rationale.

Cognitive Fitness: Beginning of a Trend

The benefits of physical exercise are well known, but how to exercise is another matter. Some people do chin-ups on their kitchen door, and others go to a cardio vascular fitness center. While the chin-ups are probably good for you (unless, of course, you break the kitchen door), you stand to gain more from a sophisticated workout. This is why we spend time and money on exercise equipment, personal trainers, and health club membership fees.

A well-designed exercise circuit takes advantage of the knowledge of human anatomy and physiology. Each exercise is designed to enhance the function of a particular muscle group or physiological system. Depending on your individual goals, you may choose a complete, well-balanced circuit or focus on a particular exercise. The workout of a college athlete getting ready for a crew meet is not the same as the exercise of his overweight, middle-aged professor concerned with his cardiovascular system and trying to ward off a heart attack.

The brain is referred to as the microcosm for a reason. Of all the biological systems, it is the most complex and diverse in function and structure. The knowledge of the brain's exquisite complexity provides a sound basis for the design of a "brain exercise circuit." Here, a particular mental exercise is designed to match a distinct cognitive function. Most of us are vaguely aware of the benefits of cognitive challenge. As with physical fitness, your mental workout can be less or more sophisticated. Your Sunday morning crossword puzzle is probably good for you; think of it as the chin-ups for the mind. But you can do much better than that.

If cognitive exercise improves and enhances the brain itself, then it is important to design a systematic workout, ensuring that *all*, or at least *most*, of the important parts of the brain are engaged. In physical fitness training, it is important to exercise various muscle groups in a balanced way. Balance is achieved through workout circuits involving diverse and carefully selected exercises. Contemporary knowledge of the brain makes it possible to design a "cognitive workout circuit" that will systematically train various parts of the brain. If undirected—in effect, random—mental exercise has a demonstrably protective effect against dementia, then a targeted, scientifically designed cognitive workout regimen should be even more beneficial.

Early symptoms of Alzheimer's disease and other primary degenerative dementias, such as Lewy body disease, are quite diverse. Memory decline, suggestive of hippocampal dysfunction, is the first sign of illness in most patients, but not in all. In some patients early decline is expressed as word-finding difficulties implicating the left temporal lobe, as spatial disorientation implicating the parietal lobes, or as the impairment of foresight, social judgment, and initiative—signs of frontal lobe dysfunction. While in general all these areas are susceptible to the effects of Alzheimer's disease, their relative vulnerability appears to be highly variable. What determines the relative vulnerability of different brain structures in different individuals?

Scientists from the Netherlands Institute for Brain Research in Amsterdam, Mirmiran, van Someren, and Swaab put forth a mind-boggling hypothesis.[59] They believe that the activation of selective brain areas throughout a lifetime may prevent or delay the degenerative effects in those parts of the brain. According to this view, someone engaged in design as a profession or hobby will protect his or her parietal lobe, someone engaged in creative writing will protect his or her temporal lobe, and someone engaged in complex decision making and planning will protect his or her frontal lobes.

The logical conclusion of this line of reasoning is provocative and striking. To protect the *whole brain* against the effects of diffuse degenerative disease, a *comprehensive cognitive fitness regimen* must be designed, engaging various parts of the brain in a balanced and scientifically grounded manner. The concept of systematic cognitive exercise as an important activity in aging and during the peak career years is still new. But it is a natural and logical extension of physical exercise. *Physical fitness* has become a household term. *Cognitive fitness* is on its way to becoming the next trend in popular culture.

Unsurprisingly, the last few years have witnessed a proliferation of companies, Web sites, and products aimed at enhancing cognition and retarding, perhaps even reversing, the cognitive decline of aging. It is increasingly possible to talk about a whole cognitive enhancement movement. Like any new concept, "cognitive fitness" has its proponents and detractors. Within a span of a few weeks toward the end of 2007 I watched a PBS program with a number of leading neuroscientists, including Michael Merzenich, and high-profile authors supporting the "cognitive fitness" movement, and read an Op-Ed page in a major newspaper lambasting it with a particularly harsh partisan zeal.[60] A more detailed review and assessment of this movement is beyond the scope of this book, but the "cognitive fitness" phenomenon is upon us, whether we like it (I do) or not.

Cognitive exercise as a way of preventing mental decline and improving mental functions is still a barely charted territory. As we move forward along this intriguing new path, we will have to develop both innovative approaches and rigorous methods to evaluate their efficacy. Ideally, one would want to examine the effects of various types of cognitive exercise on brain physiology with the methods of functional neuroimaging, and increasingly this is happening. Is there any effect at all? Are the effects global? Are they regional? Are they exercise-dependent? These are important questions to be addressed by future research in the new century and the new millennium.

14

Breaking and Entering

Inside the Black Box

Ramblings of a Dilettante

While still an undergraduate at the Moscow State University, I was attracted to the idea that for neuroscience to become a mature discipline it needed its own theoretical arm, analytical tools, and mathematics, which would do for brain research what the invention of calculus by Newton and Leibnitz did for physics. It can be argued that the importance of theoretical models is greater in neuroscience than in most other areas of scientific inquiry because the systems of interest are more complex and less linear and have a greater richness of emergent properties, given the complex patterns of interactivity that characterize the brain. While all these attributes make our field of inquiry so exciting, it imposes very severe constraints on the power of strictly experimental methods. No matter how many electrodes one implants into a poor monkey's brain, the recordings are not likely to reveal the complex neural interactions in play—they are simply too numerous, complex, and nonlinear. Our current attempts to capture such interactions in the human brain with functional neuroimaging are equally limited, for similar reasons.

With this in mind, I created for myself a special curriculum, taking courses in various branches of mathematics in addition to psychology.

My earliest interests in brain science and attempts at research revolved around modeling with formal neural networks (commonly referred to as "neural nets") as a tool. That was more than 40 years ago, before the age of computer simulations, when (at least in the Soviet Union) neural network research was a paper-and-pencil enterprise, very much in the spirit of the original work by McCulloch and Pitts.[1] Despite the severe limitations inherent in the pre-computer age, interesting results could be obtained with strictly analytical tools. I was quite taken by this work and planned to become what today would be called a "computational neuroscientist" (the birth of the actual term was still a quarter-century away).

But Moscow in the late 1960s was not the best place to pursue such interests. While several pockets of what today would be called "computational neuroscience" existed at and around Moscow State University, with the work by Nicholas Bernstein, Israel Gelfand, Michael Bongart, and a few others, this hardly amounted to a critical mass. My own mentor Alexandr Luria didn't quite know how to relate to this interest of mine. He accepted the general premise of the need for mathematical or quasi-mathematical tools in neuropsychology, but there was nothing in his own background or education or in the Zeitgeist that produced him that would have allowed him to genuinely understand, let alone, embrace it.

Over the years since those early days at the University of Moscow, particularly since my arrival in the United States, my work has become much more clinical in nature. Life is not a controlled experiment, so I will never know if I would have been a happier human being had I stuck with my early neural network and other analytical/computational interests. At a practical level, being a clinician broadens one's options and gives one the freedom from institutions that the anarchist in me has always cherished. But the early interests remained. Deep down I have always thought of my actual work as being a result of a change in circumstances rather than in interests or intellectual temperament.

In the ensuing decades, the field of computational neuroscience has grown by leaps and bounds and has expanded well beyond the point of my ability to catch up with its state-of-the-art tools. Yet I have continued to follow its development conceptually and have always tried to formulate my own ideas and theories in ways that would lend themselves to formal modeling, at least in principle. What follows are a few thoughts about possible modeling approaches that are prompted by some of the ideas expressed earlier in the book. A general reader may find this chapter too dry, arcane, and technical, and should feel free to skip it.

But a computational neuroscientist may find in it a few useful insights and ideas for neural network models and perhaps even use them to embark on the design of such models; or he or she may conclude that the next few pages are nothing more than the rambling of a dilettante; or both.

Machine in the Ghost

As we have already discussed, the brain has two fundamental propensities: to face novel situations and to utilize established knowledge. The transition from novelty to familiarity is a fundamental cycle of human cognition. It is a dynamic process that captures the essence of higher-order cognition, just like the classic reflex captures the essence of more simple behaviors. What is the nature of the complex relationship between the use of established knowledge and the acquisition of new knowledge? How are these two needs reconciled and supported in the brain? These questions have been recognized as central challenges facing cognitive and computational neuroscience and are particularly germane to the design of neural network models of the brain. The progress in uncovering the mechanisms by which the brain reconciles the ability to acquire new information with the ability to maintain previously formed neural representations without degradation has major ramifications for the design of intelligent machines and for a range of clinical applications. Before addressing these possibilities, however, we need to expand on the distinction between cognitive novelty and cognitive routines, a major theme of this book.

The brain dynamics of the novelty–familiarity cycle in the brain has not been well understood, and it remains a puzzle. Among the possible solutions to this puzzle, it has been proposed that cognitive novelty is supported by the hippocampi and cognitive routines, by the neocortex. Alternatively, it has been proposed that cognitive novelty is supported by the neocortex and cognitive routines, by the basal ganglia. While possibly capturing certain aspects of the neural mechanisms of the novelty–routinization distinction, these dichotomies fail to account for all of its essential properties.

Earlier in the book, I introduced the hypothesis linking the novelty–routinization dichotomy to hemispheric specialization (see Chapter 6). According to this formulation, the right hemisphere is particularly adept at processing novel information to which none of the mental representations available in the subject's cognitive repertoire immediately apply. The left hemisphere is particularly adept at processing routinized, familiar information with reliance on well-established mental representations and strategies. Since 1981, when the novelty–routinization hypothesis of hemispheric specialization was first published, it has found extensive support from various experimental and clinical paradigms, including cross-sectional, within-experimental learning, developmental, and brain lesion studies. More recently, a growing number of functional neuroimaging studies have provided further support to the novelty–routinization hypothesis of hemispheric specialization (see Chapter 6).

Establishing that the two hemispheres have differential relationships to novelty and familiarity is only the beginning of a more in-depth inquiry. While we have introduced an entirely new paradigm for understanding the relative roles of the two hemispheres, this alone does not elucidate the actual neural mechanisms responsible for such functional differentiation. So let's try to come up with plausible, testable, and falsifiable (in the Karl Popper sense) hypotheses to account for it.

What are the biological differences between the two hemispheres responsible for the emergence of these functional differences? As we already know, differences between the two hemispheres of the brain are pervasive in both the human and nonhuman mammalian brain at every level of observation, from the most macroscopic (gross neuroanatomical) to the molecular level. At the level of gross morphology these differences include a greater frontward protrusion of the right hemisphere and greater backward protrusion of the left hemisphere (the *Yakovlevian torque*), and differences in the size of the *planum temporale* and *frontal operculum* (both larger in the left hemisphere). At a finer level of brain wiring, disparities have been found between the cortical thicknesses of the two hemispheres (thicker in the right hemisphere than in the left hemisphere, at least in males). At the finest cytoarchitechtonic level of micro-wiring, differences have been found between the numbers of spindle cells, which are far more prolific in the right frontal lobes than in the left frontal lobes. At the level of biochemical pathways, differences were found between the projections in the two hemispheres of dopamine and norepinephrine, which are among the main chemical substances (neurotransmitters and neuromodulators) playing a central role in signal transmission in the brain. There are slightly more dopamine pathways in the left hemisphere and slightly more norepinephrine (noradrenergic) pathways in the right hemisphere. Finally, at the molecular level, asymmetries have been found between the distribution of microscopic subunits of NMDA receptors in the left and right hippocampi. The NMDA receptors play a crucial role in memory and learning, since they enable signaling between neurons that is mediated by glutamate, one of the most prevalent neurotransmitters in the brain. We also know that the hippocampi are particularly important in memory processes.

Without exception, we humans share all these assorted hemispheric differences with other mammalian species. As already discussed, this commonality poses a very serious problem for the more traditional theory of hemispheric specialization linking the left hemisphere to language and the right hemisphere to nonverbal processes, since it cannot be meaningfully applied to the nonhuman mammalian species that do not possess language. By contrast, the novelty–routinization theory of hemispheric specialization is applicable, at least in principle, to any organism capable of learning. Let us then attempt to sketch the possible formal, mechanistic models of the biological differences between the two hemispheres and think of ways to examine the emergent properties arising within such future formal models.

To this end, let's consider four factors: *(1)* structural morphological features of cortical organization, *(2)* pathway architecture, *(3)* synaptic mechanisms of long-term memory formation, and *(4)* two catecholamine neuromodulatory systems—dopaminergic and noradrenergic. We will examine how each of these factors or any combination thereof may account for the functional hemispheric differences as the emergent properties. Each of these factors or any combination thereof may be at the heart of the functional differences between the hemispheres. In fact, some interesting interactions between these factors may be in play.

Specifically, we will make the following assertions and then pose subsequent questions:

1. If one were to summarize various morphometric differences between the two hemispheres, reported in a piecemeal fashion in different studies, the following picture emerges. The overall cortical space appears to be allocated slightly differently in the two hemispheres. The left hemisphere is characterized by a slight overrepresentation of modality-specific association cortices (including the superior temporal gyrus and the premotor cortex), at the expense of heteromodal association cortices. The opposite is true for the right hemisphere: there is a slight overrepresentation of heteromodal association cortices (prefrontal, inferotemporal, and inferoparietal) at the expense of modality-specific association cortices. *Is it possible that the hemispheric differences in cortical space allocation cause information to be represented in slightly different ways in the two hemispheres and to confer differential advantages in processing novel and familiar information?*

2. In summarizing the differences between the pathway architectures of the two hemispheres, the following picture emerges. The left hemisphere is characterized by a slightly greater reliance on short local pathways than is the right hemisphere. The opposite is true for the right hemisphere: it has a slightly greater reliance on the long interregional pathways than does the left hemisphere. *Is it possible that the hemispheric differences in the pathway architecture cause information to be processed in slightly different ways in the two hemispheres and to confer differential advantages in processing novel and familiar information?*

3. The two catecholamine neuromodulatory systems are slightly asymmetric. Owing to the work of Stanley Glick and his colleagues and that of other researchers, we know that the dopaminergic (DA) system, which arises from the ventral tegmental area (VTA) and projects into the frontal lobe via the mesocortical pathway and into the temporal lobe and the hippocampus via the mesolimbic pathway, is slightly more prevalent in the left hemisphere than in the right hemisphere.[6] By contrast, the noradrenergic (NE) system, which arises from the locus coerulleus and projects via the frontal poles into extensive cortical regions, is slightly more prevalent in the right hemisphere than in the left hemisphere. The NE system is also less focal and more diffuse than the DA system. Furthermore, a certain asymmetry of specific receptor-type distribution may be present within the DA system, D2 receptors

favoring the right hemisphere.[3] *Is it possible that these differences in neuro-modulation affect the way representations are formed in the two cerebral hemispheres?*

4. Long-term memory (LTM) formation is accomplished by enhancing and stabilizing selective connectivity within a neural network. Eric Kandel and others have proposed that such selective connectivity enhancement is mediated by the growth of new synapses, which in turn is facilitated by certain neuromodulators. The relationship between LTM formation, dopamine (DA), and hemispheric specialization is particularly intriguing, and it melds into a single coherent narrative in an elegant and parsimonious way. The connection between LTM and DA was discovered by Eric Kandel and his colleagues, who have demonstrated that in the mammalian brain the growth of new synapses necessary for LTM formation is facilitated by the release of dopamine.[4] *Is it possible that this machinery of long-term memory formation is characterized by subtle differences in the two cerebral hemispheres owing to the asymmetric representation of dopamine projections?*

All these questions are amenable to direct scientific approaches, but they require different methods. Questions 3 and 4 can be best tackled through direct experimentation, by using either in vivo nonhuman mammalian models or by studying in vitro synaptic proliferation under various conditions. By contrast, questions 1 and 2 can be best tackled with computational methods. Questions 3 and 4 also call for computational methods in addition to experimental ones. We will consider these avenues of future research separately.

Dopamine, Memory, and the Bicameral Brain

Let's examine the relationship between long-term memory formation, dopamine, and hemispheric specialization. As we already know, Eric Kandel and his colleagues at Columbia University demonstrated that in the mammalian brain the growth of new synapses necessary for long-term memory formation is facilitated by the release of dopamine.[5] We also know that Stanley Glick and his associates, working at Mount Sinai Medical Center in New York, have demonstrated that dopamine is somewhat more prevalent in the left hemisphere than in the right hemisphere.[6] By way of a simple syllogism, one can conclude that long-term memory formation may be somehow facilitated and is more efficient in the left hemisphere.

The next thing to consider is the neuroanatomy of dopamine pathway distribution within the hemisphere. Unlike most other neurotransmitters and neuro-modulators, dopaminergic pathways are rather circumscribed. They are restricted basically to three sets of brain structures: *(1)* the basal ganglia, the nigrostriatal pathway projecting into them from the brain stem nucleus substantia nigra; *(2)* the mesial structures of the temporal lobe, particularly the hippocampi and the amygdala, the mesolimbic pathway projecting into them from the ventral tegmental area (VTA) found in the brain stem; *(3)* and the prefrontal cortex, the mesocortical pathway also projecting from the VTA. Among these structures, the hippocampi are most often implicated in the process of memory, particularly in episodic declarative memory. While the long-term engrams themselves are probably formed in the neocortex, the hippocampi play a critical role in facilitating the formation of such engrams, particularly in binding together their disparate components distributed across far-flung neocortical regions. This facilitation and binding is accomplished through changes in the hippocampi, and such changes in the hippocampi are facilitated by dopamine, as the work by Kandel has shown.[7,8] To the extent that the role of dopamine in long-term memory formation is expressed in the hippocampi, it is only logical to conclude that it is more efficient in the *left hippocampus*, owing to the slightly lateralized nature of dopaminergic pathways.

What is the relationship between dopamine and the emergence of hemispheric specialization in evolution? According to Kandel, the role of dopamine in long-term memory formation is not paramount throughout the whole of evolution. Quite the contrary, it becomes evident only in mammalian species. By contrast, in the giant snail *Aplysia*, long-term memory formation is facilitated by serotonin. Unlike dopamine, serotonin does not exhibit any asymmetric pattern distribution; serotonergic pathways are, for all intents and purposes, largely symmetric. According to Kandel,[9] *Aplysia* does not exhibit any lateralized asymmetries of its nervous system. So did the emergence of hemispheric specialization serve as the evolutionary basis or correlate of the transition from serotonergic to dopaminergic mediation of long-term memory formation? Or is it the other way around, the transition from serotonergic to dopaminergic mediation of long-term memory formation being the cause, and the emergence of hemispheric specialization the consequence? Or does some other more complex and less parsimonious relationship exist between the evolution of hemispheric asymmetries and the evolution of biochemical machinery of long-term memory?

In contemporary neuroscience, dopamine has been accorded a unique role in learning. It is common to talk about the role of dopamine in "reward" mechanisms,[10] about it providing the "teaching signal" in the learning processes in the neural network. Jeremy Day and colleagues have provided an impressive demonstration of how stimulus–reward pairing can affect dopamine release by shifting its timing "forward" toward predictive cues.[11]

Furthermore, the magnitude of reward-driven behavior can be modified by biochemically stimulating or suppressing dopaminergic activity.[12] But where does the instruction come from? The source of origin of the dopaminergic pathways usually implicated in these lofty functions is the ventral tegmental area, a tiny nucleus sitting in the ventral midbrain. Recording from the dopaminergic neurons found in the VTA has shown that their firing reflects complex computations pertaining to reward value predictions, cues predicting the reward and the dynamic changes of these variables over time.[13]

But the VTA is an extremely unlikely candidate for the primary site of the complex neural computation necessary for any complex adaptive decision-making. Furthermore, together with another source of dopaminergic projections, the substantia nigra, these nuclei appear to receive inputs from other structures such as the lateral habenula,[14] which is equally unlikely to be the main, let alone sole, site of neural computation at the core of complex adaptive decision-making. The underlying circuitry must be comparably complex. Rather than being the actual locus of complex neural computations inherent in reward estimates, the VTA is likely an amplifier and conveyer of the signal computed elsewhere.

Enter the prefrontal cortex and the amygdala, two other brain regions rich in dopamine. The amygdala plays a critical role in automatic, rapid, coarse, and, to a large extent, hard-wired, simple cue–based appraisal of incoming inputs in terms of their significance for survival. The prefrontal cortex provides a more elaborate, slower, learned, "cognitive" appraisal of incoming inputs according to their significance to the organism, based on assessment of a broader context.

These two structures, the prefrontal cortex and the amygdala, are the likely locations of neural computation of significance to the organism. They then send the signal to the VTA, "instructing" it to stimulate various neural structures, including the hippocampal dopaminergic pathways, which in turn facilitates the formation of long-term memories of the inputs judged as significant. This amounts to an exquisitely fine-tuned mechanism, which selects certain inputs for the privileged passage into long-term memory and denies such passage to other inputs. Let us call this mechanism the "executive-significance memory loop," or ESM. The primary information flow vector within the ESM is from the prefrontal cortex and amygdala via the VTA to the hippocampi.

While it would be naïve to link such a complex mechanism to a single neurotransmitter or neuromodulator, dopamine seems to play a particularly important role all along the ESM loop. It is mediated by the mesolimbic and mesocortical dopamine pathways. Whenever these pathways are invoked, the emphasis in the scientific literature is usually on their ascending components, but it would appear from the previous analysis that the descending components are every bit as important, since they provide the route via which the prefrontal cortex and the amygdala "command" the VTA to stimulate the dopamine pathways in the hippocampi and other structures. In a methodologically highly sophisticated fMRI study, Kimberlee D'Ardenne and her colleagues were able to image the VTA in a reward-prediction experiment. They demonstrated a direct relationship between the positive reward-prediction error and VTA activation, which in turn was correlated with activation in the ventral striatum.[15] A similar result was reported by Timothy Behrens and his colleagues.[16] Does this mean that the signal originated in the VTA, or is it possible that the VTA is an amplifier that relays to the rest of the brain the computational outcome generated in the prefrontal cortex? To answer this question it would be interesting to examine any correlation between a signal in the VTA and a signal in the prefrontal cortex in experiments like the ones conducted by D'Ardenne, Behrens, and their colleagues.[17]

According to this scenario, the mesolimbic and mesocortical pathways can be thought of as components of a single integrated memory loop. Information "worthiness" is assessed in the prefrontal cortex ("cognitively") and in the amygdala ("automatically"). If it is judged worthy of entry into long-term storage, then the signal is sent to the VTA via the descending components of the mesolimbic (from the amygdala) and mesocortical (from the prefrontal cortex) pathways to trigger phasic dopamine release via the ascending mesolimbic pathway into the hippocampi. This, in turn, facilitates the consolidation and stabilization of "worthy" memories. The mechanism proposed here clearly operates in both hemispheres, but it is probably more efficient in the left hemisphere, because of its preferential relationship with dopaminergic transmission.

The story linking together long-term memory and hemispheric asymmetries by way of dopamine helps reconcile two seemingly opposing approaches to one of the central riddles of information processing in the brain. The brain is somehow able to acquire new information without the loss of previously acquired information. It can learn how to deal with new challenges without "unlearning" how to deal with previously encountered situations. The brain can exhibit the properties of plasticity and stability at the same time. Although we take this dual ability for granted in our everyday activities as brain users, we are confounded by this ability as brain researchers. Many a serious neuroscientist has found this dual property of the brain to defy clear mechanistic explanations. The problem is particularly apparent to neural network modelers. It turns out to be very difficult to design a network capable of learning new information without paying the price of losing previously acquired information.

To resolve the dilemma, several scientists have concluded that the brain reconciles these two capabilities by having two separate systems. But what are they and where in the brain are they found? Jay McClelland and his colleagues concluded that the neocortex and the hippocampi represent the two systems in the brain supporting the two complementary abilities.[18] This idea gave rise to a whole line of research, mostly using computational methods and neural network modeling. By contrast, on the basis of my own work, I have concluded that the two complementary abilities are differentially supported by the two cerebral hemispheres.

But the foregoing discussion implies that both theories may be correct, since they are not orthogonal. A more efficient dopaminergic transmission in the left hippocampus implies that the hippocampal contribution to neural computation and long-term memory formation is more efficient in the left cerebral hemisphere than in the right cerebral hemisphere.

Neural Networks and the Bicameral Brain: Models of Novelty–Routinization Dynamics

How can one address the issues of hemispheric specialization through neural network models? Let's consider the differences in cortical space allocation and in pathway architecture. As we already know, more modality-specific association cortex exists in the left hemisphere and more heteromodal association cortex exists in the right hemisphere. We also know that signal transmission in the right hemisphere relies more on long myelinated pathways interconnecting distant regions than in the left hemisphere. By contrast, signal transmission in the left hemisphere relies more on short nonmyelinated pathways interconnecting proximal regions.

Both of these sets of hemispheric differences, those related to cortical space allocation and those related to pathway length, lend themselves well to formal modeling. What follows is a preliminary sketch of neural network models of differential cortical allocation and pathway architecture.

Cortical space allocation

First we need to create a multilayer neural network model consisting of at least four or even five layers: the input layer, two or three hidden layers, and the output layer. In this network, *input layer* corresponds to sensory cortex. It consists of several segments that correspond to different sensory modalities. Suppose we have three sensory modalities: visual, auditory, and tactile. *Hidden layer 1* also consists of several segments, each corresponding to a modality-specific association cortex and interconnected with the corresponding segment of the input layer. *Hidden layer 2* corresponds to the heteromodal association cortex and is interconnected with all the segments of hidden layer 1. We may, in fact, decide to split it into *hidden layer 2'* (corresponding to the posterior heteromodal association cortices [inferotemporal and inferoparietal]), and *hidden layer2"* (corresponding to the prefrontal cortex). Finally, *output layer* is interconnected with hidden layer 2". Of course, in a more complex, "deep" architecture, each level of this organization may be represented by a whole "stack" of layers, rather than by a single layer.

Pathway architecture

Next we must find a way of translating the notion of pathway length into the discrete terms of a formal neural network model. *Pathway length* applies both to horizontal pathways connecting neurons within the same layer and to vertical pathways connecting neurons across adjacent and, more interestingly, nonadjacent layers. One can then operationalize the pathway-length notion in a variety of ways.

Vertical pathways can be distinguished on the basis of the number of layers that the pathways "jump over": the greater the number, the longer the pathway.

This definition of vertical-pathway length is particularly interesting in a model where each layer type is represented by a whole stack of layers, rather than by a single layer.

Horizontal pathways within a hidden layer can be distinguished on the basis of projections received by the neurons with which they connect. Yet another and biologically more plausible possibility is to introduce a relatively homogeneous matrix of connections between adjacent neurons ("local pathways") and to superimpose on them another set of pathways that we will call "distal pathways." The length of such distal pathways will be defined by the number of local synaptic contacts between the adjacent neurons that they jump over. One can then vary the length of distal pathways according to this principle.

Now that we have a basic description of a multilayered neural network with different pathway types, the next step is to create a "bicameral brain" by putting together two such networks. These are our two hemispheres. We then interconnect them through horizontal pathways interfacing likewise layers. These horizontal pathways will be our corpus callosum and the anterior and posterior commissures. As a point of departure, the two networks can be exact mirror images of each other. Now we will begin to modify them in different ways by considering several possibilities.

Genetic algorithms

For starters, let's make use of "genetic algorithms," computational devices that emulate a natural-selection process. First, suppose we keep the total combined size of all the hidden layers constant, and then subject the cortical-space allocation across different layers to random variation. We can then apply a genetic algorithm to find out which allocation of cortical space across the hidden layers results in the most computationally efficient bicameral network, and for what tasks. Based on the previous discussion, our hypothesis is that the best computational outcome will be produced by the network in which the cortical-space allocation is different in the two hemispheres, one favoring hidden layer 1 (the left hemisphere), and the other favoring hidden layers 2' and 2" (the right hemisphere). By creating the model, designating a range of training tasks, and subjecting the network to a "selection process" through the application of genetic algorithms, we can subject our hypothesis to a rigorous test. Our prediction is that hemispheric differences depicted in Figure 14.1 will emerge as the most efficient architecture. We can also map out the range of tasks that benefit from such hemispheric asymmetry and those that do not.

A similar application of genetic algorithms is possible with respect to the distribution of different pathway lengths in the two hemispheres. Again, from the previous discussion, our hypothesis is that the best computational outcome will be produced by the network in which the pathway-length allocation is different in the two hemispheres, one favoring shorter pathways (the left hemisphere) and the other favoring longer pathways (the right hemisphere).

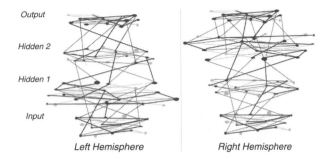

Figure 14.1 "Deep" architecture in the two hemispheres. Hidden layer 1 is larger in the left hemisphere than in the right hemisphere. Hidden layer 2 is larger in the right hemisphere than in the left hemisphere. See text for explanation. This is a heuristic representation intended to convey a general idea rather than any realistic neuroanatomical properties.

Finally, a combined cortical-space allocation and pathway-length model can be examined by varying both sets of parameters in parallel and subjecting them to the selection process with genetic algorithms. Given the previous discussion, our hypothesis is that the best computational outcome will be produced by the network with certain pairings of cortical-space allocation and pathway-length types in the two hemispheres: one favoring hidden layer 1 *and* shorter pathways (the left hemisphere), and the other favoring hidden layer 2 *and* longer pathways (the right hemisphere).

Fixed models

We can also compare the computational efficiency of two bicameral networks of identical total size, but differing by the presence or absence of design asymmetries, reflecting the previous discussion. In one of the networks the cortical-space allocation and/or pathway lengths will be exactly the same in the two hemispheres (symmetric network), and in the other network the cortical-space allocation and/or pathway lengths will be different in the two hemispheres, in keeping with our earlier description (asymmetric network). In the asymmetric network, hidden layer 1 will be larger in the left hemisphere than in the right hemisphere, whereas hidden layer 2 will be larger in the right hemisphere than in the left hemisphere (see Fig. 14.1). Likewise, in the asymmetric network short pathways will be more prolific in the left hemisphere than in the right hemisphere, and long pathways will be more prolific in the right hemisphere than in the left hemisphere.

Which of the two bicameral networks will have learning advantage and for which tasks? Our hypothesis predicts that the asymmetric network will show learning advantage over a wide range of tasks compared to the symmetric network. By comparing the two networks on a wide range of tasks, we can subject our hypothesis to a rigorous test, as well as map out the hypothesis's limitations.

Nicholas (Colly) Myers, one of United Kingdom's top software architects, the former Chief Technology Officer of Psion and Symbian and a friend of mine, proposed alternative modeling solutions to capture some of the functional differences between the two hemispheres.[19] The neural network features proposed by Colly are particularly applicable to a deep model, where hidden layer 2 is in fact a stack of layers rather than a single layer. In Colly's model, hidden layer 2 is represented by a thicker stack in the right than in the left hemisphere. Another architectural feature proposed by Colly is a difference in "receptive field" sizes in hidden layer 2 of the two hemispheres. According to this model, in the left-hemisphere neurons of hidden layer 2^i receive projections from constrained proximal neuronal groupings from hidden layer 2^{i-1}. By contrast, in the right hemisphere, neurons of hidden layer 2^i receive projections from wider-ranging neuronal groupings from hidden layer 2^{i-1}. Even though Colly's motivation was engineering more than neuroscientific, his suggestions may foreshadow some actual neuroanatomical differences between the two hemispheres.

"Lesioned" networks

Finally, we can "lesion" the asymmetric network in a variety of ways and examine the consequences. If the left hemisphere (favoring hidden layers 1 and/or short pathways) indeed excels at later stages of learning when the task is already somewhat familiar, then its damage will not interfere with early learning stages but will result in a considerable slowing of the later stages. On the other hand, if the right hemisphere (favoring hidden layers 2′ and 2″ and/or long pathways) indeed excels at dealing with novelty, then its damage will drastically slow down the learning process at early stages of exposure to an unfamiliar task. In fact, it may interfere with learning in a very global way, since the learning curve may never reach the point when the left hemisphere may be able to effectively kick in. Again, by committing ourselves to a specific, unequivocal prediction, we make our hypothesis eminently falsifiable and, thus, rigorously scientific.

"Male" and "female" networks

An interesting spin on the pathway architecture arises from the consideration of gender differences. As already discussed, a considerable body of evidence exists that cognition is less lateralized in females than in males. Particularly relevant to the subject of this book, my colleagues' and my work has shown that frontal lobe function is considerably less lateralized in females than in males, or to rephrase this, the two frontal lobes are more functionally alike ("equipotential") in females than in males.

Could these functional gender differences be a consequence of the gender differences in pathway architecture? Indeed, it has been shown that certain parts of the corpus callosum are thicker in females than in males. By contrast, some of the longitudinal fasciculi have been shown to be thicker in males than in females. Differences in bundle thickness may imply differences in the number of pathways in the bundle or greater degree of pathway myelinization, or both. Any of these functions would enhance signal transmission within the bundle. It would thus appear that interhemispheric transmission is more efficient in females, and intra-hemispheric transmission between the frontal lobes and the posterior part of the same hemisphere is more efficient in males.

What would be the functional consequences of such gender differences in path-way architecture? This, too, can be best addressed through neural network models, by comparing the functional differences between two bicameral architectures: one with enhanced horizontal pathways connecting the same layers *between* hemispheres (the "female brain"); the other one with enhanced vertical pathways connecting different layers *within* a hemisphere (the "male brain").

We also know that the Yakovlevian torque is less articulated in the female brain than in the male brain, and that the hemispheric differences in the size of the planum temporale are less pronounced in females than in males. Consequently, it is possible to conclude that the hemispheric differences in cortical-space alloca-tion across different types of neocortex are more pronounced in the male brain than in the female brain.

What would be the functional consequences of such gender differences in cortical-space allocation? This, too, can be best addressed through neural network models by comparing the functional differences between two bicameral architec-tures characterized by more or less extreme degree of hemispheric differences in relative layer sizes.

Finally, one can examine the composite effects of these gender differences by comparing "female" and "male" neural networks, combining all of the above architectural differences, on a variety of tasks.

Complicate to Simplify

Composite models

If we consider all the possible interactions between the features outlined above, then the picture becomes particularly interesting. What is the combined effect of hemispheric differences in cortical-space allocation and those in pathway archi-tecture? What is the combined effect of hemispheric differences in cortical-space allocation and of the differential dopaminergic (DA) and noradrenergic (NE) neu-romodulatory effects? What is the combined effect of hemispheric differences in pathway architecture and of the differential DA and NE neuromodulatory effects? What is the composite effect of hemispheric differences in cortical-space alloca-tion, of pathway architecture, and of the differential DA and NE neuromodulatory effects, all in the same brain?

To this end, we may explore the combined effect of the various mechanisms described above by creating a network with three sets of variables: cortical-space allocation, pathway length, and the synaptic proliferation efficiency. In this scheme of things, the left hemisphere will have preferential space allocation for hidden layer 1, emphasize short pathways, and be a relatively rapid learner (due to a more efficient long-term memory formation). By contrast, the right hemisphere will have preferential space allocation for hidden layers 2, emphasize long pathways, and be a relatively slow learner (due to a less efficient long-term memory formation).

To resolve the seeming contradiction of the "novelty" hemisphere being a slow learner and the "familiarity" hemisphere being a fast learner, consider the following. The left hemisphere is a collection of relatively specific representations, each capturing the essential properties of a particular parochial class of inputs. When the organism encounters a new class of inputs, the left hemisphere forms a new parochial representation without changing the previously formed ones. By contrast, the right hemisphere contains a composite representation of the "average" state of the world. Whenever the organism encounters a new class of inputs, this composite representation is changed somewhat, but not much. It is the composite representation of the average state of the world that the organism relies on as a *default* option whenever the new challenge does not fit any of the previously formed parochial representations—that is, until the organism forms a new parochial representation to capture the essential properties specific to the new set of inputs. This process is discussed further later in the chapter.

We can then subject this complex network to all the manipulations described above. It may very well be this complex model will yield the most interesting results.

The next step in our reasoning is to consider a preliminary sketch of computational models of differential learning rates due to differences in biochemical modulation and architectural properties.

Dynamics of learning

The novelty–routinization hypothesis of hemispheric interaction implies a leading role of the right hemipshere at early stages of dealing with a new task, and a leading role of the left hemispherc at latc stages. Does this imply a literal right-to-left hemispheric information transfer, a neural trans-callosal railroad of sorts? Not necessarily. More likely, mental representations develop interactively in both hemispheres, but the rates of their formation differ. The right hemisphere is more effective at early stages of learning a cognitive skill, but this is reversed in favor of the left hemisphere at the later stages.

We do not yet fully understand the neural machinery behind these differences, but we are in a position to formulate certain plausible hypotheses. Suppose that the left hemisphere forms and stores representations that are generic in the sense that each of them captures shared features of a whole class of specific things or situations, yet are also specific in that each such representation captures the shared properties of a relatively narrow class of situations. By definition, a huge number of such representations will be required to capture the grand sum total of one's experiences and knowledge. By contrast, the right hemisphere forms and stores much coarser representations, each of which captures the shared properties of a much broader class of situations. It stands to reason that the right hemisphere will contain fewer such representations than the left hemisphere. One may even contemplate an extreme case, whereby the association cortex of the right hemipshere does not contain specific representations at all, but rather consists of a single weakly differentiated network capturing the averaged properties of all prior experiences.

When an individual is faced with a relatively familiar cognitive task, it is likely to resonate with or be "attracted to" (to use the jargon of neural network modeling) a specific representation in the left hemisphere. But when an individual is faced with a relatively novel cognitive task, it is more likely to resonate with one of the coarser representations in the right hemisphere, precisely because these representations are less bounded and less specific. As the individual gains experience and expertise with the new type of cognitive task, very different things will be happening in the two hemipshere. In the left hemisphere a new, relatively narrow-scope representation will be formed to capture the specific properties of the new type of cognitive challenge. By contrast, the right hemisphere will react in a far less drastic way, and a mere, perhaps even subtle, updating of the larger-scale coarse network will take place.

In some sense, the way the two hemispheres represent the same data set can be compared to the two alternative representations used in descriptive statistics to summarize a data set: as a mean and standard deviation summarizing all of ther data (the right hemisphere) or as a scatter plot diagram with each point summarizing a specific subset of data (the left hemisphere). This is depicted in Figure 14.2 Clearly, the arrival of a new data set will result in the two representations being updated in very different ways. In a scatter-plot diagram a new data point will be added without erasing any of the previously entered data points (a new specific representation formed in the left hemisphere alongside the previously formed ones, which remain unperturbed). By contrast, the mean and standard deviation will be recalculated and replaced by slightly different values (an existing global coarse representation modified in the right hemipshere in its entirety).

From a mechanistic neural standpoint, this probably means that the left hemisphere is organized more like a collection of of distinctive networks, each characterized by strong internal interconnectedness but with relatively high connectivety thresholds between such local networks. In effect, the left hemisphere is characterized by a relatively high degree of resultant, a posteriori modularity. By contrast, the right hemisphere is organized more like a relatively homogeneous network.

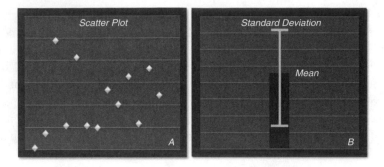

Figure 14.2 Knowledge representation in the two hemispheres. (*A*) Left hemisphere represents knowledge as a *scatter plot*—a collection of representations each capturing the specific properties of a narrow class of situations. (*B*) Right hemisphere represents knowledge as the *mean and standard deviation*—a very coarse averaging across all situations encountered by the organism. This is a heuristic representation intended to convey a general idea rather than any realistic neuroanatomical or cognitive properties.

It is not truly homogeneous, in that certain connections are stronger than others. But the contrast between strongest and weakest connections is not as well articulated in the right hemisphere as it is in the left hemisphere. It is precisely the greater degree of a posteriori modularity of the left hemisphere that makes it more efficient for dealing with familiar situations, and the relative homogeneity of the right hemisphere that makes it better suited for a broad-based search necessary for dealing with novel situations.

Differential learning rates in the two hemispheres

We now reach an interesting conclusion and explore further the paradox outlined earlier in this chapter: The right hemisphere, the novelty hemisphere, is modified by experience at a much slower rate than the left hemisphere, the hemisphere of established cognitive routines. To use the learning-rate terminology, the left hemisphere has a higher learning rate than that of the right hemisphere.

The assertion that information updating occurs in a more volatile, rapid fashion in the left hemisphere may seem counterintuitive, since the right hemisphere is the novelty hemisphere and the left hemisphere is the hemisphere of established cognitive routines. But the slow-changing right hemisphere is better suited for dealing with novelty precisely because it contains an averaged default representation capturing certain shared, and thus poorly differentiated, features of many prior experiences. When the specific knowledge about the situation at hand is lacking, you fare best by doing whatever worked in the largest number of prior experiences. But once you have figured out the properties of the specific situation at hand, you tailor your response accordingly and store the newly gained experience.

My own conclusion about the two hemispheres updating mental representations at different rates was first prompted by our experimental results on actor-centered decision making in patients with lateralized frontal lesions: damage to the left prefrontal regions produced an overly stable, almost perseverative response selection bias, whereas damage to the right prefrontal cortex produced a more "bouncy" response selection, reflecting changes in the environment.[20]

This seemingly far-fetched conclusion finds further experimental support in functional neuroimaging. According to a study by Timothy Behrens and his colleagues at Oxford University, a brain updating information in a probabilistically volatile, rapidly changing environment is characterized by a particularly high level of activation in the *left* anterior cingulate region on the mesial surface of the frontal lobe.[21] This is true both for reward-based and socially based information updating, as another, equally elegant study by Tim Behrens and his colleagues has shown.[22] To the extent that such updating is mediated by the DA system originating in VTA, these findings are also consistent with the greater prevalence of DA projections in the left hemisphere, discussed earlier.

An additional source of convergent evidence comes from computational work. Using neural network models, Stefano Fusi has demonstrated that the computational efficiency of a network will be enhanced by a variable, and not constant, rate of synaptic proliferation.[23] In other words, different learning situations call for different rates of synaptic modification. Is it possible that nature took care of this requirement by coupling two systems (hemispheres) generally similar, albeit not identical, in organization but characterized by different learning rates? Such an arrangement would benefit the combined system within a particularly broad range of learning situations by allowing it to switch on an as-needed basis between faster and slower learning rates by switching between the leading roles of one or the other hemisphere.

This set of functional considerations finds its probable biological underpinnings in the previously mentioned findings that *(a)* DA pathways are more prevalent in the left hemisphere, and *(b)* DA facilitates the formation of new synapses necessary for long-term memory formation in the mammalian brain. Therefore, the differential learning rates in the two hemispheres may be a function of the differential rate of synaptic proliferation in the two hemispheres—faster in the left hemisphere, slower in the right hemisphere.

Competitive hemispheric interaction in learning

How do the two hemispheres interact in the course of response selection? Suppose the two hemispheres arrive at different response selection choices. Then a competitive relationship exists between the two hemispheres, most likely mediated by the inhibitory pathways of the corpus callosum and the anterior comissures. Suppose also that some sort of "working memory" window keeps track of the recent history of successes and failures (let's say over i previous real-life situations or "trials" in a lab experiment). Suppose also that some "criterion of success" is set by the system, which we will call m ($0 < m < i$). Then the system operates in the following fashion: when the number of successful trials n exceeds m ($0 < m < n < i$), then the left hemisphere wins, since this implies that the specific representations that inhabit it have been adequate in guiding the decision-making process at hand. By contrast, when the number of successful trials within the "working memory window" falls short of the criterion ($0 < n < m < i$), then the right hemisphere wins, since this implies that none of the situation-specific representations housed in the left hemisphere was up to the job and the global default representation housed in the right hemisphere had to be invoked. The above discussion leads to the prediction that a neural network based on the competitive interaction described earlier will be more efficient than a neural network of equal size characterized by a homogeneous learning rate.

So in addition to introducing a paradigm shift in our thinking about the two hemispheres in broad cognitive terms, the novelty–routinization theory sets the stage for a whole program of experimental and computational research addressing the issues of underlying neural mechanisms. I hope that these preliminary ideas of computational models will encourage and stimulate further inquiry as well as actual modeling.

Further Complicate to Simplify: Front–Back, Neocortex–Hippocampi, Left–Right

The distinction between veridical and actor-centered decision making, introduced in the previous chapter, helps shed light on the nature of representations mediated by the prefrontal cortex. In a cogent review, Jacqueline Wood and Jordan Grafman discuss the relative merits of "representational" vs. "process" theories of frontal lobe functions.[24] They correctly point out that much of the scientific discourse about the prefrontal cortex emphasizes the "process" aspect, the implication being that it does not harbor any "representations." My own use of the "orchestra conductor" metaphor earlier in the book may be construed as implying a similar bias. Wood and Grafman critique this approach as insufficient, and I agree with them that the prefrontal cortex is critical for the formation of representations. But how? At a minimum, several possibilities must be considered.

First, let's consider two kinds of representations: veridical and actor centered. Veridical representations capture the relations between different aspects of the outside world; and actor-centered representations capture the relations between various goals, means, and outcomes. It may be tempting to postulate that veridical representations reside mostly in the posterior cortex and actor-centered representations reside mostly in the frontal cortex. But this would clearly be an oversimplification, since actor-centered representations involve not only actions but also things (e.g., "In order to lose weight I must stop frequenting my favorite restaurants *Petrossian* and *Russian Samovar*"), and veridical representations include not only things but also actions (as in "A cup is for *drinking* and scissors are for *cutting*"). So a simple one-to-one mapping of the veridical–actor-centered dichotomy into the posterior–frontal cortical dichotomy does not work in an absolute sense, even though it does contain a useful heuristic in a relative sense. For this heuristic to work even up to a point, the notion of the posterior cortex must be expanded by including the motor and premotor cortices, producing the "expanded posterior cortex."

There is, however, another problem. Veridical and actor-centered representations consist of essentially the same "universal set" of elements; these are just two different ways of "skinning the cat," the representation of the world being that "cat." So any theory linking veridical representations to the posterior cortex and the actor-centered representations to the prefrontal cortex would in effect imply certain re-duplication: two essentially similar sets with different metrics imposed on them mediated by two neuroanatomically distinct cortical areas. While I am in general agreement with the sentiment of the late Steven Jay Gould that evolution is dumb, how dumb can it be? It is more biologically intuitive to embrace the point of view advocated by Joaquin Fuster[25] and one to which I have subscribed in my own thinking about the brain: one extensive universal network exists with multiple circuits embedded into it through the myriad of connectivity patterns.

Two equally interesting questions can be asked about such a network: where is it housed, and how is it formed? I think that to the extent that it is neocortical (an important qualifier, since it may also include the thalamus and the striatum), the universal network inhabits the expanded posterior cortex (EPC) and perhaps also the thalamic and striatal nuclei directly connected with the EPC. What, then, is the relationship of the prefrontal cortex to cortical representations?

To understand this relationship, it may be helpful to bring the hippocampi into the discussion. The relative roles of the prefrontal cortex and the mesiotemporal-lobe hippocampal structures in the formation of long-term memories have been the subject of extensive but inconclusive debate.[26] I think their respective roles are best understood in the context of the contrast between the veridical and actor-centered knowledge; a direct parallel exists between the role of the hippocampi in the formation of veridical representations, and the role of the prefrontal cortex in the formation of actor-centered representations.

Consequently, I will put the following idea on the table: hippocampi facilitate the formation of long-term veridical store by coactivating the elements of a distributed expanded posterior-neocortical network representing certain aspects of the outside world on an ongoing basis, even long after the original externally generated sensory inputs ceased, thus enabling stable network formation in the EPC, according to the Hebbian "fire-together-wire-together" rules. This results in the formation of the veridical neural representation of the world as it is.

By contrast, the prefrontal cortex facilitates the formation of the long-term actor-centered store by coactivating the representations of goals, means, and outcomes, all of which are also components of the distributed expanded posterior-neocortical network. This results in the formation of neural representation of the ways in which the organism should act to its maximum advantage. The same substrate (EPC) is involved, but two different patterns of coactivation are imposed on it. In a sense, however, once the relationship between certain individual goals and the means toward their attainment becomes routinized, it becomes part of the veridical long-term store for the individual in question. Once this happens, the role of the prefrontal cortex abates, just as the role of the hippocampi abates in the maintenance of long-term veridical representations So the role of the prefrontal cortex is linked more to the formation of long-term actor-centered representations than to their maintenance once they have been fully, robustly formed (see discussion of the reduction of prefrontal activation with decreased task novelty and increased task familiarity, in Chapters 6 and 7). As is the case with the "liberation" of veridical knowledge from hippocampal control and its becoming exclusively neocortical, the reduction of the prefrontal contribution to the maintenance of actor-centered representations is a slow, gradual process.

We have arrived at a very interesting proposition, and I have stuck my intellectual neck out perhaps farther than I should have. Nonetheless, if the following reasoning is not wrong, it is rife with important implications. The train of thought developed in the previous paragraphs culminates in a tripartite cortical interaction: the posterior neocortex (for the purposes of this discussion it also includes motor and premotor cortex, the EPC) is the store of long-term representations; and the prefrontal cortex and hippocampi are the "meta-systems" facilitating the formation of actor-centered (facilitated by the prefrontal cortex) and veridical (facilitated by the hippocampi) long-term representations, which are ultimately stored in the posterior cortex. This tripartite relationship is depicted in Figure 14.3.

But the analogy between the formation of veridical long-term representations and the formation of actor-centered long-term representations works only to a point. First, temporal ordering is more important in actor-centered than in veridical representations, since the former tend to represent action and the latter tend to represent facts. The essentially temporal nature of the representations formed with reliance on the prefrontal cortex has been emphasized by Alexander Luria, Joaquin Fuster, and others.

Second, and perhaps even more importantly, veridical representations basically model the world as it is; their formation is usually initiated in a bottom-up fashion by sensory inputs from the outside world. This is not the case with actor-centered representations; they are initiated in a top-down fashion by an unrealized need, rather than by a certain reality. The brain constructs actor-centered representations rather than documents them. Clearly, nothing is spun entirely out of thin air, and this top-down generative process unfolds by somehow reconfiguring previously

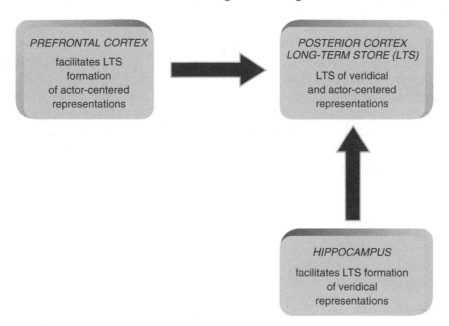

Figure 14.3 Tripartite interaction in knowledge base formation and storage. "Expanded" posterior cortex contains long-term store of both veridical and actor-centered knowledge. Hippocampi facilitate the formation of veridical long-term store. Prefrontal cortex facilitates the formation of actor-centered long-term store.

formed mental representations, many of which are part of the veridical long-term store. We all understand that this generativity is at the crux of frontal lobe function, but we don't really understand how this generative process occurs. Most existing theories of frontal lobe functions, hijacked by "working memory," sidestep the issue, even though it is clearly among the most central and profound secrets of the workings of our mind.

I believe that this is where hemispheric specialization steps in. The way in which long-term store is organized in the right hemisphere somehow lends itself better to making the jump from the known to the unknown and is more amenable to the formation of new configurations. This may be so because it is less modular (in the resultant, a posteriori sense described in Chapter 5), less broken up into very well–articulated circuits with relatively high connectivity thresholds across them. Thus connectivity is more readily permitted among diverse elements of the vast network that have no or little history of prior coactivation, through a yet-to-be-understood process that I like to refer to as "neural wandering." This process will also be facilitated by the right hemisphere's greater reliance on long myelinated pathways that mediate connectivity among distant brain regions, the myelinated pathways being fast conductors.

The neural mechanisms of generating novel constructs remain an enigma. Oddly, much more effort, in both experimental research and modeling, is directed at what happens in the brain once the construct has been generated (the emphasis on working memory being an example) than on the generative mechanisms of decision making themselves. To what extent can these mechanisms be captured by hierarchical models, and to what extent are they a product of "neural wandering" within weakly differentiated network? Most likely it is some combination of the two, but how exactly this process happens should be among the central questions of cognitive and computational neuroscience.

15

Frontal Lobes and the Leadership Paradox

Autonomy and Control in Society

In the spirit of interdisciplinary parallels adopted in this book, I am tempted to apply the analysis of brain evolution to the understanding of the momentous historical changes unfolding before us today. In science the convergence of conclusions based on vastly different sources of knowledge is highly valued. It lends credibility to predictions and points to universal principles underlying diverse complex systems. The search for such universal principles shared by superficially different systems is at the heart of the new field of complexity emerging at the cutting edge of science and philosophy. In trying to grasp history, we may be able to draw on the insights of neurobiology. A striking parallel is becoming increasingly apparent between the changing world order and the evolution of the brain.

Superficially different yet essentially similar processes are developing in eastern and western Europe. To the east, the Soviet Union has collapsed. Whereas the Communist rulers of the fallen Soviet superpower lauded their regime as the dawn of a new era, future historians will view it as the last spasm of the 400-year-old Russian Empire in its borders from the mid-nineteenth century. Farther east, a similar fate may eventually await China.

The Soviet Union disintegrated, and Russia has reconstituted itself as an imperial entity incorporating the czarist territorial acquisitions of the sixteenth and seventeenth centuries. Now its constituent ethnic groups are claiming autonomy or even outright independence. This trend took an extreme and particularly destructive form in Chechnya, but the Tatars, Bashkirs, Kalmyks, Yakuts, Ossetians, Dagestans, Ingushis, and others are also restless. Nor are the post-Soviet independent states spared from the process of disintegration, as the Abhazians, Mingrels, and South Ossetians are trying to secede from Georgia. But the fragmentation of the former Soviet Union goes even deeper; during the 1990s, the decade following the demise of the Soviet Union, some of the areas populated mostly by ethnic Russians began to claim autonomy. In the West we were hearing about the Kaliningrad Republic, the Urals Republic, and the Maritime Republic of Vladivostok.

Since then, an attempt has been under way in Russia to reverse these centrifugal processes, to recentralize the country, and even to reclaim its "sphere of influence" in some of the outlying states. Russia fought harsh punitive war with Georgia to reaffirm its influence in Georgian breakaway regions. It remains to be seen whether these efforts will bring stability and well-being to Russia or whether, to borrow the bombastic Marxist phrase so familiar to Russians of my generation, they represent a desperate, and self-defeating, attempt to "turn back the wheel of history" in the name of an imperial ideal whose time has passed. Western political scientists are becoming increasingly aware of the imminent continuing fragmentation of the Russian holdover empire and of the need for new foreign policy approaches in response to it.[1]

In the wake of the collapse of Soviet-controlled or Soviet-inspired regimes, similar changes are unfolding in central Europe. What used to be Czechoslovakia is now Czechia and Slovakia. The fallout of the collapse of Tito's Yugoslavia (a collage of former provinces of the disintegrated Ottoman Empire) with its bloody consequences is well known. Here, the process has continued fractally with Kosovo breaking away from Serbia.

In western Europe a resurgence of ethnic factionalism challenges modern nation-states. Provence and Brittany assert their autonomy in France; the Basque country and Catalonia do the same in Spain; Wallonia and Flanders, in Belgium; Northern Ireland, Scotland with its newly established Parliament, and Wales, in the United Kingdom; and northern regions, in Italy. As a result, "old tongues are flourishing in a revival of regional cultures."[2] With the blurring of national borders, semiforgotten languages—Breton in Britanny, Gaelic in Scotland, Friulian in northern Italy, Frisian and Limburgs in the Netherlands, Saami in Finland, Basque and Catalan in Spain—are experiencing an unprecedented revival. Increasingly, the claims of cultural revival go beyond a mere quest for cultural autonomy, taking the form of separatism and outright calls for independence.

In both eastern and western Europe, the stable, static, large, and modular nation-states are being replaced by smaller, more fluid political entities. While the events in the east have a clear cause and are perceived in most instances (but with notoriously bloody exceptions) as the process of liberation, the fragmentation in the west is often met with alarm and is more difficult to comprehend. The "medievalization" of Europe is viewed by many as an unwelcome return to a premodern organization.

Similar processes are taking place in Asia. In China, Tibet and the Xinjiang Uyghur region are asserting their autonomy or outright independence. East Timor has broken away from Indonesia and the Aceh region of Sumatra is trying to do the same. Following the American misadventure in Iraq, this country, as much an artifact of the collapse of the Ottoman Empire in the Middle East as Yugoslavia was in Europe, is likely to disintegrate into its constituent parts. (Anyone who would bother to Google the map of the Ottoman Empire will see three provinces—Bagdhad, Basra, and Mosul—in place of today's Iraq. Iraq was an artificial creation of British administrators trying to devise an expedient way of managing territories placed under their protectorate, very possibly while imbibing significant quantities of Scotch.)

In the United States during the presidential campaigns of the first decade of the century, the media was abuzz about the "irreconsilable division" into the "blue" and "red" states. In an intriguing *New York Times* Op-Ed piece titled "California Split" and subtitled "Divide, or Die" and "Help Democracy: Divide up the U.S.,"[3] Gar Alperovich, professor of political economy at the University of Maryland, College Park, and the author of *America Beyond Capitalism*, argued that "the United States is almost certainly too big to be a meaningful democracy." He claims that already James Madison and George F. Kennan had anticipated this concern and offers a scenario for the regionalization of the United States.

The view of modern history as one dominated by fragmentation rather than by integration may sound counterintuitive, but this is the view held by the distinguished historian Niall Ferguson.[4] As evidence, Gar Alperovitz cites the following curious statistics: "more than half of the world's 200 nations formed as breakaways after 1946."

Could it also be that what appears to be a global tendency toward fragmentation is actually a prelude toward integration, that "premodern" is also "postmodern"? One can argue that the phenomena of the East and the West represent the same natural process and the same dialectic paradox: the demise of strongly integrated nation-states and empires may be the crucial step toward a dynamic, "weakly" integrated Europe and an integrated world. The fragments resulting from this demise are the building blocks of the new order. What seems regressive is really the emergence of a new societal organization, a new spiral in societal evolution. The nature of this transition is elucidated by an analogy with the brain.

If we believe in meaningful parallels between complex systems, then we may use the knowledge of the brain to extrapolate the directions in societal changes and, to a degree, the course of history. The transition from the thalamic to the cortical principle of cerebral organization parallels the transition from the macronational to the microregional pattern of societal organization as elements of a global network. In this analogy, the nation-states are modules—autonomous, relatively self-contained entities with interactions regimented and restricted to institutional channels. Today we are witnessing their demise and transition to a new geopolitical order based on a global network comprised of microregional units of organization. The exact nature of future geopolitical entities has yet to reveal itself. Like the components of the brain, they need not be homogeneous and may combine different types of units.

Ethnic regions may become one type of unit of the new order. They are smaller than nation-states and more ancient. Yet their coexistence for the last few centuries within the nation-states and in an increasingly global economy has made them highly interdependent and interactive. A shared history has transformed them from units of isolation into units of a network. They may become the building blocks of the global politicoeconomic order transcending national borders. Paradoxically, the shift from the national to ethnic molarity of society may facilitate the shift from a parochial to a global identity, precisely because ethnicity is now less self-sufficient, self-contained, and self-absorbed than nationhood. An ethnic identity may prove easier to reconcile with a pan-European federalist identity than with a national one. As a Basque friend of mine once said, it would be easier for him to forgo his Basque identity in favor of a European identity than for a Spanish one.

Microunits based on strictly economic factors and interrelated through the flows of trade, finance, and communications may emerge as a different type of unit of the evolving new order. This is the conclusion reached by Kenchi Ohmae in *The End of the Nation State*.[5] The proliferation of multinational corporations promotes this type of organization.

The evolution of the brain teaches us the lesson that a high degree of complexity cannot be handled by rigidly organized systems. It requires distributed responsibilities and local autonomy. The arrival of the cortex on the evolutionary scene signaled a true paradigm shift in the organization of the brain. A much more dynamic, faster-working central nervous system emerged, resulting in an exponential surge in the computational power of the brain, which culminated in a conscious mind.

If we follow this analogy, the transition from a world order built of a few large autonomous geopolitical units to a network of many small, highly interdependent geopolitical units is now under way. This transition, too, is nothing short of a paradigm shift. It heralds a new societal dynamism and a quantum leap in the rate of societal change in the centuries to come. This difference is like the difference between a succession of canvases and a kaleidoscope. Far from the end of history proclaimed by some scholars, a much faster-moving history is under way.

But in the brain, the advent of the dynamic "new order" ushered in by the advent of the neocortex was balanced by the emergence of the frontal lobes, with their ability to superimpose order on an emergent dizzying multitude of possible choices. With an increasing globalization of social and economic interactions, will a similar higher-order organization emerge in the global society? What will it be? An improved version of the League of Nations and the United Nations?

Some sort of Economic Council of the Multinationals? Is the budding European Union a prototype of such a global organization of "weak" control, with Brussels as the European "prefrontal cortex"? Is a worldwide analogue of the European Union imminent? The brain analogy predicts the eventual emergence of such an organization.

My predictions about the evolution of society based on the workings of the brain may sound outlandish and far-fetched. Yet they resonate with some of the cutting-edge thinking of political scientists. My favorite newspaper, the *New York Times*, has provided me with the necessary polemic ammunition. In a review that appeared in the January 2, 1999, issue of the *New York Times* under the provocative title "As Nations Shed Roles, Is Medieval the Future?,"[6] Paul Lewis quotes Hedley Bull, the late professor of international relations at Oxford, predicting that the existing system of nation-states will be replaced by "a modern and secular equivalent of the kind of universal political organization that existed in Western Christendom in the Middle Ages."

At the close of the millennium, as fellow New Yorkers were approaching the year 2000 with the jittery anticipation of millennial frenzy, infrastructure failure, and terrorist attacks, the *New York Times* published an article titled "Could This Be the New World?". In it, Robert Kaplan outlined a doomsday scenario for the century to come: a disintegration of nation-states into a smaller city-states, with the map of the New World becoming a "hologram in constant motion" or, to use the title of his new book, "the coming anarchy."[7] But a mechanism may emerge to offset the coming anarchy through the societal equivalent of the frontal lobes.

A similar argument is made by Stephen J. Kobrin, of the University of Pennsylvania, in an article in the *Journal of International Affairs*.[8] Kobrin predicts that a "center" of universal authority is bound to emerge to complement the trends toward a growing fragmentation, fluidity, and kaleidoscopic interconnectedness of localities. He points out that most international, intergovernmental organizations were created very recently.

Which form will the postmodern secular analogue of papal authority take? This is a challenge for futurologists to ponder. The analogy with brain evolution may provide a useful, if not perfectly transparent, crystal ball.

Autonomy and Control in the Digital World

A peculiar epistemological "man–machine" relationship has developed over the last few decades. It works in both directions. Our insights into the workings of the brain have been informed by the computer analogy during much of the twentieth century, just as they were by the leading technologies of the time in centuries past. Conversely, the design of some of the most powerful computational devices was directly influenced by analogies of the brain. The first formal neural networks, designed by McCulloch and Pitts, were directly inspired by the biological neuron analogy, and the design of certain computer languages was inspired by the concept of psycholinguistic context.[9]

Do the biological evolution of the brain and the technological evolution of computers reveal similar guiding principles? If established, such principles will inform us about the ways in which various, and possibly even most, evolving complex systems cope with increasing computational demands. In the next few pages I will attempt to show that the transition from a modular principle of organization to a distributed gradiental principle of organization, which seems to characterize the evolution of the brain and society, applies also to the digital world. Furthermore, I maintain that at a late stage of the evolution of computing, a digital analogue of the frontal lobes has emerged to counterweight the digital "coming anarchy," to borrow Robert Kaplan's anxiety-provoking phrase.[10]

With this demonstration in place, the following intriguing questions arise: Do the invariant laws of evolution shared by the brain, society, and digital computing devices reflect the only intrinsically possible or optimal path of development? Or do humans recapitulate, consciously or unconsciously, their own internal organization in man-made devices and social structures? Each possibility is intriguing in its own right. In the first case, our analysis will point to some very general rules of development of complex systems. In the second case, we encounter a puzzling process of unconscious recapitulation, since neither the evolution of society nor that of the digital world has been explicitly guided by the knowledge of neuroscience.

Computer hardware has evolved from mainframe computers to personal computers to network personal computers. The mainframe computer is a "dinosaur" of the digital world. It occupied several floors of civilian or military research installations. Each mainframe computer had a complex organization and large computational power. It conducted the computation of a task from beginning to end. There were relatively few mainframe computers and the interfaces between them were sparse; they were practically isolated from one another. A digital world dominated by mainframe computers—the 1950s, 1960s, and partly 1970s—was modular in nature. Gradually, however, limited connections between large mainframe computers were created, giving rise to distributed and, ultimately, network computation.

In the 1970s personal computers (PCs) began to proliferate. While the computational power of a single PC is no match to that of a mainframe computer, there are many more PCs. Within this distributed format, a greater range and variety of tasks could be performed. The digital world was no longer dominated by large, functionally prededicated units; it was being taken over by smaller but far more numerous personal computers. To ensure that a maximum number of individual computers could interface, standardization rapidly increased. This signaled the next stage in the evolution of computational devices.

In the 1980s rapid integration of PCs and mainframe computers took place. Computational processes became distributed among numerous devices. The multitude of PCs assumed an ever-increasing range of computational tasks, thus reducing but not totally eliminating the importance of mainframe computers.

In the 1990s the Internet became ubiquitous. It provided a formal structure for creating interfaces between separate computers according to task demands, within a practically infinite range of combinatorial possibilities. The digital world was becoming increasingly like a neural net. The trend was amplified by the arrival of an entirely different class of computers, "network PCs," limited-capability devices whose main function was to provide access to the Internet. While mainframe computers continued to serve certain functions, a gradual departure from a predominantly modular to a distributed pattern of organization reshaped the digital world. In the evolution of both the brain and the digital world, a further growth of the computational power of a few self-contained centers proved to be less effective than the development of networks consisting of numerous relatively simple, smaller devices.

But the arrival of "digital anarchy" was not far behind. With the explosion in the volume of information posted on the World Wide Web, the finding of specific information required for a particular task became increasingly difficult. As in the evolution of the brain, adaptive pressures arose for the emergence of a mechanism capable of constraining the system's degrees of freedom in any specific, goal-directed situation, while preserving these degrees of freedom in principle. This signaled the invention of "search engines."

Like the frontal lobes, the search engines do not contain the exact knowledge necessary to solve the problem at hand. But like the frontal lobes, they have an aerial view of the system, enabling them to find the specific locations within the Net where this knowledge is held. And like the frontal lobes, the search engines appeared at a relatively late stage of transition of the digital world from a mostly modular to a mostly distributed "organism." Search engines provide the executive function within the Internet. They are the *digital frontal lobes*.

So it appears that strong similarities exist between the evolution of the brain, society, and man-made computational systems. Each is characterized by a transition from the modular principle of organization to the distributed, gradiental principle. At a highly evolved stage of this process, a system of "executive" control emerges, to help rein in the prospect of anarchy and chaos, which paradoxically increases with the increase of any system's complexity. The peculiar relationship between autonomy and control embodied in the executive control exerted by the frontal lobes resonates with the philosophical dilemmas considered by Hegel and Kant, and was captured in the quotable phrase coined by Frederick Engels: "Freedom is necessity recognized."[11]

16

Epilogue

By the the time I wrote this book I had lived significant portions of my life in the East and in the West, and by most realistic projections I had entered its final part—the time of integration, an executive task indeed. In retrospect, my own intellectual journey has been an amalgam and a melding of influences derived from these two worlds, and to the extent that I can claim an intellectual and scientific style of my own, it was shaped by this fusion. I am a man of the East in Western cultural cloth, so to speak. At the beginning of my life's seventh decade I am still a nomad. I run my clinical practice in New York, and do my research and lecture worldwide.

This book began with the discussion of the brain and ended with the discussion of society and history. The paradigm has been reversed; it is common in the history of ideas to use the concepts of a more mature science as a heuristic metaphor for a more embryonic one. For centuries neuroscience has been the embryonic science borrowing its metaphors from more evolved disciplines: mechanics (hydraulic pumps of the seventeenth century), electric engineering (the telephone switchboard of the early twentieth century), and computer science (the second half of the twentieth century). But now brain science is coming of age and it may be ready to offer its own heuristic metaphors to shed light on other complex systems, including society.

Brain science has always been on the border of hard science and the humanities, and it is precisely this fusion that drew me to it many years ago.

Although Descartes is often mentioned when the history of brain–mind exploration is examined, I drew my early inspiration from Descartes's contemporary and a fellow iconoclast, Baruch Spinoza.[1] Unlike Descartes, Spinoza did not believe in the duality of spirit and matter. He understood God as the fundamental laws of the universe and not as its creator, and he searched for unifying principles.

At the age of 12, browsing through my father's library, I stumbled onto a two-volume Russian translation of Spinoza's *Ethics*, the first time I had heard of the man. As I was poring through the obscure writings, I came upon his "ethics theorems proved with deductive method."[2] In my personal cognitive history, this was one of its most powerful moments. I had always been drawn to mathematics and to the humanities and history, but not particularly to natural sciences—an uncommon configuration of interests. And I was clearly interested in the life of the mind, but famously unimpressed with what little I knew at the time of psychology as a discipline. Spinoza was a revelation to me, telling me that these disparate areas could be brought together and that the seemingly inherently imprecise subjects like the mind, society, and the life of the mind in society could be approached with precise methods.

Of course, Spinoza's seventeenth-century enterprise was naive by today's standards. Nor did it exert, to my knowledge, a major influence on shaping the studies of complex systems like the brain or society into the relatively precise disciplines they have become. Many more direct and influential efforts of the kind existed, of which I was not aware at the time. But to me that early encounter with Spinoza was a formative experience; more than any single influence it encouraged my choice of psychology and neuroscience as a lifelong career.

Another intellectual encounter of comparable potency occurred much later at the Moscow State University library, where at the age of 19 I stumbled onto the classic papers by Warren McCulloch and Walter Pitts, "A Logical Calculus of the Ideas Immanent in Nervous Activity" (1943)[3] and "How We Know Universals: The Perception of Auditory and Visual Forms" (1947),[4] which laid the groundwork for formal neural network modeling of the brain. To me there was a clear intellectual continuity between Spinoza's "ethics theorems" and McCulloch and Pitts's "logical calculus." Each represented an attempt to infuse traditionally vague inquiry into the mind and the brain with precise deductive method. At that time in Russia, very little was happening in what was later called "computational neuroscience." With Luria's bemused acquiescence, my friend Yelena Artemyeva, a brilliant mathematician and a student of Andrey Kolmogorov, and I tried to introduce neural net modeling into neuropsychological research at the University of Moscow.

My subsequent life in the United States took me much farther away from basic research and toward clinical work than I had anticipated in those early years of my career. But my understanding of the brain, and the heuristic metaphor that guided that understanding, has always been informed by the early intellectual encounter with the concept of the neural net.

Following these early influences and throughout my career I have been interested, sometimes explicitly and sometimes tacitly, in general principles that transcend my own relatively narrow field of knowledge. And so it seems an intellectual full circle of sorts: my own idiosyncratic understanding of the brain produced a metaphor that was useful to me personally in understanding the cataclysmic societal phenomena through which we live. I hope that the metaphor will be useful to other people.

I believe that the discussion of the relationship between autonomy and control in various complex systems and the lessons drawn from analysis of the brain for the understanding of society is a fitting way to end this book. No complex system can succeed without an effective executive mechanism, the "frontal lobes." But the frontal lobes operate best as part of a highly distributed, interactive structure with much autonomy and many degrees of freedom.

As I was dutifully pouring through hundreds of journal articles on relevant subjects published in the years while I was working on *The New Executive Brain*, I could not help but ruminate over the state of affairs in cognitive neuroscience. My feelings are mixed. The field of cognitive neuroscience has enjoyed tremendous advances and has become embraced as a legitimate field of mainstream science. The sheer number of neuroscience papers published in *Science* and *Nature* every year attests to this progress and recognition.

These advances fall short of expectations, however. We are witnessing the advent of astoundingly powerful neuroimaging tools that have truly revolutionized our field. Yet the fundamental breakthroughs, which everyone hoped would be ushered in by the arrival of these tools, have by and large failed to materialize so far. The functional neuroimaging research has confirmed much of what had already been known (or presumed to be known) on the basis of brain lesion studies and has added precision to much of this knowledge. This is a good thing. But so far functional neuroimaging has not provided the expected quantum leap in our understanding of the brain mechanisms of cognition. The same can be said about computational neuroscience. So the feeling of exhilaration at being part of the exciting journey that cognitive neuroscience is today is mixed with a palpable sense that we have barely scratched the surface.

In our efforts to understand the brain's mechanisms we must stop looking to other disciplines to do our job for us. In order for the state-of-the-art tools of functional neuroimaging to live up to their potential and deliver on their promise, these tools and other methods must be coupled with equally compelling cognitive paradigms; such paradigms have yet to materialize. While the physicists and chemists continue to supply us with ever more powerful methodologies, we—neuropsychologists and cognitive neuroscientists— have not delivered on our side of the bargain. As a result, an oxymoronic situation prevails in the field, whereby twenty-first century neuroimaging tools are often coupled with the cognitive Zeitgeist of around the second half of the twentieth century. In effect, this is similar to what happened with neurogenomics, where failure to ask sophisticated cognitive questions has lead to misguided attempts to link specific genes to narrow cognitive traits or disorders. The fiasco of a quasi-phrenological misuse of genomics has propelled into existence "phenomics," which will hopefully do better.

It is up to cognitive neuroscientists to change this situation, but it will not happen by merely looking forward to newer and better neuroimaging or genetic technologies. If we are to succeed in a big way, we must do some very hard thinking of our own. The spectacular neuroimaging methods now available began as physics' and chemistry's innovative basic concepts. It is incumbent on us as a field to come up with equally innovative concepts intrinsic to our field.

But not enough of this activity has been happening lately. By placing our faith in the belief that the increasingly powerful methodologies proffered us on a silver plate by other disciplines will automatically offer us the Rosetta stone, we have come perilously close to abdicating our own intellectual responsibility. So, while, cognitive neuroscience has made great strides, a self-critical look is usually more productive than a self-congratulatory one, and one that is more likely to lead to constructive suggestions. So here are a few of my own, as they pertain to the integration of functional neuroimaging technologies and substantive questions emanating from our own fields.

The challenge is to design cognitive activation paradigms that would do the following:

a. Reflect state-of-the-art cognitive constructs;
b. Tap central and clinically vulnerable aspects of cognition;
c. Be strategic, rather than ad hoc, in the sense of their applicability to a wide range of clinical and normal populations; and
d. Foster long-term coherence of research themes across individual projects and populations.

The current state of cognitive neuroscience falls short of these objectives. Broadly speaking, functional neuroimaging is represented today by two different strands with considerable disconnect between them.

The first strand involves functional neuroimaging in clinical populations conducted mostly in medical environments. This work, published mostly in clinical journals, is dominated by useful and robust but dated paradigms (e.g., "oddball," "go/no-go"), which have been around since the days when the earth was flat. The second strand involves functional neuroimaging in normal subjects (and only occasionally in clinical populations) conducted mostly in psychology and cognitive neuroscience programs. This work is published mostly in neuroscience journals as well as in *Science, Nature*, and *Nature Neuroscience*. It is characterized by an abundance of imaginative and elaborate paradigms (many of them reviewed earlier in this book), but it has problems of its own:

a. The paradigms are often ad hoc, each attempting to capture an interesting but narrow aspect of cognition, thus not lending themselves to strategic thematic coherence across projects and populations. As a result, consider-able effort goes into the design of such a paradigm; then it is used in a single study, never to be used again. The field is dominated by sound bites and not by coherent themes.

b. The paradigms are often too arcane and, as a result, fragile (lacking in robust-ness); I refer to them as "Viennese cakes." The intent is admirable: to realis-tically emulate complex properties of real-life cognition. But the result is often self-defeating: the tasks are not "strategic" in the sense of being usable across projects, and they are too complex to be used in clinical populations. Many of them are too arcane to allow clear interpretation of the findings. Therefore, it is often unclear whether and to what extent the findings reflect the essential aspects of the task instead of merely the incidental aspects of the arbitrary "surface" scenarios. As a result, the tasks are "fragile"; a slight change in their incidental aspects is likely to significantly alter the findings. Furthermore, I suspect that not many of these studies would survive an attempt at replication (and such attempts are rare, since the studies are expen-sive and there is little glory in replication).

c. Certain tired fads originated as valuable constructs but now continue to dominate the field above and beyond their true utility. The opaquely defined construct of "working memory" is an example. So much effort is directed at trying to figure out how the organism holds information online that it is commonly overlooked that "holding information online" is a secondary issue. The primary issue is one of decision making: how does the organism gener-ate and select what exactly should be held online in the first place? This far more vexing neuroscientific riddle has been largely ignored by experimen-talists and computational modelers alike. Yet anyone working with clinical populations in a realistic, rather than narrowly contrived, context knows that the disruption of initiation, generativity, decision making, and selectivity central to sound executive function derails cognition to a far greater extent than does working memory deficit in a wide range of disorders involving the frontal lobes (e.g., traumatic brain injury [TBI], schizophrenia, and certain forms of dementia). Nonetheless, the field continues to cling uncritically to a few self-perpetuating notions, betraying a collective lack of imagination.

To address the above concerns, it is very important to develop a suite of innova-tive, broadly applicable cognitive activation paradigms that would satisfy the above criteria and be free of the pitfalls outlined here. They should be sensitive to central cognitive impairments in a wide range of clinical populations and should also have the potential for yielding important insights into normal neurocognitive mechanisms of the *Science* and *Nature* caliber. The design of such paradigms should be viewed as a major project. It may take many paths, will benefit from an input from many neuroscientists and neuropsychologists, and should be under-taken in a collegial and inclusive manner. My own earlier work and interests bias me in favor of two particular approaches in this quest, both touched upon in the earlier discussion.

Dynamic aspects of learning.   The process of mastering (or failure to master) a cognitive task is characterized by changes in the underlying functional neuroanatomy. As established earlier in the book, the brain regions in charge of processing a task when it is still novel are not the same as those in charge of processing the same task once it becomes familiar. These changes can often be observed within a single, brief experiment. Furthermore, an extensive body of evidence exists, some of it reviewed earlier in the book, that such changes in functional neuroanatomy over time are characterized by strong invariant properties across diverse tasks. The properties override task-specific properties and appear to be related directly to the transition from novelty to familiarity, i.e., to learning. Some of these highly invariant features involve a distinctly directional shift of cortical control from the right to the left hemisphere, and from the prefrontal cortex to the posterior cortices. Other dynamic features may be more task-specific and need to be studied further.

It is common to characterize cognitive tasks in terms of "networks" of underlying brain structures elicited with fMRI or with other neuroimaging methods. These considerations imply that these "networks" change over time. Thus, it is impossible to characterize a task through a single, static network; it is essential to characterize it as a spatiotemporal vector of changing networks. In the current state of functional neuroimaging these considerations are largely ignored, however. It is common to average the data across the whole experimental sequence on the assumption that the underlying neural network is static. This is a big mistake, since the network is usually not static, and averaging across the whole sequence is like mixing data points representing different populations. Therefore, one would be better served by segmenting the experimental sequence and averaging data separately within each segment, thus expressing the findings as a vector rather than as a single state.

A suite of cognitive activation tasks can be designed to elicit the temporal dynamics of such spatial networks as a function of learning. These tasks should be usable across a range of clinical populations (TBI, dementias, ADHD, schizophrenia), with the purpose of characterizing the underlying pathology in such dynamic spatiotemporal terms. This approach is likely to be more powerful in characterizing normal cognition, and more sensitive in characterizing pathology (as various types of aberrations of the functional neuroanatomy underlying the learning curves), since a vector by definition contains more information than a single variable.

Actor-centered decision making.   Most of our real-life cognition is directed by questions like "what should I do; what is best for me?" rather than "what is the correct answer; what is the truth?" Such questions reflect the difference between actor-centered and veridical decision making, introduced earlier in the book.

The frontal lobes and related striatal and anterior-cingulate structures are particularly central to actor-centered decision making. However, most of the cognitive activation paradigms used in clinical neuroscience are veridical rather than actor-centered and thus miss the point. This is extremely unfortunate, since, as discussed earlier in the book, the frontal lobes and actor-centered cognition are particularly vulnerable in a very broad range of disorders (TBI, ADHD, schizophrenia, and certain forms of dementia; see Chapters 10 and 12). A patient with "mild" TBI does not get into trouble in life because of his or her weak memory or perception; the patient gets into trouble because of poor decision making, bad personal choices in ambiguous environments. This is often referred to as "personality change," a misnomer because it really reflects dysfunction of the frontal lobes and its connections and, consequently, of actor-centered cognition.

A suite of cognitive activation tasks can be designed to measure actor-centered decision making. These tasks can be created de novo and/or by modifying or simplifying select "Viennese cakes," some of them reviewed earlier in the book, adapted from cognitive neuroscience (neuroeconomics, social neuroscience, etc.; see Chapter 7). The tasks should be usable across a wide range of clinical populations (TBI, dementias, ADHD, schizophrenia) with the purpose of characterizing the underlying pathology with respect to decision making in underdetermined environments, as in real life. These tasks should emphasize generativity.

The above two themes reflect my own scientific biases and interests. The resulting set of cognitive activation learning tasks should be diverse and include both actor-centered paradigms challenging the interactions between the frontal lobes and related striatal structures (e.g., selection processes in dynamic environments characterized by changing probabilistic and reward structures), and more traditional veridical paradigms challenging the interactions between posterior cortices and related thalamic structures (e.g., multisensory integration). For both types of tasks, the emphasis should be on the dynamic changes in neural network configurations over time as a function of task mastery (or its failure).

The systematic emphasis on the temporal dynamics of the neural networks underlying learning will represent an innovative and highly promising approach to characterizing both normal and abnormal cognition. It will lay the groundwork for the gradual accumulation of a suite of standardized, sophisticated, yet transparent fMRI cognitive activation packages to use across studies and populations, with results to start forming a database. Other, equally compelling themes worthy of pursuing undoubtedly exist begging for attention.

Some of the shortcomings of cognitive neuroscience alluded to earlier raise broader issues of science in modern society. First, there is the commoditization of science. Much of the ongoing research is driven by "big questions" and coherent themes. This type of research is sometimes referred to as "principled" science. But just as much research, or perhaps even more, is driven by the desire to come up with catchy, media-worthy sound bites. Without detracting from the quality of published work, one is almost forced to conclude that sound bite worthiness has become a prerequisite for getting into some of the most prestigious scientific journals today.

Such work is often referred to as "sexy" science, in tacit contrast to "principled" science. In discussions with colleagues I hear too much sexy science and not enough of the principled kind. Whatever the realities of the sociology of science, *sexy* belongs in the discussion of sex; it does not belong in the discussion of science.

We need more, programmatic research that is driven by coherent themes. In this regard, Eric Kandel's *In Search of Memory*,[5] a summary of his work, is an impressive account of a life spent in science, unique because of its intellectual coherence and logical progression. So was the work of my mentor Alexandr Luria,[6] at least during the latter part of his career. We need more of such coherence if we are to succeed in our collective enterprise as cognitive neuroscientists.

Another issue of concern is the economics of cognitive neuroscience. The introduction of high-tech neuroimaging methods has made neuroscience much more powerful, but is has also made it much more expensive. Increasingly, the focus on intellectual pursuit is supplanted by the pursuit of funding, and increasingly the accomplishments of a scientist are measured in dollars more than in ideas. A typical fMRI or PET research project today has a price tag several orders of magnitude higher than that of a paper-and pencil lesion study of 50 years ago. The capital investment into the hardware and infrastructure accounts for a large slice of the price tag, as does the permanent technical staff required for the installation. This expense often produces an ironic situation: a technology is used simply because it is there, without enough thought given to the quality of the questions asked or to the best match between the nature of the question and the technical tools thrown at it.

I once saw an advanced middle-age actor performing single-arm pushups during a high-profile award ceremony. When the question was asked why he did this, the answer was "because he could." But this is not a good rationale for conducting high-tech research. Precisely because cognitive neuroscience research today is so expensive and resource intensive the quality of the questions has become every bit as important as the quality of the answers, perhaps even more so. Yet our field, both basic cognitive neuroscience and clinical neuroscience, is replete with much ado about little, when elaborate technologies are thrown at sloppily thought-through, poorly posed, or frivolous questions of marginal significance. Again, we are reminded of the need to ensure the caliber and rigor of thought guiding our work, and the need for coherent, big themes.

References and Notes

Chapter 1: Introduction

1. A. Damasio, *Descartes' Error: Emotion, Reason, and the Human Brain* (New York: Putnam Publishing Group, 1994).
2. R. A. Barkley, *ADHD and the Nature of Self-Control* (New York: Guilford Press, 1997).
3. E. Goldberg, "Tribute to Alexandr Romanovich Luria," in *Contemporary Neuropsychology and the Legacy of Luria*, ed. E. Goldberg (Hillsdale, NJ: Lawrence Erlbaum Associates, 1990), 1–9.
4. S. Sontag, *Illness as Metaphor and AIDS and Its Metaphors* (New York: Doubleday Books, 1990).

Chapter 2: An End and a Beginning: A Dedication

1. Following the demise of the Soviet Union, streets and public places named after the Soviet demigods and memorable dates were changed, in most instances given their prerevolutionary names.

Chapter 3: The Brain's Chief Executive: The Frontal Lobes at a Glance

1. For the transformation of military leadership throughout history, see J. Keegan, *The Mask of Command* (New York: Penguin, 1989).
2. Napoleon's chronic illness had no direct relationship to his brain. Quite the opposite, it entailed greatly inflamed hemorrhoids. For further reading, see A. Neumayr, *Dictators in the Mirror of Medicine: Napoleon, Hitler, Stalin*, trans. D. J. Parent (Bloomington, IL: Medi-Ed Press, 1995).
3. F. Tilney, *The Brain: From Ape to Man* (New York: Hoeber, 1928).
4. J. Jaynes, *The Origin of Consciousness in the Breakdown of the Bicameral Mind* (New York: Houghton Mifflin, 1990).

5. Quoted in W. E. Wallace, *Michelangelo: The Complete Sculpture, Painting, Architecture* (Southport, CT: Hugh Lauter Levin Associates, 1998).
6. J. D. Wallis, K. C. Anderson, and E. K. Miller, "Single neurons in prefrontal cortex encode abstract rules," *Nature* 411 (2001): 953–6.
7. K. Shima, M. Isoda, H. Mushiake, and J. Tanji, "Categorization of behavioural sequences in the prefrontal cortex," *Nature* 445 (2007): 315–8.
8. S. Pinker, *The Language Instinct* (New York: Harper Perennial Library, 1995).
9. M. T. Ullman, "A neurocognitive perspective on language: the declarative/procedural model," *Nat Rev Neurosci* 2 (2001): 717–26.
10. P. Hagoort, L. Hald, M. Bastiaansen, and K. M. Petersson, "Integration of word meaning and world knowledge in language comprehension," *Science* 304 (2004): 438–41.

Chapter 4: Architecture of the Brain: A Primer

1. M. Wang, S. Vijayraghavan, and P. S. Goldman-Rakic, "Selective D2 receptor actions on the functional circuitry of working memory," Science 303 (2004): 853–6.
2. S. Vijayraghavan, M. Wang, S. G. Birnbaum, G. V. Williams, and A. F. T. Arnsten, "Inverted-U dopamine D1 receptor actions on prefrontal neurons engaged in working memory," *Nat Neurosci* 10 (2007): 376–84.
3. H. F. Clarke, J. W. Dalley, H. S. Crofts, T. W. Robbins, and A. C. Roberts, "Cognitive inflexibility after prefrontal serotonin depletion," *Science* 304 (2004): 878–80.
4. For a more thorough review see A. Parent, *Carpenter's Human Neuroanatomy*, 9th ed. (Baltimore: Williams & Wilkins, 1995). (Revised edition of M. B. Carpenter and J. Satin, *Human Neuroanatomy*, 8th ed., 1983.)
5. H. W. Magoun, "The ascending reticular activating system," *Res Publ Assoc Nerv Ment Dis* 30 (1952).
6. Thorough review on this topic can be found in D. Oakley and H. Plotkin, eds., *Brain, Behavior and Evolution* (Cambridge, UK: Cambridge University Press, 1979).
7. Again, for a more thorough review see A. Parent, *Carpenter's Human Neuroanatomy*, 9th ed. (Baltimore: Williams & Wilkins, 1995).
8. Ibid.
9. J. LeDoux, *The Emotional Brain: The Mysterious Underpinnings of Emotional Life* (New York: Touchstone Books, 1998).
10. J. Grafman, I. Litvan, S. Massaquoi, M. Stewart, A. Sirigu, and M. Hallett, "Cognitive planning deficit in patients with cerebellar atrophy," *Neurology* 42 (1992): 1493–1496.
11. H. C. Leiner, A. L. Leiner, and R. S. Dow, "Reappraising the cerebellum: what does the hindbrain contribute to the forebrain?" *Behav Neurosci* 103 (1989): 998–1008.
12. N. Ramnani, "The primate cortico-cerebellar system: anatomy and function," *Nat Rev Neurosci* 7 (2006): 511–22.
13. In D. Oakley and H. Plotkin, eds., *Brain, Behavior and Evolution* (Cambridge, UK: Cambridge University Press, 1979).
14. B. L. McNaughton and R. G. M Morris, "Hippocampal synaptic enhancement and information storage," *Trends Neurosci* 10 (1987): 408–15; B. L. McNaughton, "Associative pattern competition in hippocampal circuits: new evidence and new questions," *Brain Res Rev* 16 (1991): 202–4.
15. B. Milner, "Cues to the cerebral organization of memory," in *Cerebral Correlates of Conscious Experience*, eds. P. Buser and A. Rougeul-Buser (Amsterdam: Elsevier, 1978), 139–53.
16. K. L. Hoffman and B. L. McNaughton, "Coordinated reactivation of distributed memory traces in primate neocortex," *Science* 297 (2002): 2070–3.

17. T. Maviel, T. P. Durkin, F. Menzaghi, and B. Bontempi, "Sites of neocortical reorganization critical for remote spatial memory," *Science* 305(5680) (2004): 96–9.

18. M. Remondes and E. M. Schuman, "Role for a cortical input to hippocampal area CA1 in the consolidation of a long-term memory," *Nature* 431(7009) (2004): 699–703.

19. R. A. Poldrack, J. Clark, and E. J. Pare-Blagoev, et al., "Interactive memory systems in the human brain," *Nature* 414(6863) (2001): 546–50.

20. In C. H. Hockman, ed., *Limbic System Mechanisms and Autonomic Function* (Springfield, IL: Charles C. Thomas, 1972).

21. C. S. Carter, M. M. Botvinick, and J. D. Cohen, "The contribution of the anterior cingulate cortex to executive processes in cognition," *Rev Neurosci* 10 (1999): 49–57.

22. K. E. Stephan, J. C. Marshall, K. J. Friston, J. B. Rowe, A. Ritzl, K. Zilles, and G. R. Fink, "Lateralized cognitive processes and lateralized task control in the human brain," *Science* 301 (2003): 384–6.

23. In D. Oakley and H. Plotkin, eds., *Brain, Behavior and Evolution* (Cambridge, UK: Cambridge University Press, 1979).

24. K. Brodmann, *Vergleichende Lokalisationslehre der Grosshinrinde in ihren Prinzipien dargestellt auf Grund des Zellenbaues* (Leipzig: Barth, 1909). Cited in J. M. Fuster, *The Prefrontal Cortex: Anatomy, Physiology, and Neuropsychology of the Frontal Lobe*, 3rd ed. (Philadelphia: Lippincott–Raven, 1997).

25. G. W. Roberts, P. N. Leigh, and D. R. Weinberger, *Neuropsychiatric Disorders* (London: Wolfe, 1993).

26. J. M. Fuster, *The Prefrontal Cortex: Anatomy, Physiology, and Neuropsychology of the Frontal Lobe*, 3rd ed. (Philadelphia: Lippincott–Raven, 1997).

27. In A. W. Campbell, *Histological Studies on the Localization of Cerebral Function* (Cambridge, UK: Cambridge University Press, 1905). Cited in J. M. Fuster, *The Prefrontal Cortex: Anatomy, Physiology, and Neuropsychology of the Frontal Lobe*, 3rd ed. (Philadelphia: Lippincott–Raven, 1997).

28. J. H. Jackson, "Evolution and dissolution of the nervous system," *Croonian Lecture. Selected Papers* 2, Br Med J. 1884 April 5; 1(1214): 660–663. London.

29. A. R. Luria, *Higher Cortical Functions in Man* (New York: Basic Books, 1966).

30. A. Damasio, "The frontal lobes," in *Clinical Neuropsychology*, eds. K. Heilman and E. Valenstein (New York: Oxford University Press, 1993), 360–412.

31. J. M. Fuster, *The Prefrontal Cortex: Anatomy, Physiology, and Neuropsychology of the Frontal Lobe*, 3rd ed. (Philadelphia: Lippincott–Raven, 1997).

32. P. S. Goldman-Rakic, "Circuitry of primate prefrontal cortex and regulation of behavior by representational memory," in *Handbook of Physiology: Nervous System, Higher Functions of the Brain*, Part 1, ed. F. Plum (Bethesda, MD: American Physiological Association, 1987), 373–417.

33. D. T. Stuss and D. F. Benson, *The Frontal Lobes* (New York: Raven Press, 1986).

34. W. J. Nauta, "Neural associations of the frontal cortex," *Acta Neurobiol Exp* 32 (1972): 125–40.

35. E. K. Miller, "The prefrontal cortex and cognitive control," *Nat Rev Neurosci* 1 (2000): 59–65.

36. Ibid.

37. Y. Tsushima, Y. Sasaki, and T. Watanabe, "Greater disruption due to failure of inhibitory control on an ambiguous distractor," *Science* 314 (2006): 1786–8.

38. J. H. Jackson, "Evolution and dissolution of the nervous system," *Croonian Lecture. Selected Papers* 2, Br Med J. 1884 April 5; 1(1214): 660–663. London.

39. J. M. Fuster, *Cortex and Mind: Unifying Cognition* (New York: Oxford University Press, 2003).

40. J. Hawkins and S. Blakeslee, *On Intelligence* (New York: Times Books, 2004).

Chapter 5: The Orchestra's Front Row: The Cortex

1. F. J. Gall, *Sur le fonctions du cerveau*, 6 vols. (Paris, 1822–1823).
2. K. Kleist, *Gehirnpathologie* (Leipzig: Barth, 1934).
3. J. M. Gold, K. F. Berman, C. Randolph, T. E. Goldberg, and D. Weinberger, "PET valida-tion of a novel prefrontal task: delayed response alteration," *Neuropsychology* 10 (1996): 3–10; R. J. Haier, B. V. Siegel, Jr., A. MacLachlan, E. Soderling, S. Lottenberg, and M. S. Buchsbaum, "Regional glucose metabolic changes after learning a complex visu-ospatial/motor task: a positron emission tomographic study," *Brain Res* 570 (1992): 134–43; M. E. Raichle, J. A. Fiez, T. O. Videen, A. M. MacLeod, J. V. Pardo, P. T. Fox, and S. E. Petersen, "Practice-related changes in human brain functional anatomy during non-motor learning," *Cereb Cortex* 4 (1994): 8–26.
4. J. A. Fodor, "Precis of the modularity of mind," *Behav Brain Sci* 8 (1985): 1–42.
5. E. Goldberg, "Rise and fall of modular orthodoxy," *J Clin Exp Neuropsychol* 17, (1995): 193–208; E. Goldberg, "From neuromythology to neuroscience. *Cortex and Mind: Unifying Cognition*, by Joaquin Fuster," *J Int Neuropsychol Soc* 10 (2004): 470–1.
6. G. Aston-Jones and J. D. Cohen, "An integrative theory of locus coeruleus-norepinephrine function: adaptive gain and optimal performance," *Annu Rev Neurosci* 28 (2005): 403–50.
7. J. R. Binder, J. A. Frost, T. A. Hammeke, S. M. Rao, and R. W. Cox, "Function of the left planum temporale in auditory and linguistic processing," *Brain* 119 (1996): 1239–47.
8. J. Shaplesk, S. L. Rossell, P. W. R. Woodruff, and A. S. David, "The planum temporale: a systematic, quantitative review of its structural, functional and clinical significance," *Brain Res Rev* 29 (1999): 26–49.
9. A. R. Damasio, H. Damasio, and G. W. Van Hoesen, "Prosopagnosia: anatomical basis and behavioral mechanisms," *Neurology* 32 (1982): 331–41; A. R. Damasio, "Prosopagnosia," *Trends Neurosci* 8 (1985): 132–5.
10. M. Takamura, "Prosopagnosia: a look at the laterality and specificity issues using evi-dence from neuropsychology and neurophysiology," *The Harvard Brain*, Spring (1996): 9–13.
11. E. Goldberg, "Gradiental approach to neocortical functional organization," *J Clin Exp Neuropsychol* 11 (1989): 489–517; E. Goldberg, "Higher cortical functions in humans: the gradiental approach," in *Contemporary Neuropsychology and the Legacy of Luria*, ed. E. Goldberg (Hillsdale, NJ: Lawrence Erlbaum Associates, 1990), 229–76.
12. K. R. Ridderinkhof, M. Ullsperger, E. A. Crone, and S. Nieuwenhuis, "The role of the medial frontal cortex in cognitive control," *Science* 306 (2004): 443–7.
13. E. Goldberg, "Gradiental approach to neocortical functional organization," *J Clin Exp Neuropsychol* 11 (1989): 489–517.
14. E. Goldberg, "Higher cortical functions in humans: the gradiental approach," in *Contemporary Neuropsychology and the Legacy of Luria*, ed. E. Goldberg (Hillsdale, NJ: Lawrence Erlbaum Associates, 1990), 229–76.
15. E. Goldberg, "Rise and fall of modular orthodoxy," *J Clin Exp Neuropsychol* 17 (1995): 193–208.
16. J. L. McClelland, B. L. McNaughton, and R. C. O'Reilly, "Why there are complementary learning systems in the hippocampus and neocortex: insights from the successes and failures of connectionist models of learning and memory," *Psychol Rev* 102 (1995): 419–57.
17. S. L. Thompson-Schill, M. D'Esposito, G. K. Aguirre, and M. J. Farah, "Role of left infe-rior prefrontal cortex in retrieval of semantic knowledge: a reevaluation," *Proc Natl Acad Sci USA* 94 (1997): 14792–7.
18. O. W. Sacks, "Scotoma: forgetting and neglect in science," in *Hidden Histories of Science*, ed. R. B. Silver (New York: New York Review, 1996), 141–87.

19. E. S. Lein, M. J. Hawrylycz, N. Ao, et al., "Genome-wide atlas of gene expression in the adult mouse brain," *Nature* 445, (2007): 168–176.
20. For review see K. Heilman and E. Valenstein, eds., *Clinical Neuropsychology* (New York: Oxford University Press, 1993).
21. E. Goldberg, "Associative agnosias and the functions of the left hemisphere," *J Clin Exp Neuropsychol* 12 (1990): 467–484.
22. E. Goldberg, "Gradiental approach to neocortical functional organization," *J Clin Exp Neuropsychol* 11 (1989): 489–517.
23. A. Martin, L. G. Ungerleider, and J. V. Haxby, "Category specificity and the brain: the sensory/motor model of semantic representation of objects," in *The New Cognitive Neuroscience*, ed. M. S. Gazzaniga (Cambridge, MA: MIT Press, 1999).
24. A. Martin, C. L. Wiggs, L. G. Ungerleider, and J. V. Haxby, "Neural correlates of category-specific knowledge," *Nature* 379(6566) (1996): 649–52.
25. E. K. Warrington and T. Shallice, "Category-specific semantic impairments," *Brain* 107 (1984): 829–54; R. A. McCarthy and E. K. Warrington, "Evidence for modality-specific meaning systems in the brain," *Nature* 334(6181) (1988): 428–30.
26. E. Goldberg, "Gradiental approach to neocortical functional organization," *J Clin Exp Neuropsychol* 11 (1989): 489–517.
27. E. Goldberg and D. Tucker, "Motor perseverations and long-term memory for visual forms," *J Clin Neuropsychol* 1 (1979): 273–88.
28. E. Goldberg, "Varieties of perseveration: comparison of two taxonomies," *J Clin Exp Neuropsychol* 8 (1986): 710–26; E. Goldberg and R. M. Bilder, "The frontal lobes and hierarchical organization of cognitive control," in E. Perecman, ed., *The Frontal Lobes Revisited* (Hillsdale, NJ: Lawrence Erlbaum Associates, 1987): 159–88.
29. E. Goldberg, "Varieties of perseveration: comparison of two taxonomies," *J Clin Exp Neuropsychol* 8 (1986): 710–26.
30. E. Koechlin, G. Basso, P. Pietrini, S. Panzer, and J. Grafman, "The role of the anterior prefrontal cortex in human cognition," *Nature* 399 (1999): 148–51.
31. J. Hoffman, D. Badre, T. Berg-Kirkpatrick, F. Krienen, J. Cooney, and M. D'Esposito, "Dissociating levels of cognitive control in frontal cortex hierarchy: evidence from patients with focal lesions," *Cogn Neurosci Soc* (2007): 263.
32. E. Koechlin, C. Ody, and F. Kouneiher, "The architecture of cognitive control in the human prefrontal cortex," *Science* 302 (2003): 1181–5.
33. E. Koechlin and A. Hyafil, "Anterior prefrontal function and the limits of human decision-making," *Science* 318 (2007): 594–8.
34. N. Ramnani and A. M. Owen, "Anterior prefrontal cortex: insights into function from anatomy and neuroimaging," *Nat Rev Neurosci* 5 (2004): 184–94.
35. Ibid.
36. J. A. Fodor, "Precis of the modularity of mind," *Behav Brain Sci* 8 (1985): 1–42.
37. E. Goldberg, "Gradiental approach to neocortical functional organization," *J Clin Exp Neuropsychol* 11 (1989): 489–517; E. Goldberg, "Higher cortical functions in humans: the gradiental approach," in *Contemporary Neuropsychology and the Legacy of Luria*, ed. E. Goldberg (Hillsdale, NJ: Lawrence Erlbaum Associates, 1990), 229–76; E. Goldberg, "Rise and fall of modular orthodoxy," *J Clin Exp Neuropsychol* 17 (1995): 193–208.
38. W. S. McCulloch and W. Pitts, "A logical calculus of the ideas immanent in nervous activity. 1943 classical article," *Bull Math Biol* 52 (1990): 99–115.
39. E. Goldberg, "Gradiental approach to neocortical functional organization," *J Clin Exp Neuropsychol* 11 (1989): 489–517.
40. D. Oakley and H. Plotkin, eds., *Brain, Behavior and Evolution* (Cambridge, UK: Cambridge University Press, 1979).

41. T. E. J. Behrens, H. Johansen-Berg, M. W. Woolrich, et al., "Non-invasive mapping of connections between human thalamus and cortex using diffusion imaging," *Nat Neurosci* 6 (2003): 750–7.

Chapter 6: Novelty, Routines, and Cerebral Hemispheres

1. P. Broca, "Remarques sur le siège de la faculté du language articule," *Bull Soc Anthrop* 6 (1861).
2. C. Wernicke, *Der aphasische Symptomencomplex* (Breslau, 1874).
3. M. LeMay, "Morphological cerebral asymmetries of modern man, fossil man, and nonhuman primate," *Ann N Y Acad Sci* 280 (1976): 349–66.
4. S. Chance, M. M. Esiri, and T. J. Crow, "Macroscopic brain asymmetry is changed along the antero-posterior axis in schizophrenia," *Schizophr Res* 74, (2005): 163–70; T. R. Barricka, C. E. Mackayb, S. Primac, F. Maesd, D. Vandermeulend, T. J. Crowb, and N. Roberts, "Automatic analysis of cerebral asymmetry: an exploratory study of the relationship between brain torque and planum temporale asymmetry," *Neuroimage* 24 (2005): 678–91.
5. M. C. de Lacoste, D. S. Horvath, and D. J. Woodward, "Possible sex differences in the developing human fetal brain," *J Clin Exp Neuropsychol* 13 (1991): 831–46.
6. M. LeMay, "Morphological cerebral asymmetries of modern man, fossil man, and nonhuman primate," *Ann N Y Acad Sci* 280 (1976): 349–66.
7. M. C. Diamond, "Rat forebrain morphology: right–left; male–female; young–old; enriched–impoverished," in *Cerebral Laterality in Nonhuman Species*, ed. S. D. Glick (New York: Academic Press, 1985); M. C. Diamond, G. A. Dowling, and R. E. Johnson, "Morphologic cerebral cortical asymmetry in male and female rats," *Exp Neurol* 71 (1981): 261–8.
8. N. Geschwind and W. Levitsky, "Human brain: left–right asymmetries in temporal speech region," *Science* 161(837) (1968): 186–7; T. R. Barrick, C. E. Mackay, S. Prima, et al., "Automatic analysis of cerebral asymmetry: an exploratory study of the relationship between brain torque and planum temporale asymmetry," *Neuroimage* 24 (2005): 678–91.
9. M. LeMay and N. Geschwind, "Hemispheric differences in the brains of great apes," *Brain Behav Evol* 11 (1975): 48–52.
10. P. J. Gannon, R. L. Holloway, D. C. Broadfield, and A. R. Braun, "Asymmetry of chimpanzee planum temporale: humanlike pattern of Wernicke's brain language area homolog," *Science* 279(5348) (1998): 220–2.
11. T. R. Barricka, C. E. Mackayb, S. Primac, F. Maesd, D. Vandermeulend, T. J. Crowb, and N. Roberts, "Automatic analysis of cerebral asymmetry: an exploratory study of the relationship between brain torque and planum temporale asymmetry," *Neuroimage* 24 (2005): 678–91.
12. T. Klingberg, C. J. Vaidya, J. D. E. Gabrieli, M. E. Moseley, and M. Hedehus, "Myelination and organization of the frontal white matter in children: a diffusion tensor MRI study," *Neuroreport* 10 (1999): 2817–21.
13. A. Louilot and M. Le Moal, "Lateralized interdependence between limbicotemporal and ventrostriatal dopaminergic transmission," *Neuroscience* 59 (1994): 495–500.
14. E. Morice, C. Denis, A. Macario, B. Giros, and M. Nosten-Bertrand, "Constitutive hyperdopaminergia is functionally associated with reduced behavioral lateralization," *Neuropsychopharmacology* 30 (2004): 575–81.
15. S. D. Glick, *Cerebral Lateralization in Non-Human Species* (Orlando, FL: Academic Press, 1985).
16. S. Sandu, P. Cook, and M. C. Diamond, "Rat cortical estrogen receptors: male–female, right–left," *Exp Neurol* 92 (1985): 186–96.

17. S. D. Glick, R. C. Meibach, R. D. Cox, and S. Maayani, "Multiple and interrelated functional asymmetries in rat brain," *Life Sci* 25 (1979): 395–400.

18. S. A. Sholl and K. L. Kim, "Androgen receptors are differentially distributed between right and left cerebral hemispheres of the fetal male rhesus monkey," *Brain Res* 516 (1990): 122–6.

19. R. Kawakami, Y. Shinohara, Y. Kato, H. Sugiyama, R. Shigemoto, and I. Ito, "Asymmetrical allocation of NMDA receptor epsilon-2 subunits in hippocampal circuitry," *Science* 300 (2003): 990–4.

20. A. Cowey, "Sensory and non-sensory visual disorders in man and monkey," *Phil Trans R Soc Lond B* 298 (1982): 3–13; C. R. Hamilton and J. S. Lund, "Visual discrimination of movement: midbrain or forebrain?" *Science* 170 (1970): 1428–30; C. R. Hamilton, S. B. Tieman, and W. S. Farell, Jr., "Cerebral dominance in monkeys?" *Neuropsychologia* 12 (1974): 193–8; C. R. Hamilton, "Lateralization for orientation in split-brain monkeys," *Behav Brain Res* 10 (1983): 399–403; C. R. Hamilton and B. A. Vermeire, "Complementary hemispheric specialization in monkeys," *Science* 242 (1988): 1691–4; C. R. Hamilton and B. A. Vermeire, "Cognition, not handedness, is lateralized in monkeys," *Behav Brain Sci* 11 (1988): 723–5; C. R. Hamilton and B. A. Vermeire, "Functional lateralization in monkeys," in *Cerebral Laterality: Theory and Research* (Hillsdale, NJ: Lawrence Erlbaum Associates, 1991).

21. K. M. Kendrick, A. P. da Costa, A. E. Leigh, M. R. Hinton, and J. W. Peirce, "Sheep don't forget a face," *Nature* 414 (2001): 165–6.

22. E. Goldberg, *The Wisdom Paradox: How Your Mind Can Grow Stronger as Your Brain Grows Older* (New York: Gotham Books, 2005).

23. E. Bates, "Plasticity, localization and language development," in *Changing Nervous System: Neurobehavioral Consequences of Early Brain Disorders*, ed. S. H. Bronan (New York: Oxford University Press, 1999): 214–53.

24. E. Goldberg and L. D. Costa, "Hemisphere differences in the acquisition and use of descriptive systems," *Brain Lang* 14 (1981). 144–73.

25. H. Simon, *The Sciences of the Artificial* (Cambridge, MA: MIT Press, 1996).

26. S. Grossberg, ed., *Neural Networks and Natural Intelligence* (Cambridge, MA: MIT Press, 1988).

27. M. S. Jog, Y. Kubota, C. I. Connolly, V. Hillegaart, and A. M. Graybiel, "Building neural representations of habits," *Science* 286 (1999): 1745–9.

28. E. Goldberg, *The Wisdom Paradox: How Your Mind Can Grow Stronger as Your Brain Grows Older* (New York: Gotham Books, 2005).

29. Ibid.

30. E. Goldberg, R. Harner, M. Lovell, K. Podell, and S. Riggio, "Cognitive bias, functional cortical geometry, and the frontal lobes: laterality, sex, and handedness," *J Cogn Neurosci* 6 (1994): 276–96.

31. S. Fusi, M. Annunziato, D. Badoni, A. Salamon, and D. J. Amit, "Spike-driven synaptic plasticity: theory, simulation, VLSI implementation," *Neural Comp* 12 (2000): 2227–58.

32. E. Goldberg and L. D. Costa, "Hemisphere differences in the acquisition and use of descriptive systems," *Brain Lang* 14 (1981): 144–73. For relevant computational models using formal neural nets, see S. Grossberg, ed., *Neural Networks and Natural Intelligence* (Cambridge, MA: MIT Press, 1988); R. A. Jacobs and M. I. Jordan, "Computational consequences of a bias toward short connections," *J Cogn Neurosci* 4 (1992): 323–36; R. A. Jacobs, M. I. Jordan, and A. G. Barto, "Task decomposition through competition in a modular connectionist architecture: the what and where vision tasks," *Cogn Sci* 15 (1991): 219–50.

33. G. Vallortigara and R. J. Andrew, "Differential involvement of right and left hemisphere in individual recognition in the domestic chick," *Behav Processes* 33, (1994): 41–58;

G. Vallortigara and L. J. Rogers, "Survival with an asymmetrical brain: advantages and disadvantages of cerebral lateralization," *Behav Brain Sci* 28 (2005): 575–633; G. Vallortigara, L. J. Rogers, and A. Bisazza, "Possible evolutionary origins of cognitive brain lateralization," *Brain Res Rev* 30 (1999): 164–75; G. Vallortigara, "Comparative neuropsychology of the dual brain: a stroll through animals' left and right perceptual worlds," *Brain Lang* 73 (2000): 189–219.

34. E. Goldberg and L. D. Costa, "Hemisphere differences in the acquisition and use of descriptive systems," *Brain Lang* 14 (1981): 144–73.

35. R. W. Sperry, M. S. Gazzaniga, and J. E. Bogen, "Interhemispheric relationships: the neocortical commisures; syndromes of hemisphere disconnection," in *Handbook of Clinical Neurology*, Vol. 4, eds. P. J. Vinken and G. W. Bruyn (Amsterdam: North-Holland Publishing Company, 1969).

36. B. P. Rourke, *Nonverbal Learning Disabilities: The Syndrome and the Model* (New York: Guilford Press, 1989).

37. For review see S. Springer and G. Deutsch, *Left Brain, Right Brain: Perspective from Cognitive Neuroscience*, 5th ed. (New York: W. H. Freeman & Co., 1997).

38. T. G. Bever and R. J. Chiarello, "Cerebral dominance in musicians and nonmusicians," *Science* 185(150) (1974): 537–9.

39. C. A. Marzi and G. Berlucchi, "Right visual field superiority for accuracy of recognition of famous faces in normals," *Neuropsychologia* 15 (1977): 751–6.

40. A. Martin, C. L. Wiggs, and J. Weisberg, "Modulation of human medial temporal lobe activity by form, meaning, and experience," *Hippocampus* 7 (1997): 587–93.

41. R. Henson, T. Shallice, and R. Dolan, "Neuroimaging evidence for dissociable forms of repetition priming," *Science* 287(5456) (2000): 1269–72.

42. J. M. Gold, K. F. Berman, C. Randolph, T. E. Goldberg, and D. R. Weinberger, "PET validation of a novel prefrontal task: delayed response alteration," *Neuropsychology* 10 (1996): 3–10.

43. R. Shadmehr and H. H. Holcomb, "Neural correlates of motor memory consolidation," *Science* 277(5327) (1997): 821–5.

44. R. J. Haier, B. V. Siegel Jr., A. MacLachlan, E. Soderling, S. Lottenberg, and M. S. Buchsbaum, "Regional glucose metabolic changes after learning a complex visuospatial/motor task: a positron emission tomographic study," *Brain Res* 570 (1992): 134–43.

45. G. S. Berns, J. D. Cohen, and M. A. Mintun, "Brain regions responsive to novelty in the absence of awareness," *Science* 276(5316) (1997): 1272–5.

46. M. E. Raichle, J. A. Fiez, T. O. Videen, A. M. MacLeod, J. V. Pardo, P. T. Fox, and S. E. Petersen, "Practice-related changes in human brain functional anatomy during nonmotor learning," *Cereb Cortex* 4 (1994): 26.

47. J. Crinion, R. Turner, A. Grogan, et al., "Language control in the bilingual brain," *Science* 312 (2006): 1537–40.

48. E. Tulving, H. J. Markowitsch, F. E. Craik, R. Hiabib, and S. Houle, "Novelty and familiarity activations in PET studies of memory encoding and retrieval," *Cereb Cortex* 6 (1996): 71–9.

49. R. D. Newman-Norlund, H. T. van Schie, A. M. van Zuijlen, and H. Bekkering, "The mirror neuron system is more active during complementary compared with imitative action," *Nat Neurosci* 10 (2007): 817–8; K. Vogeley, et al., "Theory of mind and self perspective in the human brain—a fMRI study," *Cognitive Neuroscience Society Meeting* (2001): C28.

50. N. D. Daw, J. P. O'Doherty, P. Dayan, B. Seymour, and R. J. Dolan, "Cortical substrates for exploratory decisions in humans," *Nature* 441 (2006): 876–9.

51. H. R. Heekeren, S. Marrett, P. A. Bandettini, and L. G. Ungerleider, "A general mechanism for perceptual decision-making in the human brain," *Nature* 431 (2004): 859–62.

52. Y. Kamiya, M. Aihara, M. Osada, C. Ono, K. Hatakeyama, H. Kanemura, et al., "Electrophysiological study of lateralization in the frontal lobes," *Jpn J Cogn Neurosci* 3 (2002): 188–191.

53. E. Goldberg, R. Harner, M. Lovell, K. Podell, and S. Riggio, "Cognitive bias, functional cortical geometry, and the frontal lobes: laterality, sex, and handedness," *J Cogn Neurosci* 6 (1994): 276–96.

54. W. R. Staines, M. Padilla, and R. T. Knight, "Frontal–parietal event-related potential changes associated with practising a novel visuomotor task," *Brain Res Cogn Brain Res* 13 (2002): 195–202.

55. J. O'Doherty, P. Dayan, J. Schultz, R. Deichmann, K. Friston, and R. J. Dolan, "Dissociable roles of ventral and dorsal striatum in instrumental conditioning," *Science* 304 (2004): 452–4.

56. D. M. Tucker and P. A. Williamson, "Asymmetric neural control systems in human self-regulation," *Psychol Rev* 91 (1984): 185–215; E. Goldberg, R. Harner, M. Lovell, K. Podell, and S. Riggio, "Cognitive bias, functional cortical geometry, and the frontal lobes: laterality, sex, and handedness," *J Cogn Neurosci* 6 (1994): 276–96; N. D. Daw, J. P. O'Doherty, P. Dayan, B. Seymour, and R. J. Dolan, "Cortical substrates for exploratory decisions in humans," *Nature* 441 (2006): 876–9.

57. S. R. Chamberlain, U. Muller, A. D. Blackwell, L. Clark, T. W. Robbins, and B. J. Sahakian, "Neurochemical modulation of response inhibition and probabilistic learning in humans," *Science* 311 (2006): 861–3.

58. S. Grossberg, *Neural Networks and Natural Intelligence* (Cambridge, MA: MIT Press, 1988).

59. E. Goldberg, R. Harner, M. Lovell, K. Podell, and S. Riggio, "Cognitive bias, functional cortical geometry, and the frontal lobes: laterality, sex, and handedness," *J Cogn Neurosci* 6 (1994): 276–96.

60. L. Metzger, M. W. Gilbertson, and S. P. Orr, "Electrophysiology of PTSD," in *Neurophysiology of PTSD*, eds. J. Vasterling and C. R. Brewin (New York: Guilford Press, 2005).

61. L. Vygotsky, *Thought and Language*, ed. A. Kozulin (Cambridge, MA: MIT Press, 1986).

62. J. Jaynes, *The Origin of Consciousness in the Breakdown of the Bicameral Mind* (New York: Houghton Mifflin, 1990).

63. For tests review see M. D. Lezak, D. B. Howieson, and D. W. Loring, eds., *Neuropsychological Assessment*, 4th ed. (New York: Oxford University Press, 2004).

64. K. E. Stephan, J. C. Marshall, K. J. Friston, et al., "Lateralized cognitive processes and lateralized task control in the human brain," *Science* 301 (2003): 384–6.

65. E. Goldberg and W. Barr, "Three possible mechanisms of unawareness of deficit, in *Awareness of Deficit: Theoretical and Clinical Issues*, eds. G. Prigatano and D. Schacter (New York: Oxford University Press, 1991): 152–75.

66. E. Goldberg, "Associative agnosias and the functions of the left hemisphere," *J Clin Exp Neuropsychol* 12 (1990): 467–84.

67. R. M. Bauer and A. R. Rubens, "Agnosia," in *Clinical Neuropsychology*, 2nd ed., eds. K. M. Heilman and E. Valenstein (New York: Oxford University Press, 1985): 187–242.

68. H. Hécaen and M. I. Albert, *Human Neuropsychology* (New York: John Wiley & Sons, 1978).

69. H. Hécaen and J. de Ajuruguerra, *Les toubles mentaux au course du tumeurs intracraniennes* (Paris: Masson et Cie, 1956).

70. H. Hoff and O. Pötzl, "Über ein neues parieto-occipitales Syndrom. *Journal der Psychiatrie und Neurologie* 52 (1935): 173–218.

71. H. Hécaen, M. C. Goldblum, M. C. Masure, and A. M. Ranier, "Une novelle observation d'agnostic d'object. Deficit de l'association, ou de la cate'gorization specifique de la modalite' visuelle?" *Neuropsychologia* 12 (1974): 447–64.

72. W. von Stauffenberg, "Klinische und anatomische Beiträge für Kenntnis der apraxischen, agnostischen, und apraletiachen Symptome," *Zeitschrift für die gesammte Neurologie und Psychiatrie* 93 (1918): 71.

73. J. M. Nielsen, "Unilateral cerebral dominance as related to mind blindness: minimal lesion capable of causing visual agnosia for objects," *Arch Neurol Psychiatry* 38 (1937): 108–35.

74. J. M. Nielsen, *Agnosia, Apraxia, Aphasia: Their Value in Cerebral Localization*, 2nd ed. (New York: Hoebner, 1946).

75. C. Foix, "Sur une variété de troubles bilateraux de la sensibilié par lésion unilaterale de cerveau," *Rev Neurol (Paris)* 29 (1922): 322–31.

76. K. Goldstein, "Über korticale Sensibilitätstörungen," *Neurologisches Zentralblatt* 19 (1916): 825–7.

77. J. Lhermitte and J. de Ajuriaguerra, "Asymbolie tactile et hallucinations du toucher. Étude anatomoclinique," *Rev Neurol (Paris)* (1938): 492–5.

78. P. Faglioni, H. Spinnler, and L. A. Vignolo, "Contrasting behavior of right and left hemisphere–damaged patients on a discriminative and a semantic task of auditory recognition," *Cortex* 5 (1969): 366–89.

79. K. Kleist, "Gehirnpatologische und lokalizatorische Ergebnisse über Hörstörungen, Gerausch-Taubheiten und Amusien," *Monatschrift für Psychiatrie und Neurologie* 68 (1928): 853–60.

80. H. Spinnler and L. A. Vignolo, "Impaired recognition of meaningful sounds in aphasia," *Cortex* 2 (1966): 337–48.

81. L. A. Vignolo, "Auditory agnosia," *Phil Trans R Soc Lond B* 298 (1982): 49–57.

82. A. R. Damasio, "Prosopagnosia," *Trends Neurosci* 8 (1985): 132–5.

83. Benton and Van Allen (1968)

84. A. R. Damasio, H. Damasio, and G. W. Van Hoesen, "Prosopagnosia: anatomical basis and behavioral mechanisms," *Neurology* 32 (1982): 331–41.

85. J. C. Meadows, "Disturbed perception of colours associated with localized cerebral lesions," Brain 97 (1974): 615–624.

86. E. De Renzi, A. Pieczulo, and L. A. Vignolo, "Ideational apraxia: a quantitative study," *Neuropsychologia* 6 (1969): 41–52.

87. E. K. Warrington, "Neuropsychological studies of object recognition," *Phil Trans R Soc Lond B* 298 (1982): 16–33.

88. E. K. Warrington and M. James, An experimental investigation of of facial recognition in patients with unilateral cerebral lesion. Cortex 3 (1967): 317-326; E. K. Warrington and M. James, Disorders of visual perception in patients with localized cerebral lesions. Neuropsychologia 5 (1967): 252-266.

89. E. K. Warrington and M. James, "Visual apperceptive agnosia: a clinico-anatomical study of three cases," *Cortex* 24 (1988): 13–32.

90. E. K. Warrington and A. M. Taylor, "A contribution of the right parietal lobe to object recognition," *Perception* 7 (1973): 695–705.

91. P. Faglioni H. Spinnler, and L. A. Vignolo, "Contrasting behavior of right and left hemisphere–damaged patients on a discriminative and a semantic task of auditory recognition," *Cortex* 5(4) (1969): 366–389.

92. For review see A. R. Luria, *Higher Cortical Functions in Man* (New York: Basic Books, 1980).

93. E. Goldberg and R. M. Bilder, "The frontal lobes and hierarchical organization of cognitive control," in *The Frontal Lobes Revisited*, ed. E. Perecman (New York: Psychology Press, 1987): 159–88.

94. R. C. O'Reilly, "Biologically based computational models of high-level cognition," *Science* 314(5796) (2006): 91–4.

95. Ibid.

96. Ibid.

97. Z. C. Xu, G. Ling, R. N. Sahr, and B. S. Neal-Beliveau, "Asymmetrical changes of dopamine receptors in the striatum after unilateral dopamine depletion," *Brain Res* 1038 (2005): 163–70.

98. R. C. O'Reilly and Y. Munakata, *Computational Explorations in Cognitive Neuroscience* (Cambridge, MA: MIT Press, 2000).

99. E. Goldberg, *The Wisdom Paradox: How Your Mind Can Grow Stronger as Your Brain Grows Older* (New York: Gotham Books, 2005).

100. E. Goldberg, K. Podell, R. Bilder, and J. Jaeger, *The Executive Control Battery* (Melbourne, Australia: Psych Press, 2000).

101. Ibid.

Chapter 7: The Conductor: A Closer Look at the Frontal Lobes

1. M. E. Raichle, J. A. Fiez, T. O. Videen, A. M. MacLeod, J. V. Pardo, P. T. Fox, and S. E. Petersen, "Practice-related changes in human brain functional anatomy during non-motor learning," *Cereb Cortex* 4 (1994): 8–26.

2. J. N. Wood and J. Grafman, "Human prefrontal cortex: processing and representational perspectives," *Nat Rev Neurosci* 4 (2003): 139–47.

3. J. M. Gold, K. F. Berman, C. Randolph, T. F. Goldberg, and D. Weinberger, "PET validation of a novel prefrontal task: delayed response alteration," *Neuropsychology* 10 (1996): 3–10.

4. A. R. McIntosh, M. N. Rajah, and N. J. Lobaugh, "Interactions of prefrontal cortex in relation to awareness in sensory learning," *Science* 284 (1999): 1531–3.

5. Y. Kamiya, M. Aihara, M. Osada, C. Ono, K. Hatakeyama, H. Kanemura, et al., "Electrophysiological study of lateralization in the frontal lobes," *Jpn J Cogn Neurosci* 3 (2002): 188–191.

6. I. G. Dobbins, D. M. Schnyer, M. Verfaellie, and D. L. Schacter, "Cortical activity reductions during repetition priming can result from rapid response learning," *Nature* 428 (2004): 316–9.

7. D. J. Freedman, M. Riesenhuber, T. Poggio, and E. K. Miller, "Categorical representation of visual stimuli in the primate prefrontal cortex," *Science* 291 (2001): 312–6.

8. C. F. Jacobsen, "Functions of the frontal association area in primates," *Arch Neurol Psychiatry* 33 (1935): 558–69; C. F. Jacobsen and H. W. Nissen, "Studies of cerebral function in primates: IV. The effects of frontal lobe lesion on the delayed alternation habit in monkeys," *J Comp Physiol Psychol* 23 (1937): 101–12.

9. A. R. Luria, *Higher Cortical Functions in Man* (New York: Basic Books, 1966).

10. P. S. Goldman-Rakic, "Circuitry of primate prefrontal cortex and regulation of behavior by representational memory," in *Handbook of Physiology: Nervous System, Higher Functions of the Brain*, Part 1, ed. F. Plum (Bethesda, MD: American Physiological Association, 1987), 373–417.

11. J. M. Fuster, *The Prefrontal Cortex: Anatomy, Physiology, and Neuropsychology of the Frontal Lobe*, 3rd ed. (Philadelphia: Lippincott–Raven, 1997).

12. T. Klingberg, *The Overflowing Brain: Information Overload and the Limits of Working Memory* (New York: Oxford, 2008).

13. J. M. Fuster, "Temporal organization of behavior (Introduction)," *Hum Neurobiol* 4 (1985): 57–60.

14. S. G. Birnbaum, P. X. Yuan, M. Wang, S. Vijayraghavan, A. K. Bloom, D. J. Davis, et al., "Protein kinase C overactivity impairs prefrontal cortical regulation of working memory," *Science* 306 (2004): 882–4.

15. S. Vijayraghavan, M. Wang, S. G. Birnbaum, G. V. Williams, and A. F. T. Arnsten, "Inverted-U dopamine D1 receptor actions on prefrontal neurons engaged in working memory," *Nat Neurosci* 10 (2007): 376–84; M. Wang, S. Vijayraghavan, and P. S. Goldman-Rakic, "Selective D2 receptor actions on the functional circuitry of working memory," *Science* 303 (2004): 853–6.

16. J. B. Rowe, I. Toni, O. Josephs, R. S. Frackowiak, and R. E. Passingham, "The prefrontal cortex: response selection or maintenance within working memory?" *Science* 288 (2000): 1656–60.

17. B. A. Kuhl, N. M. Dudukovic, I. Kahn, and A. D. Wagner, "Decreased demands on cognitive control reveal the neural processing benefits of forgetting," *Nat Neurosci* 10 (2007): 908–14.

18. B. E. Depue, T. Curran, and M. T. Banich, "Prefrontal regions orchestrate suppression of emotional memories via a two-phase process," *Science* 317 (2007): 215–9.

19. D. C. Delis, J. H. Kramer, E. Kaplan, and B. A. Ober, *California Verbal Learning Test: Adult Version* (San Antonio, TX: The Psychological Corporation, 1987).

20. E. A. Hazlett, M. S. Buchsbaum, L. A. Jeu, I. Nenadic, M. B. Fleischman, L. Shihabuddin, et al., "Hypofrontality in unmedicated schizophrenia patients studied with PET during performance of a serial verbal learning task," *Schizophr Res* 43 (2000): 33–46.

21. J. H. Jackson, "Evolution and dissolution of the nervous system," *Croonian Lecture. Selected Papers* 2 (1884).

22. S. Funahashi, C. J. Bruce, and P. S. Goldman-Rakic, "Mnemonic coding of visual space in the monkey's dorsolateral prefrontal cortex," *J Neurophysiol* 61 (1989): 331–49.

23. S. M. Courtney, L. G. Ungerleider, K. Keil, and J. V. Haxby, "Object and spatial visual working memory activate separate neural systems in human cortex," *Cereb Cortex* 6 (1996): 39–49.

24. S. Funahashi, C. J. Bruce, and P. S. Goldman-Rakic, "Mnemonic coding of visual space in the monkey's dorsolateral prefrontal cortex," *J Neurophysiol* 61 (1989): 331–49.

25. E. Koechlin, G. Basso, P. Pietrini, S. Panzer, and J. Grafman, "The role of the anterior prefrontal cortex in human cognition," *Nature* 399 (1999): 148–51.

26. C. Sanchez, S. Meek, M. Phillips, V. Nair, A. Craig, L. Jelsone, et al., "Anterior cingulate and prefrontal activity as correlates of attention switching and consideration of multiple relations during truthful and deceptive responses: a bold imaging study," presented at Cognitive Neuroscience Society Annual Meeting, New York, NY, May 5–8, 2007.

27. E. Koechlin, C. Ody, and F. Kouneiher, "The architecture of cognitive control in the human prefrontal cortex," *Science* 302 (2003): 1181–5.

28. D. J. Amit, S. Fusi, and V. Yakovlev, "Paradigmatic working memory (attractor) cell in IT cortex," *Neural Comput* 9 (1997): 1071–92; G. Mongillo, O. Barak, and M. Tsodyks, "Synaptic theory of working memory," *Science* 319 (2008): 1543–6; C. K. Machens, R. Romo, and C. D. Brody, "Flexible control of mutual inhibition: a neural model of two-interval discrimination," *Science* 307 (2005): 1121–4.

29. D. J. Amit, "The Hebbian paradigm reintegrated: local reverberations as internal representations," *Behav Brain Sci* 18 (1994): 617–26; G. Mongillo, O. Barak, and M. Tsodyks, "Synaptic theory of working memory," *Science* 319 (2008): 1543–6.

30. E. Goldberg, R. Harner, M. Lovell, K. Podell, and S. Riggio, "Cognitive bias, functional cortical geometry, and the frontal lobes: laterality, sex, and handedness," *J Cogn Neurosci* 6 (1994): 276–96.

31. K. Vogeley, K. Podell, J. Kukolja, L. Schilbach, E. Goldberg, K. Zilles, et al., "Recruitment of the left prefrontal cortex in preference-based decisions in males (fMRI study)," presented at the Ninth Annual Meeting of the Organization for Human Brain Mapping, New York, NY, 2003.

32. B. Pesaran, M. J. Nelson, and R. A. Andersen, "Free choice activates a decision circuit between frontal and parietal cortex," 453 (2008): 406–9.

33. J. N. Wood, D. D. Glynn, B. C. Phillips, and M. D. Hauser, "The perception of rational, goal-directed action in nonhuman primates," *Science* 317 (2007): 1402–5.

34. E. Herrmann, J. Call, M. V. Hernandez-Lloreda, B. Hare, and M. Tomasello, "Humans have evolved specialized skills of social cognition: the cultural intelligence hypothesis," *Science* 317 (2007): 1360–6.

35. C. Zimmer, "Sociable, and smart," *New York Times* (March 4, 2008): F1–F4.

36. E. Goldberg, A. Kluger, T. Griesing, L. Malta, M. Shapiro, and S. Ferris, "Early diagnosis of frontal-lobe dementias," presented at the Eighth Congress of the International Psychogeriatric Association, Jerusalem, Israel, August 17–22, 1997.

37. For review see B. Reisberg, ed., *Alzheimer's Disease* (New York: Free Press, 1983).

38. A. Verdejo-Garcia, R. Vilar-Lopez, M. Perez Garcia, K. Podell, and E. Goldberg, "Altered adaptive but not veridical decision-making in substance dependent individuals," *J Int Neuropsychol Soc* 12 (2006): 90–9.

39. E. Goldberg, *The Wisdom Paradox: How Your Mind Can Grow Stronger as Your Brain Grows Older* (New York: Gotham Books, 2005).

40. R. C. O'Reilly, "Biologically based computational models of high-level cognition," *Science* 314 (2006): 91–4.

41. R. C. O'Reilly and Y. Munakata, *Computational Explorations in Cognitive Neuroscience* (Cambridge, MA: MIT, 2000).

42. H. C. Lau, R. D. Rogers, P. Haggard, and R. E. Passingham, "Attention to intention," *Science* 303(5661) (2004): 1208–10.

43. E. Goldberg, K. Podell, R. Bilder, and J. Jaeger, *The Executive Control Battery* (Melbourne, Australia: Psych Press, 2000).

44. CNN, *Supreme Court bars executing mentally retarded.* CNN.com/Law Center. Retrieved July 8, 2008, from http://archives.cnn.com/2002/LAW/06/20/scotus.executions

45. P. W. Glimcher, *Decisions, Uncertainty, and the Brain: The Science of Neuroeconomics* (Cambridge, MA: MIT, 2003).

46. D. Marchiori and M. Warglien, "Predicting human interactive learning by regret-driven neural networks," *Science* 319 (2008): 1111–3.

47. CNN, *Transcript: March 21, 2008.* CNN Newsroom. Retrieved July 8, 2008, from http://transcripts.cnn.com/TRANSCRIPTS/0803/21/cnr.02.html

48. M. Botvinick, L. E. Nystrom, K. Fissell, C. S. Carter, and J. D. Cohen, "Conflict monitoring versus selection-for-action in anterior cingulate cortex," *Nature* 402 (1999): 179–81; J. G. Kerns, J. D. Cohen, A. W. MacDonald, 3rd, R. Y. Cho, V. A. Stenger, and C. S. Carter, "Anterior cingulate conflict monitoring and adjustments in control," *Science* 303 (2004): 1023–6.

49. S. Ito, V. Stuphorn, J. W. Brown, and J. D. Schall, "Performance monitoring by the anterior cingulate cortex during saccade countermanding," *Science* 302 (2003): 120–2.

50. T. Paus, "Primate anterior cingulate cortex: where motor control, drive and cognition interface," *Nat Rev Neurosci* 2 (2001): 417–24.

51. V. Van Veen and C. S. Carter, "A PDP model of conflict and anterior cingulate activity in the go-change task," presented at the Cognitive Neuroscience Society Annual Meeting, New York, NY, May 5–8, 2008.

52. J. W. Brown and T. S. Braver, "Learned predictions of error likelihood in the anterior cingulate cortex," *Science* 307 (2005): 1118–21.

53. F. A. Mansouri, M. J. Buckley, and K. Tanaka, "Mnemonic function of the dorsolateral prefrontal cortex in conflict-induced behavioral adjustment," *Science* 318 (2007): 987–90.

54. M. Botvinick, L. E. Nystrom, K. Fissell, C. S. Carter, and J. D. Cohen, "Conflict monitoring versus selection-for-action in anterior cingulate cortex," *Nature* 402 (1999): 179–81.

54. J. G. Kerns, J. D. Cohen, A. W. MacDonald, 3rd, R. Y. Cho, V. A. Stenger, and C. S. Carter, "Anterior cingulate conflict monitoring and adjustments in control," *Science* 303 (2004): 1023–6.

55. K. Samejima, Y. Ueda, K. Doya, and M. Kimura, "Representation of action-specific reward values in the striatum," *Science* 310 (2005): 1337–40.

56. M. Hsu, M. Bhatt, R. Adolphs, D. Tranel, and C. F. Camerer, "Neural systems responding to degrees of uncertainty in human decision-making," *Science* 310 (2005): 1680–3.

57. S. M. Tom, C. R. Fox, C. Trepel, and R. A. Poldrack, "The neural basis of loss aversion in decision-making under risk," *Science* 315 (2007): 515–8.

58. J. W. Kable and P. W. Glimcher, "The neural correlates of subjective value during intertemporal choice," *Nat Neurosci* 10 (2007): 1625–33.

59. S. M. McClure, D. I. Laibson, G. Loewenstein, and J. D. Cohen, "Separate neural systems value immediate and delayed monetary rewards," *Science* 306 (2004): 503–7.

60. M. Pessiglione, L. Schmidt, B. Draganski, R. Kalisch, H. Lau, R. J. Dolan, and C. D. Frith, "How the brain translates money into force: a neuroimaging study of subliminal motivation," *Science* 316 (2007): 904–6.

61. L. Tremblay and W. Schultz, "Relative reward preference in primate orbitofrontal cortex," *Nature* 398 (1999): 704–8; M. Watanabe, "Neurobiology. Attraction is relative not absolute," *Nature* 398 (1999): 661, 663.

62. D. Kahneman and A. Tversky, "On the psychology of prediction," *Psychol Rev* 80 (1973): 237–51.

63. B. De Martino, D. Kumaran, B. Seymour, and R. J. Dolan, "Frames, biases, and rational decision-making in the human brain," *Science* 313 (2006): 684–7.

64. A. G. Sanfey, J. K. Rilling, J. A. Aronson, L. E. Nystrom, and J. D. Cohen, "The neural basis of economic decision-making in the Ultimatum Game," *Science* 300 (2003): 1755–8.

65. D. Knoch, A. Pascual-Leone, K. Meyer, V. Treyer, and E. Fehr, "Diminishing reciprocal fairness by disrupting the right prefrontal cortex," *Science* 314 (2006): 829–32.

66. D. J. de Quervain, U. Fischbacher, V. Treyer, M. Schellhammer, U. Schnyder, A. Buck, and E. Fehr, "The neural basis of altruistic punishment," *Science* 305 (2004): 1254–8.

67. B. King-Casas, D. Tomlin, C. Anen, C. F. Camerer, S. R. Quartz, and P. R. Montague, "Getting to know you: reputation and trust in a two-person economic exchange," *Science* 308 (2005): 78–83.

68. T. Singer, B. Seymour, J. P. O'Doherty, K. E. Stephan, R. J. Dolan, and C. D. Frith, "Empathic neural responses are modulated by the perceived fairness of others," *Nature* 439 (2006): 466–9.

69. C. Padoa-Schioppa and J. A. Assad, "The representation of economic value in the orbitofrontal cortex is invariant for changes of menu," *Nat Neurosci* 11 (2008): 95–102.

Chapter 8: Emotion and Cognition

1. J. LeDoux, *The Emotional Brain: The Mysterious Underpinnings of Emotional Life* (New York: Touchstone Books, 1998).
2. K. Goldstein, *The Organism* (New York: American Books, 1939); A. R. Luria, *Higher Cortical Functions in Man* (New York: Basic Books, 1966).
3. A. R. Luria, *Higher Cortical Functions in Man* (New York: Basic Books, 1966).
4. Ibid.
5. A. Damasio, *Descartes' Error; Emotion, Reason, and the Human Brain* (New York: Putnam Publishing Group, 1994).
6. R. Jorge, R. Robinson, S. Arndt, A. Forrester, F. Geisler, and S. Starkstein, "Comparison between acute- and delayed-onset depression following traumatic brain injury," *J Neuropsychiatry Clin Neurosci* 5 (1993): 43–9.
7. T. D. Wager, J. K. Rilling, E. E. Smith, A. Sokolik, K. L. Casey, R. J. Davidson, S. M. Kosslyn, R. M. Rose, and J. D. Cohen, "Placebo-induced changes in fMRI in the anticipation and experience of pain," *Science* 303 (2004): 1162–7.
8. R. Jorge, R. Robinson, S. Arndt, A. Forrester, F. Geisler, and S. Starkstein, "Comparison between acute- and delayed-onset depression following traumatic brain injury," *J Neuropsychiatry Clin Neurosci* 5 (1993): 43–9; R. E. Jorge and S. E. Starkstein, "Pathophysiologic aspects of major depression following traumatic brain injury," *J Head Trauma Rehabil* 20 (2005): 475–87; H. S. Levin, S. R. McCauley, C. P. Josic, C. Boake, S. A. Brown, H. S. Goodman, S. G. Merritt, and S. I. Brundage, "Predicting depression following mild traumatic brain injury," *Arch Gen Psychiatry* 62 (2005): 523–8.
9. K. S. LaBar and R. Cabeza, "Cognitive neuroscience of emotional memory," *Nat Rev Neurosci* 7 (2006): 54–64.
10. R. Jorge, R. Robinson, S. Arndt, A. Forrester, F. Geisler, and S. Starkstein, "Comparison between acute- and delayed-onset depression following traumatic brain injury," *J Neuropsychiatry Clin Neurosci* 5 (1993): 43–9.
11. M. Koenigs, L. Young, R. Adolphs, D. Tranel, F. Cushman, M. Hauser, and A. Damasio, "Damage to the prefrontal cortex increases utilitarian moral judgements," *Nature* 446 (2007): 908–11.
12. E. Grantham, "Prefrontal lobotomy for relief of pain, with a report of a new operative technique," *J Neurosurg* 8 (1951): 405–10.
13. R. Davidson, (1995). "Cerebral asymmetry, emotion, and affective style," in *Brain Asymmetry*, eds. R. Davidson and K. Hugdahl (Cambridge, MA: MIT Press, 1995): 361–88; T. D. Wager, J. K. Rilling, E. E. Smith, A. Sokolik, K. L. Casey, R. J. Davidson, S. M. Kosslyn, R. M. Rose, and J. D. Cohen, "Placebo-induced changes in fMRI in the anticipation and experience of pain," *Science* 303 (2004): 1162–7.
14. A. G. Sanfey, J. K. Rilling, J. A. Aronson, L. E. Nystrom, and J. D. Cohen, "The neural basis of economic decision-making in the Ultimatum Game," *Science* 300 (2003): 1755–8.
15. D. Knoch, A. Pascual-Leone, K. Meyer, V. Treyer, and E. Fehr, "Diminishing reciprocal fairness by disrupting the right prefrontal cortex," *Science* 314 (2006): 829–32; D. J. de Quervain, U. Fischbacher, V. Treyer, M. Schellhammer, U. Schnyder, A. Buck, and E. Fehr, "The neural basis of altruistic punishment," *Science* 305 (2004): 1254–8.
16. B. E. Depue, T. Curran, and M. T. Banich, "Prefrontal regions orchestrate suppression of emotional memories via a two-phase process," *Science* 317 (2007): 215–9.
17. M. C. Anderson, K. N. Ochsner, B. Kuhl, J. Cooper, E. Robertson, S. W. Gabrieli, G. H. Glover, and J. D. Gabrieli, "Neural systems underlying the suppression of unwanted memories," *Science* 303 (2004): 232–5.

18. M. Koenigs, E. D. Huey, V. Raymont, B. Cheon, J. Solomon, E. M. Wassermann, and J. Grafman, "Focal brain damage protects against post-traumatic stress disorder in combat veterans," *Nat Neurosci* 11 (2008): 232–7.

19. A. Newberg and J. Iversen, "The neural basis of the complex mental task of meditation: neurotransmitter and neurochemical considerations," *Med Hypotheses* 61 (2003): 282–91.

20. N. I. Eisenberger, M. D. Lieberman, and K. D. Williams, "Does rejection hurt? An fMRI study of social exclusion," *Science* 302 (2003): 290–2.

21. M. Koenigs, L. Young, R. Adolphs, D. Tranel, F. Cushman, M. Hauser, and A. Damasio, "Damage to the prefrontal cortex increases utilitarian moral judgements," *Nature* 446 (2007): 908–11.

22. R. Davidson, "Cerebral asymmetry, emotion, and affective style," in *Brain Asymmetry*, eds. R. Davidson and K. Hugdahl (Cambridge, MA, MIT Press, 1995): 361–88.

23. Ibid.

24. R. J. Davidson, K. M. Putnam, and C. L. Larson, "Dysfunction in the neural circuitry of emotion regulation—a possible prelude to violence," *Science* 289 (2000): 591–4.

25. Ibid.

26. S. Maren and G. J. Quirk, "Neuronal signalling of fear memory," *Nat Rev Neurosci* 5 (2004): 844–52.

27. M. G. Baxter and E. A. Murray, "The amygdala and reward," *Nat Rev Neurosci* 3 (2002): 563–73.

28. R. J. Davidson, K. M. Putnam, and C. L. Larson, "Dysfunction in the neural circuitry of emotion regulation—a possible prelude to violence," *Science* 289 (2000): 591–4.

29. Ibid.

30. S. L. Andersen and M. H. Teicher, "Serotonin laterality in amygdala predicts performance in the elevated plus maze in rats," *Neuroreport* 10 (1999): 3497–3500.

31. M. G. Baxter and E. A. Murray, "The amygdala and reward," *Nat Rev Neurosci* 3 (2002): 563–73; I. G. Dobbins, D. M. Schnyer, M. Verfaellie, and D. L. Schacter, "Cortical activity reductions during repetition priming can result from rapid response learning," *Nature* 428 (2004): 316–9.

32. D. Mobbs, P. Petrovic, J. L. Marchant, D. Hassabis, N. Weiskopf, B. Seymour, R. J. Dolan, and C. D. Frith, "When fear is near: threat imminence elicits prefrontal-periaqueductal gray shifts in humans," *Science* 317 (2007): 1079–83.

33. E. Goldberg, *The Wisdom Paradox: How Your Mind Can Grow Stronger as Your Brain Grows Older* (New York: Gotham Books, 2005).

34. T. Sharot, A. M. Riccardi, C. M. Raio, and E. A. Phelps, "Neural mechanisms mediating optimism bias," *Nature* 450 (2007): 102–5.

35. K. S. LaBar and R. Cabeza, "Cognitive neuroscience of emotional memory," *Nat Rev Neurosci* 7 (2006): 54–64; T. Sharot, A. M. Riccardi, C. M. Raio, and E. A. Phelps, "Neural mechanisms mediating optimism bias," *Nature* 450 (2007): 102–5.

36. E. Goldberg, *The Wisdom Paradox: How Your Mind Can Grow Stronger as Your Brain Grows Older* (New York: Gotham Books, 2005).

37. M. Pessiglione, B. Seymour, G. Flandin, R. J. Dolan, and C. D. Frith, "Dopamine-dependent prediction errors underpin reward-seeking behaviour in humans," *Nature* 442 (2006): 1042–5.

38. M. J. Frank, L. C. Seeberger, and C. O'Reilly R, "By carrot or by stick: cognitive reinforcement learning in parkinsonism," *Science* 306 (2004): 1940–3.

39. M. G. Baxter and E. A. Murray, "The amygdala and reward," *Nat Rev Neurosci* 3 (2002): 563–73.

Chapter 9: Different Lobes for Different Folks: Decision-Making Styles and the Frontal Lobes

1. J. Talairach and P. Tournoux, *Co-planar Stereotaxic Atlas of the Human Brain* (New York: Thieme, 1988).
2. R. P. Ebstein, O. Novick, R. Umansky, B. Priel, Y. Osher, D. Blaine, E. R. Bennett, L. Nemanov, M. Katz, and R. H. Belmaker, "Dopamine D4 receptor (D4DR) exon III polymorphism associated with the human personality trait of novelty seeking," *Nat Genet* 12 (1996): 78–80.
3. D. M. Amodio, J. T. Jost, S. L. Master, and C. M. Yee, "Neurocognitive correlates of liberalism and conservatism," *Nat Neurosci* 10 (2007): 1246–7.
4. E. Goldberg, R. Harner, M. Lovell, K. Podell, and S. Riggio, "Cognitive bias, functional cortical geometry, and the frontal lobes: laterality, sex, and handedness," *J Cogn Neurosci* 6 (1994): 276–96.
5. M. LeMay, "Morphological cerebral asymmetries of modern man, fossil man, and nonhuman primate," *Ann N Y Acad Sci* 280 (1976): 349–66.
6. M. C. Diamond, "Rat forebrain morphology: right–left; male–female; young–old; enriched–impoverished," in *Cerebral Laterality in Nonhuman Species*, ed. S. D. Glick (New York: Academic Press, 1985); M. C. Diamond, G. A. Dowling, and R. E. Johnson, "Morphologic cerebral cortical asymmetry in male and female rats," *Exp Neurol* 71 (1981): 261–8; S. D. Glick, R. C. Meibach, R. D. Cox, and S. Maayani, "Multiple and interrelated functional asymmetries in rat brain," *Life Sci* 25 (1979): 395–400; S. D. Glick, D. A. Ross, and L. B. Hough, "Lateral asymmetry of neurotransmitters in human brain," *Brain Res* 234 (1982): 53–63.
7. J. M. Allman, A. Hakeem, J. M. Erwin, E. Nimchinsky, and P. Hof, "The anterior cingulate cortex. The evolution of an interface between emotion and cognition," *Ann N Y Acad Sci* 935 (2001): 107–17.
8. S. D. Glick, D. A. Ross, and L. B. Hough, "Lateral asymmetry of neurotransmitters in human brain," *Brain Res* 234 (1982): 53–63; S. Sandu, P. Cook, and M. C. Diamond, "Rat cortical ostrogen receptors: male–female, right–left," *Exp Neurol* 92 (1985): 186–96.
9. S. D. Glick, D. A. Ross, and L. B. Hough, "Lateral asymmetry of neurotransmitters in human brain," *Brain Res* 234 (1982): 53–63.
10. E. Goldberg, K. Podell, R. Bilder, and J. Jaeger, *Executive Control Battery (ECB)* (Melbourne, Australia: Psych Press, 2000).
11. E. Goldberg, K. Podell, and M. Lovell, "Lateralization of frontal lobe functions and cognitive novelty," *J Neuropsychiatry Clin Neurosci* 6 (1994): 371–8; K. Podell, M. Lovell, M. Zimmerman, and E. Goldberg, "The Cognitive Bias Task and lateralized frontal lobe functions in males", *J Neuropsychiatry Clin Neurosci* 7 (1995): 491–501.
12. R. K. Heaton, G. J. Chelune, J. L. Talley, G. G. Kay, and G. Curtiss, *Wisconsin Card Sorting Test Manual* (Odessa, FL: Psychological Assessment Resources, 1993).
13. For review see E. Goldberg, R. Harner, M. Lovell, K. Podell, and S. Riggio, "Cognitive bias, functional cortical geometry, and the frontal lobes: laterality, sex, and handedness," *J Cogn Neurosci* 6 (1994): 276–96; S. Springer and G. Deutsch, *Left Brain, Right Brain: Perspective from Cognitive Neuroscience*, 5th ed. (New York: W. H. Freeman & Co: 1997); D. W. Lewis and M. C. Diamond, "The influence of the gonadal steroids on the assymetry of the cerebral cortex," in *Brain Assymetry*, eds. R. J. Davidson and K. Hugdahl (Cambridge, MA: MIT Press, 1995): 31–50.
14. K. S. Kendler and D. Walsh, "Gender and schizophrenia: results of an epidemiologically based family study," *Br J Psychiatry* 167 (1995): 184–92.
15. E. Shapiro, A. K. Shapiro, and J. Clarkin, "Clinical psychological testing in Tourette's syndrome," *J Pers Assess* 38 (1974): 464–78.

16. S. L. Andersen and M. H. Teicher, "Sex differences in dopamine receptors and their relevance to ADHD," *Neurosci Biobehav Rev* 24 (2000): 137–41.

17. S. K. Min, S. K. An, D. I. Jon, and J. D. Lee, "Positive and negative symptoms and regional cerebral perfusion in antipsychotic-naive schizophrenic patients: a high-resolution SPECT study," *Psychiatry Res* 90 (1999): 159–68; R. E. Gur, S. M. Resnick, and R. C. Gur, "Laterality and frontality of cerebral blood flow and metabolism in schizophrenia: relationship to symptom specificity," *Psychiatry Res* 27 (1989): 325–34.

18. P. Flor-Henry, "The obsessive-compulsive syndrome: reflection of fronto-caudate dysregulation of the left hemisphere?" *Encephale* 16 (special issue) (1990): 325–9.

19. L. Baving, M. Laucht, and M. H. Schmidt, "Atypical frontal brain activation in ADHD: preschool and elementary school boys and girls," *J Am Acad Child Adolesc Psychiatry* 38 (1999): 1363–71.

20. E. Goldberg, R. Harner, M. Lovell, K. Podell, and S. Riggio, "Cognitive bias, functional cortical geometry, and the frontal lobes: laterality, sex, and handedness," *J Cogni Neurosci* 6 (1994): 276–96.

21. D. Kimura, "Sex differences in cerebral organization for speech and praxic functions," *Can J Psychol* 37 (1983): 19–35.

22. F. B. Wood, D. L. Flowers, and C. E. Naylor, "Cerebral laterality in functional neuroimaging," in *Cerebral Laterality: Theory and Research. The Toledo Symposium*, ed. F. L. Kittle (Hillsdale, NJ: Lawrence Erlbaum Associates, 1991), 103–15.

23. B. A. Shaywitz, S. E. Shaywitz, K. R. Pugh, R. T. Constable, P. Skudlarski, R. K. Fulbright, R. A. Bronen, J. M. Fletcher, D. P. Shankweiler, and L. Katz, "Sex differences in the functional organization of the brain for language," *Nature* 373(6515) (1995): 607–9.

24. S. F. Witelson, "The brain connection: the corpus callosum is larger in left-handers," *Science* 229 (1985): 665–8; M. Habib, D. Gayraud, A. Oliva, J. Regis, G. Salamon, and R. Khalil, "Effects of handedness and sex on the morphology of the corpus callosum: a study with brain magnetic resonance imaging," *Brain Cogn* 16 (1991): 41–61.

25. J. Harasty, K. L. Double, G. M. Halliday, J. J. Krill, and D. A. McRitchie, "Language-associated cortical regions are proportionally larger in the female brain," *Arch Neurol* 54 (1997): 171–6; J. Harasty, "Language processing in both sexes: evidence from brain studies," *Brain* 123 (2000): 404–6.

26. M. Mishkin and K. H. Pribram, "Analysis of the effects of frontal lesions in monkeys: I. Variations of delayed alterations," *J Comp Physiol Psychol* 48 (1955): 492–5; M. Mishkin and K. H. Pribram, "Analysis of the effects of frontal lesions in the monkey: II. Variations of delayed response," *J Comp Physiol Psychol* 49 (1956): 36–40.

27. E. Goldberg, R. Harner, M. Lovell, K. Podell, and S. Riggio, "Cognitive bias, functional cortical geometry, and the frontal lobes: laterality, sex, and handedness," *J Cogn Neurosci* 6 (1994): 276–96.

28. J. Bradshaw and L. Rogers, *The Evolution of Lateral Assymetries, Language, Tool Use, and Intellect* (San Diego: Academic Press, 1993).

29. M. D. Diaz Palarea, M. C. Gonzalez, and M. Rodriguez, "Behavioral lateralization in the T-maze and monoaminergic brain asymmetries," *Physiol Behav* 40 (1987): 785–9.

30. S. Springer and G. Deutsch, *Left Brain, Right Brain: Perspective from Cognitive Neuroscience*, 5th ed. (New York: W. H. Freeman & Co., 1997).

31. Ibid.

32. Mortimer Mishkin, personal communication, 1994.

33. J. D. Wallis, K. C. Anderson, and E. K. Miller, "Single neurons in prefrontal cortex encode abstract rules," *Nature* 411 (2001): 953–6.

34. E. Goldberg, R. Harner, M. Lovell, K. Podell, and S. Riggio, "Cognitive bias, functional cortical geometry, and the frontal lobes: laterality, sex, and handedness," *J Cogn Neurosci* 6 (1994): 276–96.

35. R. P. Ebstein, O. Novik, R. Umansky, B. Priez, Y. Osher, D. Blaine, E. R. Bennett, L. Nemanov, M. Katz, and R. M. Bellmaker, "Dopamine D4 receptor (D4DR) exon III polymorphism associated with the human personality trait of novelty seeking," *Nat Genet* 12 (1996): 78–80; J. Benjamin, L. Li, C. Patterson, B. D. Greenberg, D. L. Murphy, and D. H. Hamer, "Population and familial association between the D4 dopamine receptor gene and measures of novelty seeking," *Nat Genet* 12 (1996): 81–4.

36. J. W. Dalley, T. D. Fryer, L. Brichard, E. S. Robinson, D. E. Theobald, K. Laane, et al., "Nucleus accumbens D2/3 receptors predict trait impulsivity and cocaine reinforcement," *Science* 315 (2007): 1267–70.

37. A. Koestler, *The Thirteenth Tribe* (New York: Random House, 1976).

38. D. L. Orsini and P. Satz, "A syndrome of pathological left-handedness: correlates of early left hemisphere injury," *Arch Neurol* 43 (1986): 333–7; P. Satz, P. Cook, and M. C. Diamond, "The pathological left-handedness syndrome," *Brain Cogn* 4 (1985): 27–46.

39. G. Rajkowska and P. S. Goldman-Rakic, "Cytoarchitectonic definition of prefrontal areas in the normal human cortex: II. Variability in locations of areas 9 and 46 and relationship to the Talairach Coordinate System," *Cereb Cortex* 5 (1995): 323–7; G. Rajkowska and P. S. Goldman-Rakic, "Cytoarchitectonic definition of prefrontal areas in the normal human cortex: I. Remapping of areas 9 and 46 using quantitative criteria," *Cereb Cortex* 5 (1995): 307–22.

40. H. E. Gardner, *Multiple Intelligences. The Theory in Practice* (New York: Basic Books, 1993).

41. D. Goleman, *Emotional Intelligence* (New York: Bantam Books, 1997).

42. S. J. Gould, *The Mismeasure of Man* (New York: W. W. Norton, 1981).

43. S. F. Witelson, D. L. Kigar, and T. Harvey, "The exceptional brain of Albert Einstein," *Lancet* 353(9170) (1999): 2149–53.

44. C. D. Frith and U. Frith, "Interacting minds: a biological basis," *Science* 286 (5445) (1999): 1692–5.

45. Ibid.

46. G. G. Gallup Jr., "Absence of self-recognition in a monkey (*Macaca fascicularis*) following prolonged exposure to a mirror," *Dev Psychobiol* 10 (1977): 281–4; M. D. Hauser, J. Kralik, C. Botto-Mahan, M. Garrett, and J. Oser, "Self-recognition in primates: phylogeny and the salience of species-typical features," *Proc Natl Acad Sci USA* 92 (1995): 10811–4.

47. M. D. Hauser, J. Kralik, C. Botto-Mahan, M. Garrett, and J. Oser, "Self-recognition in primates: phylogeny and the salience of species-typical features," *Proc Natl Acad Sci USA* 92 (1995): 10811–4.

48. C. D. Frith and U. Frith, "Interacting minds: a biological basis," *Science* 286(5445) (1999): 1692–5.

49. J. Jaynes, *The Origin of Consciousness in the Breakdown of the Bicameral Mind* (New York: Houghton Mifflin, 1990).

50. Ibid.

Chapter 10: When the Leader Is Wounded

1. A. Damasio, *Descartes' Error; Emotion, Reason, and the Human Brain* (New York: Putnam Publishing Group, 1994).

2. E. Goldberg, "Introduction: the frontal lobes in neurological and psychiatric conditions," *Neuropsychiatry Neuropsychol Behav Neurol* 5 (1992): 231–2.

3. Ibid.
4. A. Lilja, S. Hagstadius, J. Risberg, L. G. Salford, and G. J. W. Smith, "Frontal lobe dynamics in brain tumor patients: a study of regional cerebral blood flow and affective changes before and after surgery," *J Neuropsychiatry Neuropsychol Behav Neurol* 5, n4 (1992): 294–300.
5. M. S. Nobler, H. A. Sakheim, I. Prohovnik, J. R. Moeller, S. Mukherjee, D. B. Schur, J. Prudic, and D. P. Devanand, "Regional cerebral blood flow in mood disorders: III. Treatment and clinical response," *Arch Gen Psychiatry* 51 (1994): 884–97.
6. J. Risberg, "Regional cerebral blood flow measurements by ^{133}Xe-inhalation: methodology and applications in neuropsychology and psychiatry," *Brain Lang* 9 (1980): 9–34.
7. W. G. Honer, I. Prohovnik, G. Smith, and L. R. Lucas, "Scopolamine reduces frontal cortex perfusion," *J Cereb Blood Flow Metab* 8 (1988): 635–41.
8. E. Goldberg, A. Kluger, T. Griesing, L. Malta, M. Shapiro, and S. Ferris, "Early diagnosis of frontal-lobe dementias," presented at the Eighth Congress of the International Psychogeriatric Association, August, 17–22, 1997, Jerusalem, Israel.
9. E. Goldberg, "Introduction: the frontal lobes in neurological and psychiatric conditions," *Neuropsychiatry Neuropsychol, Behav Neurol* 5 (1992): 231–2.
10. J. H. Jackson, "Evolution and dissolution of the nervous system," *Croonian Lecture. Selected Papers* 2 (1884).
11. A. R. Luria, *Higher Cortical Functions in Man* (New York: Basic Books, 1966).
12. E. Goldberg and L. D. Costa, "Qualitative indices in neuropsychological assessment: an extension of Luria's approach to executive deficit following prefrontal lesion," in *Neuropsychological Assessment of Neuropsychiatric Disorders*, eds. I. Grant and K. M. Adams (New York: Oxford University Press, 1985), 48–64.
13. See K. Heilman and E. Valenstein, eds., *Clinical Neuropsychology* (New York: Oxford University Press, 1993).
14. E. Moniz, "Essai d'un traitement chirurgical de certaines psychoses," *Bull Acad Natl Med* 115 (1936): 385–92.
15. See K. Heilman and E. Valenstein, eds., *Clinical Neuropsychology* (New York: Oxford University Press, 1993).
16. Dr. Robert Iacono, personal communication, January 2000.
17. C. S. Carter, M. M. Botvinick, and J. D. Cohen, "The contribution of the anterior cingulate cortex to executive processes in cognition," *Rev Neurosci* 10 (1999): 49–57.
18. A. Ploghaus, I. Tracey, J. S. Gati, S. Clare, R. S. Menon, P. M. Matthews, and J. N. Rawlings, "Dissociating pain from its anticipation in the human brain," *Science* 284(5422) (1999): 1979–81.
19. T. D. Wager, J. K. Rilling, E. E. Smith, A. Sokolik, K. L. Casey, R. J. Davidson, S. M. Kosslyn, R. M. Rose, and J. D. Cohen, "Placebo-induced changes in fMRI in the anticipation and experience of pain," *Science* 303 (2004): 1162–7.
20. Ibid.
21. T. Singer, B. Seymour, J. O'Doherty, H. Kaube, R. J. Dolan, and C. D. Frith, "Empathy for pain involves the affective but not sensory components of pain," *Science* 303 (2004): 1157–62.
22. N. I. Eisenberger, M. D. Lieberman, and K. D. Williams, "Does rejection hurt? An fMRI study of social exclusion," *Science* 302 (2003): 290–2.
23. N. Fujii and A. M. Graybiel, "Representation of action sequence boundaries by macaque prefrontal cortical neurons," *Science* 301 (2003): 1246–9.
24. P. Mychack, J. H. Kramer, K. B. Boone, and B. L. Miller, "The influence of right frontotemporal dysfunction on social behavior in frontotemporal dementia," *Neurology* 56 (2001): 11S-15S.

25. D. H. Ingvar, "'Memory of the future: an essay on the temporal organization of conscious awareness," *Hum Neurobiol* 4 (1985): 127–36.
26. P. H. Rudebeck, M. J. Buckley, M. E. Walton, and M. F. Rushworth, "A role for the macaque anterior cingulate gyrus in social valuation," *Science* 313 (2006): 1310–2.
27. S. M. McClure, D. I. Laibson, G. Loewenstein, and J. D. Cohen, "Separate neural systems value immediate and delayed monetary rewards," *Science* 306 (2004): 503–7.
28. R. N. Cardinal, D. R. Pennicott, C. L. Sugathapala, T. W. Robbins, and B. J. Everitt, "Impulsive choice induced in rats by lesions of the nucleus accumbens core," *Science* 292 (2001): 2499–501.
29. From E. Goldberg and L. D. Costa, "Qualitative indices in neuropsychological assessment: an extension of Luria's approach to executive deficit following prefrontal lesion," in *Neuropsychological Assessment of Neuropsychiatric Disorders*, eds. I. Grant and K. M. Adams (New York: Oxford University Press, 1985), 55.
30. F. Lhermitte, "Utilization behavior and its relationship to lesions of the frontal lobes," *Brain* 106 (1983): 237–55.
31. For more detailed description see M. D. Lezak, *Neuropsychological Assessment*, 3rd ed. (New York: Oxford University Press, 1995).
32. P. Goldman-Rakic, personal communication, February 1991.
33. K. Brodmann, "Neue Ergebnisse über die vergleichende histologische Lokalisation der Grosshirnrinde mit besonderer Berücksichtigung des Stirnhirns," *Anat Anz* 41 (1912; Suppl): 157–216. Cited in J. M. Fuster, *The Prefrontal Cortex: Anatomy, Physiology, and Neuropsychology of the Frontal Lobe*, 3rd ed. (Philadelphia: Lippincott–Raven, 1997).
34. R. A. Barkley, *ADHD and the Nature of Self-Control* (New York: Guilford Press, 1997).
35. J. W. de Fockert, G. Rees, C. D. Frith, and N. Lavie, "The role of working memory in visual selective attention," *Science* 291 (2001): 1803–6.
36. S. L. Rauch, M. A. Jenike, N. M. Alpert, L. Baer, H. G. Breiter, C. R. Savage, and A. J. Fischman, "Regional cerebral blood flow measured during symptom provocation in obsessive-compulsive disorder using oxygen 15 labeled carbon dioxide and positron emission tomography," *Arch Gen Psychiatry* 51 (1994): 62–70.
37. A. R. Luria, *Higher Cortical Functions in Man* (New York: Basic Books, 1966).
38. E. Goldberg and D. Tucker, "Motor perseverations and long-term memory for visual forms," *J Clin Neuropsychol* 1 (1979): 273–88.
39. J. B. Rowe, I. Toni, O. Josephs, R. S. Frackowiak, and R. E. Passingham, "The prefrontal cortex: response selection or maintenance within working memory?" *Science* 288 (2000): 1656–60.
40. H. Tomita, M. Ohbayashi, K. Nakahara, I. Hasegawa, and Y. Miyashita, "Top-down signal from prefrontal cortex in executive control of memory retrieval," *Nature* 401 (1999): 699–703.
41. D. A. Grant and E. A. Berg, "A behavioral analysis of degree of reinforcement and ease of shifting to new responses in a Weigl-type card-sorting problem," *J Exp Psychol* 38 (1948): 404–11.
42. K. Nakahara, T. Hayashi, S. Konishi, and Y. Miyashita, "Functional MRI of macaque monkeys performing a cognitive set-shifting task," *Science* 295 (2002): 1532–6.
43. For review see K. Heilman and E. Valenstein, eds., *Clinical Neuropsychology* (New York: Oxford University Press, 1993).
44. E. Goldberg and W. B. Barr, "Three possible mechanisms of unawareness deficit," in *Awareness of Deficit after Brain Injury*, eds. G. Prigatano and D. Schacter (New York: Oxford University Press, 1991), 152–75.
45. Ibid.

46. K. R. Ridderinkhof, M. Ullsperger, E. A. Crone, and S. Nieuwenhuis, "The role of the medial frontal cortex in cognitive control," *Science* 306 (2004): 443–7.
47. A. W. MacDonald, 3rd, J. D. Cohen, V. A. Stenger, and C. S. Carter, "Dissociating the role of the dorsolateral prefrontal and anterior cingulate cortex in cognitive control," *Science* 288 (2000): 1835–8.

Chapter 11: Social Maturity, Morality, Law, and the Frontal Lobes

1. H. Oppenheim, "Zur Pathologie der Grosshirngeschwulste," *Arch Psychiatry* 21 (1889): 560.
2. L. Tremblay and W. Schultz, "Relative reward preference in primate orbitofrontal cortex," *Nature* 398 (1999): 704–8.
3. B. De Martino, D. Kumaran, B. Seymour, and R. J. Dolan, "Frames, biases, and rational decision-making in the human brain," *Science* 313 (2006): 684–7.
4. M. Koenigs, E. D. Huey, V. Raymont, B. Cheon, J. Solomon, E. M. Wassermann, and J. Grafman, "Focal brain damage protects against post-traumatic stress disorder in combat veterans," *Nat Neurosci* 11 (2008): 232–7.
5. A. Schore, *Affect Regulation and the Origin of the Self: The Neurobiology of Emotional Development* (Hillsdale, NJ: Lawrence Erlbaum Associates, 1999).
6. K. Shima, M. Isoda, H. Mushiake, and J. Tanji, "Categorization of behavioural sequences in the prefrontal cortex," *Nature* 445 (2007): 315–8.
7. S. W. Anderson, A. Bechara, H. Damasio, D. Tranel, and A. R. Damasio, "Impairment of social and moral behavior related to early damage in human prefrontal cortex," *Nat Neurosci* 2 (1999): 1032–7.
8. M. Koenigs, L. Young, R. Adolphs, D. Tranel, F. Cushman, M. Hauser, and A. Damasio, "Damage to the prefrontal cortex increases utilitarian moral judgements," *Nature* 446 (2007): 908–11.
9. G. Miller, "Neurobiology: the roots of morality," *Science* 320 (2008): 734–7.
10. M. Koenigs, L. Young, R. Adolphs, D. Tranel, F. Cushman, M. Hauser, and A. Damasio, "Damage to the prefrontal cortex increases utilitarian moral judgements," *Nature* 446 (2007): 908–11; D. Talmi and C. Frith, "Neurobiology: feeling right about doing right," *Nature* 446 (2007): 865–6.
11. M. I. Posner and M. K. Rothbart, "Attention, self-regulation and consciousness," *Philos Trans R Soc Lond B Biol Sci* 353(1377) (1998): 1915–27.
12. S. Ito, V. Stuphorn, J. W. Brown, and J. D. Schall, "Performance monitoring by the anterior cingulate cortex during saccade countermanding," *Science* 302 (2003): 120–2.
13. P. H. Rudebeck, M. J. Buckley, M. E. Walton, and M. F. Rushworth, "A role for the macaque anterior cingulate gyrus in social valuation," *Science* 313 (2006): 1310–2.
14. K. Matsumoto, W. Suzuki, and K. Tanaka, "Neuronal correlates of goal-based motor selection in the prefrontal cortex," *Science* 301 (2003): 229–32.
15. D. C. Turner, M. R. Aitken, D. R. Shanks, B. J. Sahakian, T. W. Robbins, C. Schwartzbauer, et al., "The role of the lateral frontal cortex in causal associative learning: exploring preventative and super-learning," *Cereb Cortex*, 14(8) (2004): 872–80.
16. W. T. Fitch and M. D. Hauser, "Computational constraints on syntactic processing in a nonhuman primate," *Science*, 303 (2004): 377–80.
17. N. Camille, G. Coricelli, J. Sallet, P. Pradat-Diehl, J. R. Duhamel, and A. Sirigu, "The involvement of the orbitofrontal cortex in the experience of regret," *Science* 304(5674) (2005): 1167–70.
18. P. I. Yakovlev and A. R. Lecours, "The myelogenetic cycles of regional maturation of the brain," in *Regional Development of the Brain in Early Life*, ed. A. Minkowski (Oxford: Blackwell, 1967), 3–70.

19. F. I. M. Craik and E. Bialystok, "Cognition through the lifespan: mechanisms of change," *Trends Cogn Sci* 10 (2006): 131–8.
20. K. Powell, "Neurodevelopment: how does the teenage brain work?" *Nature* 442 (2006): 865–7.
21. Ibid.
22. W. Golding, *Lord of the Flies*, rpt (Mattituck, NY: Amereon House, 1999).
23. J. Volavka, *Neurobiology of Violence* (Washington, DC: American Psychiatric Press, 1995); A. Raine, *The Psychopathology of Crime: Criminal Behavior as a Clinical Disorder* (San Diego: Academic Press, 1993).
24. E. Goldberg, R. M. Bilder, J. E. Hughes, S. P. Antin, and S. Mattis, "A reticulo-frontal disconnection syndrome," *Cortex* 25 (1989): 687–95.
25. A. Raine, M. Buchsbaum, and L. LaCasse, "Brain abnormalities in murderers indicated by positron emission tomography," *Biol Psychiatry* 42 (1997): 495–508.
26. A. Raine, T. Lencz, S. Bihrle, L. LaCasse, and P. Colletti, "Reduced prefrontal gray matter volume and reduced autonomic activity in antisocial personality disorder," *Arch Gen Psychiatry* 57 (2000): 119–27; discussion 128–9.
27. A. R. Luria, *Higher Cortical Functions in Man* (New York: Basic Books, 1966).
28. E. Goldberg, K. Podell, R. Bilder, and J. Jaeger, *The Executive Control Battery* (Melbourne, Australia: Psych Press, 2000); E. Goldberg, K. Podell, R. Bilder, and J. Jaeger, *Test for Bedomning av Exekutive Dysfunktion*, (Stockholm, Sweden: Psykologiforlaget AB, 1997).
29. For test description see M. D. Lezak, *Neuropsychological Assessment*, 3rd ed. (New York: Oxford University Press, 1995).
30. O. W. Sacks, *The Man Who Mistook His Wife for a Hat: And Other Clinical Tales* (New York: Touchstone Books, 1998).
31. E. Goldberg, *The Wisdom Paradox: How Your Mind Can Grow Stronger as Your Brain Grows Older* (New York: Gotham Books, 2005)
32. A. Snyder, *What Makes a Champion! Fifty Extraordinary Individuals Share Their Insights* (New York: Penguin Books, 2002).

Chapter 12: Fateful Disconnections

1. N. Geshwind, "Disconnexion syndromes in animals and man," *Brain* 88 (1965): 237–94.
2. S. J. Gould, *The Mismeasure of Man* (New York: W. W. Norton, 1981).
3. A. Parent, *Carpenter's Human Neuroanatomy*, 9th ed. (Baltimore: Williams & Wilkins, 1995).
4. E. Goldberg, R. M. Bilder, J. E. Hughes, S. P. Antin, and S. Mattis, "A reticulo-frontal disconnection syndrome," *Cortex* 25 (1989): 687–95.
5. E. K. Miller, "The prefrontal cortex and cognitive control," *Nat Rev Neurosci* 1 (2000): 59–65.
6. E. Goldberg, *The Wisdom Paradox: How Your Mind Can Grow Stronger as Your Brain Grows Older* (New York: Gotham Books, 2005).
7. E. Goldberg, S. P. Antin, R. M. Bilder Jr., L. J. Gerstman, J. E. Hughes, and S. Mattis, "Retrograde amnesia: possible role of mesencephalic reticular activation in long-term memory," *Science* 213(4514) (1981): 1392–4.
8. For review see H. S. Nasrallah, ed., *Handbook of Schizophrenia* (New York: Elsevier, 1991).
9. E. Kraepelin, *Dementia Praecox and Paraphrenia* (Edinburgh: E. S Livingstone, 1919/1971), Vol. 4, p. 219.
10. K. F. Berman, R. F. Zec, and D. R. Weinberger, "Physiologic dysfunction of dorsolateral prefrontal cortex in schizophrenia: II. Role of neuroleptic treatment, attention, and mental

effort," *Arch Gen Psychiatry* 43 (1986): 126–35; D. R. Weinberger, K. F. Berman, and R. F. Zec, "Physiologic dysfunction of dorsolateral prefrontal cortex in schizophrenia: I. Regional cerebral blood flow evidence," *Arch Gen Psychiatry* 43 (1986): 114–24.

11. B. Milner, "Effects of different brain lesions in card sorting: the role of the frontal lobes," *Arch Neurol* 9 (1963): 100–10; D. R. Weinberger, K. F. Berman, and R. F. Zec, "Physiologic dysfunction of dorsolateral prefrontal cortex in schizophrenia: I. Regional cerebral blood flow evidence," *Arch Gen Psychiatry* 43 (1986): 114–24.

12. G. Franzen and D. H. Ingvar, "Absence of activation in frontal structures during psychological testing of chronic schizophrenics," *J Neurol Neurosurg Psychiatry* 38 (1975): 1027–32; M. S. Buchsbaum, L. E. DeLisi, H. H. Holcomb, J. Cappelletti, A. C. King, J. Johnson, E. Hazlett, S. Dowling-Zimmerman, R. M. Post, and J. Morihisa, "Anteroposterior gradients in cerebral glucose use in schizophrenia and affective disorders," *Arch Gen Psychiatry* 41 (1984): 1159–66.

13. D. R. Weinberger and K. F. Berman, "Speculation on the meaning of cerebral metabolic hypofrontality in schizophrenia," *Schizophr Bull* 14 (1988): 157–68.

14. E. Valenstein, *The Great and Desperate Cures* (New York: Basic Books, 1986).

15. J. R. Stevens, "An anatomy of schizophrenia?" *Arch Gen Psychiatry* 29 (1973): 177–89; S. Matthysse, "Dopamine and the pharmacology of schizophrenia: the state of the evidence," *J Psychiatr Res* 11 (1974): 107–13; D. A. Lewis, T. Hashimoto, and D. W. Volk, "Cortical inhibitory neurons and schizophrenia," *Nat Rev Neurosci* 6 (2005): 312–24.

16. For review see J. R. Cooper, F. E. Bloom, and R. H. Roth, *The Biochemical Basis of Neuropharmacology*, 7th ed. (New York: Oxford University Press, 1996).

17. M. Carlsson and A. Carlsson, "Schizophrenia: a subcortical neurotransmitter imbalance syndrome?" *Schizophr Bull* 16 (1990): 425–32.

18. For review see J. R. Cooper, F. E. Bloom, and R. H. Roth, *The Biochemical Basis of Neuropharmacology*, 7th ed. (New York: Oxford University Press, 1996).

19. E. S. Gershon and R. O. Rieder, "Major disorders of mind and brain," *Sci Am* 267 (1992): 126–33.

20. B. Kolb and I. Q. Whishaw, *Fundamentals of Human Neuropsychology*, 4th ed. (New York: W. H. Freeman & Co., 1995).

21. E. Goldberg. (1991), "Schizophrenia and stored memories," *Behav Brain Sci* 14 (1991): 30.

22. E. K. Miller, "The prefrontal cortex and cognitive control," *Nat Rev Neurosci* 1 (2000): 59–65; S. Chance, M. M. Esiri, and T. J. Crow, "Macroscopic brain asymmetry is changed along the antero-posterior axis in schizophrenia," *Schizophr Res* 74 (2005): 163–70; T. R. Barricka, C. E. Mackayb, S. Primac, F. Maesd, D. Vandermeulend, T. J. Crowb, and N. Roberts, "Automatic analysis of cerebral asymmetry: an exploratory study of the relationship between brain torque and planum temporale asymmetry," *Neuroimage* 24 (2005): 678–91; S. Silverstein, M. Hatashita-Wong, L. Schenkel, S. Wilkniss, I. Kovacs, A. Feher, et al., "Reduced top-down influences in contour detection in schizophrenia," *Cogn Neuropsychiatry* 11 (2006): 112—32; M. Kim, T. Ha, and J. S. Kwon, "Neurological abnormalities in schizophrenia and obsessive-compulsive disorder," *Curr Opin Psychiatry* 17 (2004): 215–20; T. J. Crow, P. Paez, and S. A. Chance, "Callosal misconnectivity and the sex difference in psychosis," *Int Rev Psychiatry* 19 (2007): 449–57; T. J. Crow, "Nuclear schizophrenic symptoms as a window on the relationship between thought and speech," *Br J Psychiatry* 173 (1998): 303–9; M. Ising, T. Dietl, G. Dirlich, L. Vogl, T. Pollmächer, T. Nickel, et al., "Long-latency somatosensory potentials in high risk probands for affective disorders," *J Psychiatr Res* 38 (2004): 219–21.

23. National Institute of Neurological Disorders and Stroke, *Interagency Head Injury Task Force Report* (Bethesda, MD: National Institutes of Health, 1989).

24. J. C. Masdeu, H. Abdel-Dayem, and R. L. Van Heertum, "Head trauma: use of SPECT," *J Neuroimaging* 5 (1995; Suppl 1): S53–7.

25. J. Burns, D. Job, M. E. Bastin, H. Whalley, T. Macgillivray, E. C. Johnstone, et al., "Structural disconnectivity in schizophrenia: a diffusion tensor magnetic resonance imaging study," *Br J Psychiatry* 182 (2003): 439–43.

26. E. Goldberg and D. Bougakov, "Novel approaches to the diagnosis and treatment of frontal lobe dysfunction," in *International Handbook of Neuropsychological Rehabilitation*, eds. A.-L. Christensen and B. P. Uzzel (New York: Kluwer Academic/Plenum Publishers, 2000), 93–112.

27. Ibid.

28. R. A. Barkley, *ADHD and the Nature of Self-Control* (New York: Guilford Press, 1997).

29. T. Klingberg, *The Overflowing Brain: Information Overload and the Limits of Working Memory* (New York: Oxford, 2008).

30. T. J. Buschman and E. K. Miller, "Top-down versus bottom-up control of attention in the prefrontal and posterior parietal cortices," *Science* 315 (2007): 1860–2.

31. For review of relevant anatatomical structures see A. Parent, *Carpenter's Human Neuroanatomy*, 9th ed. (Baltimore: Williams & Wilkins, 1995). (Revised edition of M. B. Carpenter and J. Satin, *Human Neuroanatomy*, 8th ed., 1983.)

32. T. J. Buschman and E. K. Miller, "Top-down versus bottom-up control of attention in the prefrontal and posterior parietal cortices," *Science* 315 (2007): 1860–2.

33. J. H. Jensen, A. Ramani, H. Lu, and K. Kaczynski, "Diffusional kurtosis imaging: the quantification of non-gaussian water diffusion by means of magnetic resonance imaging," *Magn Reson Med* 53 (2005): 1432–40.

34. From *Possible Poetry*, Toby's unpublished collection of poems written as a teenager on the streets of Sydney. Reprinted with the author's permission.

35. G. G. Tourette, "Étude sur une affection nerveuse caractérisée par de l'incoordination motice accompagnée d'écholalie et de copralalie," *Arch Neurol* 9 (1885).

36. C. W. Bazil, "Seizures in the life and works of Edgar Allan Poe," *Arch Neurol* 56 (1999): 740–3; E. A. Poe, *The Complete Tales and Poems of Edgar Allan Poe* (New York: Barnes & Noble Books, 1989).

37. E. Shapiro, A. K. Shapiro, and J. Clarkin, "Clinical psychological testing in Tourette's syndrome," *J Pers Assess* 38 (1974): 464–78.

38. D. M. Sheppard, J. L. Bradshaw, R. Purcell, and C. Pantelis, "Tourette's and comorbid syndromes: obsessive compulsive and attention deficit hyperactivity disorder. A common etiology?" *Clin Psychol Rev* 19 (1999): 531–52.

39. O. W. Sacks, "Tourette's syndrome and creativity," *BMJ* 305 (1992): 1515–6.

40. J. W. Brown and T. S. Braver, "Learned predictions of error likelihood in the anterior cingulate cortex," *Science* 307 (2005): 1118–21.

41. J. M. Welch, J. Lu, R. M. Rodriguiz, N. C. Trotta, J. Peca, J. Ding, C. Feliciano, M. Chen, J. P. Adams, J. Luo, S. M. Dudek, R. J. Weinberg, N. Calakos, W. C. Wetsel, and G. Feng, "Cortico-striatal synaptic defects and OCD-like behaviours in Sapap3-mutant mice," 448 (2007): 894–900.

42. L. Handler, *Twitch and Shout: A Touretter's Tale* (New York: Plume, 1999).

43. J. Lauwereyns, K. Watanabe, B. Coe, and O. Hikosaka, "A neural correlate of response bias in monkey caudate nucleus," *Nature* 418 (2002): 413–7.

44. F. Lhermitte, "Utilization behavior and its relationship to lesions of the frontal lobes," *Brain* 106 (1983): 237–55.

45. Ibid.

46. N. D. Daw, J. P. O'Doherty, P. Dayan, B. Seymour, and R. J. Dolan, "Cortical substrates for exploratory decisions in humans," *Nature* 441 (2006): 876–9.

47. A. Pasupathy and E. K. Miller, "Different time courses of learning-related activity in the prefrontal cortex and striatum," *Nature* 433 (2005): 873–6.

48. J. LeDoux, *The Emotional Brain: The Mysterious Underpinnings of Emotional Life* (New York: Touchstone Books, 1998).

49. K. Samejima, Y. Ueda, K. Doya, and M. Kimura, "Representation of action-specific reward values in the striatum," *Science* 310 (2005): 1337–40.

50. M. Hsu, M. Bhatt, R. Adolphs, D. Tranel, and C. F. Camerer, "Neural systems responding to degrees of uncertainty in human decision-making," *Science* 310 (2005): 1680–3.

51. D. J. de Quervain, U. Fischbacher, V. Treyer, M. Schellhammer, U. Schnyder, A. Buck, and E. Fehr, "The neural basis of altruistic punishment," *Science* 305 (2004): 1254–8.

52. H. E. Atallah, D. Lopez-Paniagua, J. W. Rudy, and R. C. O'Reilly, "Separate neural substrates for skill learning and performance in the ventral and dorsal striatum," *Nat Neurosci* 10 (2007): 126–31.

53. Ibid.

54. T. D. Barnes, Y. Kubota, D. Hu, D. Z. Jin, and A. M. Graybiel, "Activity of striatal neurons reflects dynamic encoding and recoding of procedural memories," *Nature* 437 (2005): 1158–61.

55. H. H. Yin and B. J. Knowlton, "The role of the basal ganglia in habit formation," *Nat Rev Neurosci* 7 (2006): 464–76.

56. Ibid.

Chapter 13: "What Can You Do for Me?"

1. E. Goldberg, L. J. Gerstman, S. Mattis, J. E. Hughes, C. A. Sirio, and R. M. Bilder Jr., "Selective effects of cholinergic treatment on verbal memory in posttraumatic amnesia," *J Clin Neuropsychol* 4 (1982): 219–34.

2. S. A. Areosa and F. Sherriff, "Memantine for dementia," *Cochrane Database Syst Rev* 3 (2003): CD003154.

3. V. M. Polyakov, L. I. Moskovichyute, and E. G. Simernitskaya, "Neuropsychological analysis of the role in brain functional organization in man," in *Modern Problems in Neurobiology*, ed. (Tbilisi: 1986), 329–30; O. A. Krotkova, T. A. Karaseva, and L. I. Moskovichyute, "Lateralization features of the dynamics of higher mental functions following endonasal glutamic acid electrophoresis," *Zh Vopr Neirokhir Im N N Burdenko*, no. 3 (1982): 48–52; N. K. Korsakova and L. I. Moskovichyute, *Subcortical Structures and Psychological Processes* (Moscow: Moscow University Publishing House, 1985); L. I. Moskovitchyute, M. Mimura, and M. Albert, "Selective effect of dopamine on apraxia," presented at the AAN Annual Meeting, May 1–7, 1994, Washington, D.C.

4. B. H. Dobkin and R. Hanlon, "Dopamine agonist treatment of anterograde amnesia from a mediobasal forebrain injury," *Ann Neurol* 33 (1993): 313–6.

5. D. E. Hobson, E. Pourcher, and W. R. Martin, "Ropinirole and pramipexole, the new agonists," *Can J Neurol Sci* 26 (1999; Suppl 2): S27–33.

6. E. D. Ross and R. M. Stewart, "Akinetic mutism from hypothalamic damage: successful treatment with dopamine agonists," *Neurology* 31 (1981): 1435–39; B. H. Dobkin and R. Hanlon, "Dopamine agonist treatment of antegrade amnesia from a mediobasal forebrain injury," *Ann Neurol* 33 (1993): 313–6.

7. M. F. Kraus and P. Maki, "The combined use of amantadine and L-dopa/carbidopa in the treatment of chronic brain injury," *Brain Inj* 11 (1997): 455–60; M. F. Kraus and P. M. Maki, "Effect of amantadine hydrochloride on symptoms of frontal lobe dysfunction in brain injury: case studies and review," *J Neuropsychiatry Clin Neurosci* 9 (1997): 222–30.

8. J. Wolper, *Schizophrenia could be treated with fewer side effects.* eFlux Media. Retrieved August 30, 2008, from http://www.efluxmedia.com/news_Schizophrenia_Could_Be_Treated_with_Fewer_Side_Effects_08288.html (2007).

9. M. J. Farah, J. Illes, R. Cook-Deegan, H. Gardner, E. Kandel, P. King, E. Parens, B. Sahakian, and P. R. Wolpe, "Neurocognitive enhancement: what can we do and what should we do?" *Nat Rev Neurosci* 5 (2004): 421–5.

10. Memory Pharmaceuticals, *About Us: Scientific Advisory Board.* Retrieved August 30, 2008, from http://www.memorypharma.com/a_advisoryboard.html (2008).

11. B. Sahakian and S. Morein-Zamir, "Professor's little helper," *Nature* 450 (2007): 1157–9.

12. M. E. Rettmann, J. L. Prince, and S. M. Resnick, "Analysis of sulcal shape changes associated with aging," Human Brain Mapping Conference, New York, NY, June 18–23, 2003, #929

13. S. N. Burke and C. A. Barnes, "Neural plasticity in the ageing brain," *Nat Rev Neurosci* 7 (2006): 30–40.

14. M. Ballmaier, M. Kumar, V. Elderkin-Thompson, et al., "Cortical abnormalities in elderly depressed patients," Human Brain Mapping Conference, New York, NY, June 18–23, 2003, #735; S. Grieve, R. Clark, and E. Gordon, "Brain volume and regional tissue distribution in 193 normal subjects using structural MRI: the effect of gender, handedness and age," Human Brain Mapping Conference, New York, NY, June 18–23, 2003, #1203; D. Rex and A. Toga, "Age, gender, and handedness influences on relative tissue volumes in the human brain," Human Brain Mapping Conference, New York, NY, June 18–23, 2003, #930; Y. Taki, R. Goto, et al. (2003). Voxel based morphometry of age-related structural change of gray matter for each decade in normal male subjects," Human Brain Mapping Conference, New York, NY, June 18–23, 2003, #1228.

15. E. Goldberg, *The Wisdom Paradox: How Your Mind Can Grow Stronger as Your Brain Grows Older* (New York: Gotham Books, 2005).

16. Ibid

17. M. E. Rettmann, J. L. Prince, and S. M. Resnick, "Analysis of sulcal shape changes associated with aging, Human Brain Mapping Conference, New York, NY, June 18–23, 2003, #929.

18. S. Grieve, R. Clark, and E. Gordon, "Brain volume and regional tissue distribution in 193 normal subjects using structural MRI: the effect of gender, handedness and age, Human Brain Mapping Conference, New York, NY, June 18–23, 2003, #1203.

19. L. A. Leigland, L. E. Schulz, and J. S. Janowsky, "Age-related changes in emotional memory," *Neurobiol Aging* 25 (2004): 1117–24.

20. Y. Taki, R. Goto, et al., "Voxel based morphometry of age-related structural change of gray matter for each decade in normal male subjects," Human Brain Mapping Conference, New York, NY, June 18–23, 2003, #1228.

21. M. Ballmaier, M. Kumar, V. Elderkin-Thompson, et al., "Cortical abnormalities in elderly depressed patients," Human Brain Mapping Conference, New York, NY, June 18–23, 2003. #735.

22. S. Ramon y Cajal, "Textura del sistema nervioso del hombre y de los vertebrados" (Aragon, Spain: Gobierno de Aragon, Departamento de Educacion y Cultura, 2002).

23. S. A. Goldman and F. Nottebohm, "Neuronal production, migration, and differentiation in a vocal control nucleus of the adult female canary brain," *Proc Natl Acad Sci USA* 80 (1983): 2390–4.

24. J. Altman, "Are new neurons formed in the brains of adult mammals?" *Science* 135 (1962): 1127–8.

25. E. Gould, P. Tanapat, B. S. McEwen, G. Flugge, and E. Fuchs, "Proliferation of granule cell precursors in the dentate gyrus of adult monkeys is diminished by stress," *Proc Natl Acad Sci USA* 95 (1998): 3168–71.

26. E. Gould, A. J. Reeves, M. S. Graziano, and C. G. Gross, "Neurogenesis in the neocortex of adult primates," *Science* 286(5439) (1999): 548–52.

27. P. S. Eriksson, E. Perfilieva, T. Bjork-Eriksson, A. M. Alborn, C. Nordborg, D. A. Peterson, et al., "Neurogenesis in the adult human hippocampus," *Nat Med* 4 (1998): 1313–7.

28. A. Sahay and R. Hen, "Adult hippocampal neurogenesis in depression," *Nat Neurosci* 10 (2007): 1110–5.

29. E. Gould, "How widespread is adult neurogenesis in mammals?" *Nat Rev Neurosci* 8 (2007): 481–8.

30. Ibid.

31. Ibid.

32. R. Katzman, R. Terry, R. DeTeresa, T. Brown, P. Davies, P. Fuld, X. Renbing, and A. Peck, "Clinical, pathological, and neurochemical changes in dementia: a subgroup with preserved mental status and numerous neocortical plaques," *Ann Neurol* 23 (1988): 138–44.

33. J. E. Brody, "Mental reserves keep brains agile," *New York Times* (December 11, 2007): F7.

34. R. Katzman, "Education and the prevalence of dementia and Alzheimer's disease," *Neurology* 43 (1993): 13–20.

35. M. S. Albert, K. Jones, C. R. Savage, L. Berkman, T. Seeman, D. Blazer, and J. W. Rowe, "Predictors of cognitive change in older persons: MacArthur studies of successful aging," *Psychol Aging* 10 (1995): 578–89.

36. D. A. Snowdon, S. J. Kemper, J. A. Mortimer, L. H. Greiner, D. R. Wekstein, and W. R. Markesbery, "Linguistic ability in early life and cognitive function and Alzheimer's disease in late life: findings from the Nun Study [see comments]," *JAMA* 275 (1996): 528–32.

37. Ibid.

38. E. A. Maguire, D. G. Gadian, I. S. Johnsrude, C. D. Good, J. Ashburner, R. S. Frakowiak, and C. D. Frith, "Navigation-related structural change in the hippocampi of taxi drivers," *Proc Natl Acad Sci USA* 97 (2000): 4398–4403.

39. B. L. McNaughton, "Associative pattern competition in hippocampal circuits: new evidence and new questions," *Brain Res Rev* 16 (1991): 202–4; B. L. McNaughton and R. G. M Morris, "Hippocampal synaptic enhancement and information storage," *Trends Neurosci* 10 (1987): 408–15.

40. D. W. Green, J. Crinion, and C. J. Price, "Exploring cross-linguistic vocabulary effects on brain structures using voxel-based morphometry," *Bilingualism: Language and Cognition* 10 (2007): 189–99.

41. P. Schneider, M. Scherg, H. G. Dosch, H. J. Specht, A. Gutschalk, and A. Rupp, "Morphology of Heschl's gyrus reflects enhanced activation in the auditory cortex of musicians," *Nat Neurosci* 5 (2002): 688–94.

42. D. Golden, "Building a better brain," *Life* (July 1994), 62–70.

43. A. Damasio, *Descartes' Error: Emotion, Reason, and the Human Brain* (New York: Putnam Publishing Group, 1994); A. Damasio, *The Feeling of What Happens: Body and Emotion in the Making of Consciousness* (New York: Harcourt Brace, 1999).

44. J. W. Rowe and R. L. Kahn, *Successful Aging* (New York: Pantheon, 1998).

45. R. Katzman, "The prevalence and malignancy of Alzheimer's disease: a major killer," *Arch Neurol* 33 (1976): 217.

46. A. Newell and H. A. Simon, *Human Problem Solving* (Englewood Cliffs, NJ: Prentice-Hall, 1972); H. A. Simon, P. Langley, G. Bradshaw, and J. Zykow, *Scientific Discovery: Exploration of the Creative Process* (Cambridge, MA: MIT Press, 1987).

47. R. J. Hamm, M. D. Temple, D. M. O'Dell, B. R. Pike, and B. G. Lyeth, "Exposure to environmental complexity promotes recovery of cognitive function after traumatic brain injury," *J Neurotrauma* 13 (1996): 41–7.

48. B. Kolb, *Brain Plasticity and Behavior* (Mahwah, NJ: Lawrence Erlbaum Associates, 1995).

49. W. D. Heiss, J. Kessler, R. Mielke, B. Szelies, and K. Herholtz, "Long-term effects of phosphatidylserine, pyritinol, and cognitive training in Alzheimer's disease: a neuropsychological, EEG, and PET investigation," *Dementia* 5 (1994): 88–98.

50. G. Kempermann, H. G. Kuhn, and F. H. Gage, "More hippocampal neurons in adult mice living in an enriched environment," *Nature* 386(6624) (1997): 493–5.

51. Ibid.

52. Ibid.

53. F. Dellu, W. Mayo, M. Valee, M. Le Moaz, and H. Simon, "Facilitation of cognitive performance in aged rats by past experience depends on the type of information processing involved: a combined cross-sectional and longitudinal study," *Neurobiol Learn Mem* 67 (1997): 121–8.

54. N. Milgram, E. Head, S. Zicker, C. Ikeda-Douglas, H. Murphey, B. Muggenburg, et al., "Learning ability in aged beagle dogs is preserved by behavioral enrichment and dietary fortification: a two-year longitudinal study," *Neurobiol Aging* 26 (2005): 77–90.

55. K. W. Schaie and S. L. Willis, "Can decline in adult intellectual functioning be reversed?" *Dev Psychol* 22 (1986): 223.

56. S. L. Willis, S. L. Tennstedt, M. Marsiske, K. Ball, J. Elias, K. M. Koepke, et al., "Long-term effects of cognitive training on everyday functional outcomes in older adults," *JAMA* 296 (2006): 2805–14.

57. H. W. Mahncke, B. B. Connor, J. Appelman, O. N. Ahsanuddin, J. L. Hardy, R. A. Wood, et al., "Memory enhancement in healthy older adults using a brain plasticity-based training program: a randomized, controlled study," *Proc Natl Acad Sci USA* 103 (2006): 12523–8.

58. W. D. Heiss, J. Kessler, R. Mielke, B. Szelies, and K. Herholz, "Long-term effects of phosphatidylserine, pyritinol, and cognitive training in Alzheimer's disease: a neuropsychological, EEG, and PET investigation," *Dementia* 5 (1994): 88–98.

59. M. Mirmiran, E. J. van Someren, and D. F. Swaab, "Is brain plasticity preserved during aging and in Alzheimer's disease?" *Behav Brain Res* 78 (1996): 43–8.

60. S. Aamodt and S. Wang, "Exercise on the brain," *New York Times* (November 8, 2007): A33.

Chapter 14: Breaking and Entering: Inside the Black Box

1. W. S. McCulloch and W. Pitts, "A logical calculus of the ideas immanent in nervous activity. 1943 classical article," *Bull Math Biol* 52 (1990): 99–115.

2. Z. C. Xu, G. Ling, R. N. Sahr, and B. S. Neal-Beliveau, "Asymmetrical changes of dopamine receptors in the striatum after unilateral dopamine depletion," *Brain Res* 1038 (2005): 163–70.

4. Y. Y. Huang and E. R. Kandel, "D1/D5 receptor agonists induce a protein synthesis-dependent late potentiation in the CA1 region of the hippocampus," *Proc Natl Acad Sci USA* 92 (1995): 2446–50.

5. Ibid.

6. S. D. Glick, D. A. Ross, and L. B. Hough, "Lateral asymmetry of neurotransmitters in human brain," *Brain Res* 234 (1982): 53–63.

7. E. Kandel, *In Search of Memory: The Emergence of a New Science of Mind* (W. W. Norton and Company, 2007).

8. A. Hersi, J. Richard, P. Gaudreau, and R. Quirion, "Local modulation of hippocampal acetylcholine release by dopamine D1 receptors: a combined receptor autoradiography and in vivo dialysis study," *J Neurosci* 15 (1995): 7150–7.

9. E. Kandel, personal communication.

10. K. D'Ardenne, S. M. McClure, L. E. Nystrom, and J. D. Cohen, "BOLD responses reflecting dopaminergic signals in the human ventral tegmental area," *Science* 319 (2008): 1264–7.

11. J. J. Day, M. F. Roitman, R. M. Wightman, and R. M. Carelli, "Associative learning mediates dynamic shifts in dopamine signaling in the nucleus accumbens," *Nat Neurosci* 10 (2007): 1020–8.

12. M. Pessiglione, B. Seymour, G. Flandin, R. J. Dolan, and C. D. Frith, "Dopamine-dependent prediction errors underpin reward-seeking behaviour in humans," *Nature* 442 (2006): 1042–5.

13. M. R. Roesch, D. J. Calu, and G. Schoenbaum, "Dopamine neurons encode the better option in rats deciding between differently delayed or sized rewards," *Nat Neurosci* 10 (2007): 1615–24; N. D. Daw, "Dopamine: at the intersection of reward and action," *Nat Neurosci* 10 (2007): 1505–7.

14. M. Matsumoto and O. Hikosaka, "Lateral habenula as a source of negative reward signals in dopamine neurons," *Nature* 447(7148) (2007): 1111–5.

15. K. D'Ardenne, S. M. McClure, L. E. Nystrom, and J. D. Cohen, "BOLD responses reflecting dopaminergic signals in the human ventral tegmental area," *Science* 319 (2008): 1264–7.

16. T. E. Behrens, M. W. Woolrich, M. E. Walton, and M. F. Rushworth, "Learning the value of information in an uncertain world," *Nat Neurosci* 10 (2007): 1214–21.

17. D'Ardenne, S. M. McClure, L. E. Nystrom, and J. D. Cohen, "BOLD responses reflecting dopaminergic signals in the human ventral tegmental area," *Science* 319 (2008): 1264–7; T. E. Behrens, M. W. Woolrich, M. E. Walton, and M. F. Rushworth, "Learning the value of information in an uncertain world," *Nat Neurosci* 10 (2007): 1214–21.

18. J. L. McClelland, B. L. McNaughton, and R. C. O'Reilly, "Why there are complementary learning systems in the hippocampus and neocortex: insights from the successes and failures of connectionist models of learning and memory," *Psychol Rev* 102 (1995): 419–57.

19. Nicholas Myers, personal communication.

20. E. Goldberg, K. Podell, R. Harner, M. Lovell, and S. Riggio. "Cognitive bias, functional cortical geometry, and the frontal lobes: laterality, sex, and handedness." *J Cogn Neurosci* 6 (1994): 274-94.

21. T. E. Behrens, M. W. Woolrich, M. E. Walton, and M. F. Rushworth, "Learning the value of information in an uncertain world," *Nat Neurosci* 10 (2007): 1214–21.

22. T. J. Behrens, L. T. Hunt, M. W. Woolrich, and M. F. Rushworth, "Associative learning of social value." *Nature* 456 (2008): 245–9.

23. S. Fusi, M. Annunziato, D. Badoni, A. Salamon, and D. J. Amit, "Spike-driven synaptic plasticity: theory, simulation, VLSI implementation," *Neural Comp* 12 (2000): 2227–58.

24. J. N. Wood and J. Grafman, "Human prefrontal cortex: processing and representational perspectives," *Nat Rev Neurosci* 4 (2003): 139–47.

25. J. M. Fuster, *Memory in the Cerebral Cortex: An Empirical Approach to Neural Networks in the Human and Nonhuman Primate*, 3rd ed. (Cambridge, MA: MIT, 1999).

26. J. S. Simons and H. J. Spiers, "Prefrontal and medial temporal lobe interactions in long-term memory," *Nat Rev Neurosci* 4 (2003): 637–48.

Chapter 15: Frontal Lobes and the Leadership Paradox

1. S. Nunn and A. N. Stulberg, "The many faces of modern Russia," *Foreign Affairs* 79, no. 2 (2000): 45–62.
2. M. Simons, "In new Europe, a lingual hodgepodge," *The New York Times* (October 17, 1999): A4.
3. G. Alperovich, "California split: divide, or die; help democracy, divide up the US," *New York Times* (February 10, 2007): A10.
4. N. Ferguson, *The War of the World: Twentieth Century Conflict and the Descent of the West* (New York: Penguin Press, 2006).
5. K. Ohmae, *The End of the Nation State: The Rise of Regional Economies* (New York: Free Press, 1995).
6. P. Lewis, "As nations shed roles, is medieval the future?" *The New York Times* (January 2, 1999): B7, B9.
7. R. D. Kaplan, *Coming Anarchy: Shattering the Dreams of the Post Cold War* (New York: Random House, 2000).
8. S. J. Kobrin, "Back to the future: neo-medievalism and post-modern digital world," *Journal of International Affairs* 51, no. 2 (1998): 361–86.
9. W. S. McCulloch and W. Pitts, "A logical calculus of the ideas immanent in nervous activity: 1943 classical article," *Bull Math Biol* 52 (1990): 99–115.
10. R. D. Kaplan, *Coming Anarchy: Shattering the Dreams of the Post Cold War* (New York: Random House, 2000).
11. E. D. Tucker, ed., *The Marx-Engels Reader*, 2nd ed. (New York: W. W. Norton, 1978). As an ideological slogan in the old Soviet Union, this phrase acquired a distinctly sadistic twist, vaguely akin to "Arbeit Macht Frei" (German for "work liberates," a sign on the gates of Auschwitz). In 1968, the year of the suppressed Prague Spring, a grim joke circulated around Moscow that then-president of Czechoslovakia, General Svoboda ("svoboda" meaning "freedom" in Russian), had been renamed General Poznannaya Neobhodimostj ("General Recognized Necessity").

Chapter 16: Epilogue

1. B. Spinoza, *Ethics*, trans. A. Boyle (London: Everyman, 1997).
2. Ibid.
3. W. S. McCulloch and W. Pitts, "A logical calculus of the ideas immanent in nervous activity: 1943 classical article," *Bull Math Biol* 52 (1990): 99–115.
4. W. Pitts and W. S. McCulloch, "How we know universals: the perception of auditory and visual forms," *Bull Math Biophys* 9 (1947): 127–47.
5. E. Kandel, *In Search of Memory: The Emergence of a New Science of Mind* (W. W. Norton and Company, 2007).
6. A. R. Luria, *Higher Cortical Functions in Man* (New York: Basic Books, 1966).

Index

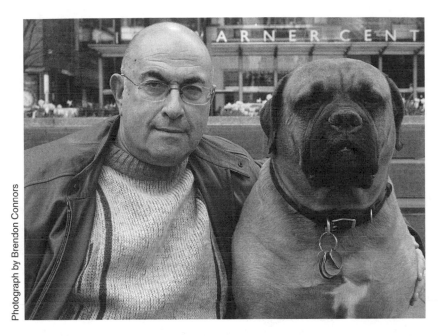

Elkhonon Goldberg, Ph.D., is the author of *The Executive Brain* and *The Wisdom Paradox*, and is a Clinical Professor of Neurology at New York University School of Medicine. He divides his time between research in cognitive neuroscience, clinical practice in neuropsychology, and teaching worldwide. He and his bullmastiff Brit live in New York City.

www.elkhonongoldberg.com